Respiratory Disorders and Behavioral Medicine

Edited by

Adrian A. Kaptein
Unit of Psychology
Leiden University Medical Center
Leiden, The Netherlands

and

Thomas L. Creer
Professor Emeritus of Psychology
Department of Psychology
Ohio University
Athens, Ohio, USA

MARTIN DUNITZ

Front cover image created by Astrid Beumer

First published in the United Kingdom in 2002 by:

Martin Dunitz Ltd
The Livery House
7–9 Pratt Street
London NW1 0AE

Tel: +44 (0) 20 7482 2202
Fax: +44 (0) 20 7267 0159
E-mail: info@dunitz.co.uk
Website: http://www.dunitz.co.uk

A CIP record for this book is available from the British Library.

ISBN: 90–5823–240–9

Distributed in the USA by
Fulfilment Center
Taylor & Francis
7625 Empire Drive, Florence, KY 41042, USA
Toll Free Tel.: +1 800 634 7064 E-mail: cserve@routledge_ny.com

Distributed in Canada by
Taylor & Francis
74 Rolark Drive, Scarborough, Ontario M1R 4G2, Canada
Toll Free Tel.: +1 877 226 2237 E-mail: tal_fran@istar.ca

Distributed in the rest of the world by
ITPS Limited
Cheriton House, North Way, Andover, Hampshire SP10 5BE, UK
Tel.: +44 (0)1264 332424 E-mail: reception@itps.co.uk

Composition by Wearset Ltd, Boldon, Tyne and Wear
Printed and bound in Great Britain by Biddles Ltd, Guildford and King's Lynn

Contents

List of Contributors v

Preface vii
Adrian A. Kaptein and Thomas L. Creer

Dedication ix

List of Figures x

List of Tables xii

1 Respiratory disorders and behavioral research 1
Adrian A. Kaptein

2 Epidemiology of asthma 19
Peter J. Gergen and Herman E. Mitchell

3 A family asthma management approach to behavioral assessment and treatment in children with asthma 45
Mary D. Klinnert and Bruce G. Bender

4 Chronic obstructive pulmonary disease: Behavioral assessment and treatment 85
Robert M. Kaplan and Andrew L. Ries

5 Symptom perception in asthma 117
Simon Rietveld and Walter Everaerd

6 Self-management and respiratory disorders: Guiding patients from health counseling and self-management perspectives 139
Ilse Mesters, Thomas L. Creer and Frans Gerards

7 Neuropsychological and psychiatric side effects of medications used to treat asthma and allergic rhinitis 175
Bruce G. Bender and Henry Milgrom

8 Compliance and respiratory disorders 197
Deirdre A. Levstek Caplin

9 Quality of life in respiratory disease 233
Michael E. Hyland

10 Cystic fibrosis: A biopsychosocial perspective 255
Kathryn E. Gustafson and Melanie J. Bonner

11 Respiratory disorders and their treatment 283
Thomas L. Creer and John A. Winder

12 Smoking cessation and chronic pulmonary disease 317
Russ VanCott Reynolds

13 Future issues in behavioral science research with respiratory disorders 335
Michele Hindi-Alexander, Gregory Fritz and Thomas L. Creer

14 Future directions of research on respiratory disorders 359
Thomas L. Creer

Index 395

List of Contributors

Bruce G. Bender
Department of Psychiatry
University of Colorado School of Medicine;
Department of Pediatrics
National Jewish Medical and Research Center
1400 Jackson Street
Denver, Colorado 80206
USA

Melanie J. Bonner
Division of Medical Psychology
Department of Psychiatry and Behavioral Science
Duke University Medical Center
DUMC-3362
Durham, North Carolina 27710
USA

Deirdre A. Levstek Caplin
Department of Pediatrics
University of Utah
Salt Lake City, Utah 84132
USA

Thomas L. Creer
Professor Emeritus of Psychology
Department of Psychology
Ohio University
Athens, Ohio 45701
USA

Walter Everaerd
Department of Psychology
University of Amsterdam
Roetersstraat 15
1018 WB Amsterdam
The Netherlands

Gregory Fritz
Division of Child & Adolescent Psychiatry
Rhode Island Hospital
Brown University School of Medicine
Providence, Rhode Island 02903
USA

Frans Gerards
Department of Health Education and Health Promotion
Maastricht University
PO Box 616
6200 MD Maastricht
The Netherlands

Peter J. Gergen
Center for Primary Care and Research
Agency for Healthcare Research and Quality
6010 Executive Blvd., Room 201
Rockville, Maryland 20852
USA

Kathryn E. Gustafson
Division of Medical Psychology
Department of Psychiatry and Behavioral Science
Duke University Medical Center
DUMC-3362
Durham, North Carolina 27710
USA

Michele Hindi-Alexander
National Institutes of Health
Risk, Prevention and Health Behavior
Two Rockledge Center
6701 Rockledge Drive
Bethesda, Maryland 20892–7848
USA

Michael E. Hyland
Department of Psychology
University of Plymouth
Drake Circus
Plymouth PL4 8AA
United Kingdom

Robert M. Kaplan
Department of Family and Preventive Medicine
University of California San Diego
School of Medicine
9500 Gilman Drive
La Jolla, California 92093–0628
USA

Adrian A. Kaptein
Unit of Psychology
Leiden University Medical Center
PO Box 1251
2340 BG Oegstgeest
The Netherlands

Mary D. Klinnert
Department of Pediatrics
National Jewish Medical and Research Center
1400 Jackson Street
Denver, Colorado 80206
USA

Ilse Mesters
Department of Health Education and Health Promotion
Maastricht University
PO Box 616
6200 MD Maastricht
The Netherlands

Henry Milgrom
Department of Pediatrics and Medicine
University of Colorado
Health Sciences Center
Denver, Colorado
USA

Herman E. Mitchell
Rho Federal Systems Division
University of North Carolina
School of Public Health
100 Eastowne Drive
Chapel Hill, North Carolina 27514
USA

Andrew L. Ries
Division of Pulmonary and Critical Care Medicine
Department of Medicine
University of California San Diego
School of Medicine
9500 Gilman Drive
La Jolla
California 92093–0628
USA

Simon Rietveld
Department of Psychology
University of Amsterdam
Roetersstraat 15
1018 WB Amsterdam
The Netherlands

Russ VanCott Reynolds
BWXT Y12, LLC
Occupational Health
P.O. Box 2009
Bldg 9706–2, MS 8103
Oak Ridge, Tennessee 37831
USA

John A. Winder
Toledo Center for Clinical Research
5860 Alexis Road, Suite B
Sylvania, Ohio 43560
USA

Preface

Respiratory disorders are major contributors to morbidity and mortality rates throughout the world. Asthma, chronic obstructive pulmonary disease (COPD), cystic fibrosis, and tuberculosis have a substantial impact on the daily functioning of millions of afflicted patients and their families. Their plight, in turn, has major consequences throughout society in general. Research by medical and behavioral scientists has clearly shown how the behavior of patients with respiratory disorders is closely linked to the initiation and maintenance of these conditions. A superficial examination of the contents of major health psychology or behavioral medicine journals indicates that respiratory conditions are underrepresented compared with other disorders such as cardiology problems or cancer. One reason may be that those medical and behavioral scientists working with respiratory conditions tend to publish in journals such as the *American Journal of Respiratory and Critical Care Medicine*, where findings can be read by a broader array of scientists. While the latter is laudatory, the authors still have a nagging feeling that not enough attention is focused on topics described in the chapters of this book.

As editors of the book, we feel there is an urgent need to stimulate research on behavioral and medical aspects of respiratory disorders by producing a book that will cover major theoretical issues and empirical findings on these conditions. One of us (Thomas L. Creer) has written a brief introduction to each chapter in order to establish a framework for that chapter. The contributors and editors of the book have all been active in research on behavioral aspects of asthma, COPD, cystic fibrosis, and tuberculosis. One cannot fail to be impressed when comparing where we were 20 years ago to where we are now. In Europe and North America, there has been a sharp increase in both the quantity and quality of research on respiratory conditions. Much of this has been fostered by such organizations as the European Respiratory Society and the American Thoracic Society; patient organizations, governmental agencies, and pharmaceutical and health care companies have also generated interest in research with respiratory disorders. We feel that exciting opportunities lie ahead for interdisciplinary work in the area; psychologists, physicians, nurses, health educators, physiotherapists and, the most important group of all, patients will benefit from this work.

The editors are grateful to those who contributed chapters to the book. They were a joy to work with. We thank them for their work, their dedication, and their patience. The editors express their wish that the book will be instrumental in furthering the cause of interdisciplinary research in respiratory disorders. If this goal is attained, the consequence can only be a better quality of life for the patients with whom we all work.

Adrian A. Kaptein
Thomas L. Creer

Dedication

The book is dedicated to the memory of Elliott Middleton, Jr., M.D., who was one of the first to recognize and encourage interdisciplinary research among medical and behavioral scientists.

List of Figures

Figure 1.1 Papers on CVD, CA, COPD, and asthma published in *Health Psychology*, 1990–1999.

Figure 1.2 Lung disease (obstructive) and quality of life (MEDLINE 1975–1999).

Figure 4.1 Disease burden estimated using disability-adjusted life years showing rank order of 15 major causes of death in the world, 1990–2020.

Figure 4.2 Disability adjusted life years for diarrhea, HIV and tobacco use; projections for 1990–2020.

Figure 4.3 Relationship between disability and COPD.

Figure 4.4 Cumulative self-reported walking in five groups.

Figure 4.5 Percent of initial exercise endurance for five groups at three months.

Figure 4.6 Change in quality of well-being for three treatment groups (combined into 'treated' line) and two control groups (combined into 'control' line).

Figure 4.7 Results of treadmill endurance exercise tests for patients in the rehabilitation and education groups at baseline and for 12 months of follow up.

Figure 4.8 Kaplan–Meier proportional estimate survival curves: upper median QWB scores versus lower median QWB scores.

Figure 4.9 Survival of 78 males for high versus low social support satisfaction.

Figure 4.10 Survival of 32 females for high versus low social support satisfaction.

Figure 4.11 Correlations between categories of self-efficacy and FEV1.0.

Figure 4.12 Relationship between diffusing capacity (DLCL) and tertile of self-efficacy.

Figure 4.13 Mean self-efficacy for walking by years of survival.

Figure 4.14 Regression of compliance on exercise. Each 0.35 unit change in compliance resulted in a one minute change in exercise endurance.

Figure 4.15 Changes in exercise endurance among rehabilitation and education patients who increased or decreased in depression.

Figure 4.16 Changes in VO_{2Max} as a function of initial depression for rehabilitation and education patients.

Figure 6.1 Definitions of self management.

Figure 7.1 SALT. Mean response time (in seconds) to alarms for days 1 and 3 of each treatment period.

Figure 7.2 Mean (SE) years of survival on the simulation for patient groups receiving diphenhydramine (DIP), acrivastine + pseudoephedrine (A + P), placebo (PLA), and non-treated normal controls (NOR), during training and examination sessions.

Figure 9.1 The causal sequence model of quality of life.

Figure 10.1 Transactional stress and coping model of adjustment to chronic illness.

Figure 12.1 Progression of COPD from smoking onset through mortality.

Figure 14.1 Reciprocal determinism model.

List of Tables

Table 3.1 Behavorial domains assessed in FAMSS interview
Table 3.2 Areas of family asthma management to be assessed in FAMSS interview
Table 3.3 Case illustration: FAMSS multidimensional assessment
Table 6.1 Definitions of self-management
Table 7.1 Parent questionnaire problem scales from a blinded comparison of theophylline and placebo
Table 7.2 Psychological test scores from a blinded comparison of theophylline and placebo
Table 8.1 Four major problems with current definitions of compliance
Table 8.2 Typical methods of compliance measurement
Table 8.3 Factors reported to affect compliance for patients with respiratory diseases
Table 8.4 Suggestions for health care professionals to assist patients with respiratory care
Table 8.5 Improvements to traditional self-management training
Table 9.1 Relationship of two components of quality of life, problems and evaluations, the shuttle walking test and neuroticism in COPD patients
Table 9.2 Correlations between four different quality of life construct scores from the Living with Asthma Questionnaire and mean PEF taken at different times of the day
Table 9.3 Summary of respiratory-specific measures of quality of life
Table 11.1 Asthma questionnaire
Table 11.2 COPD questionnaire
Table 11.3 Common symptoms of tuberculosis
Table 11.4 Medications used to treat asthma and COPD
Table 11.5 Types of preventive, controller or maintenance medications
Table 12.1 Smoking cessation program components for COPD patients

1
Respiratory disorders and behavioral research

Adrian A. Kaptein

> *As the fish that thrusts its jaw to water draw*
> *so I some air do seek to snare,*
> *and like the weanling goat upon the nipple I suck,*
> *but it is not milk so sweet I crave, but air, so pure*
>
> (*Horowitz, 1996*)

Kleinman (1988) hit the nail on the head with his plea for health care workers to listen to the stories patients tell about their symptoms and the complaints they voice regarding their illnesses. There is overwhelming evidence that attests to the impact of patient responses to the medical management of asthma or chronic obstructive pulmonary disease (COPD). A recent series of papers in *Thorax*, for example, outlined the association between asthma patients' self-management skills, medical management, and the most serious outcome of this condition, death (Bucknall *et al.*, 1999; Burr *et al.*, 1999). At the same time, reviews of the effects of self-management skills in asthma and COPD describe the positive consequences of these skills on outcomes such as hospital admission, psychological well-being, and school and work absenteeism (e.g., Devine, 1996; Devine & Pearcy, 1996).

How patients with respiratory disorders – or any somatic disorder for that matter – manage their illness is determined in part by how patients perceive their illness, including the cognitive representation of symptoms, causes, consequences, duration, and cure or lack thereof (Leventhal *et al.*, 1997). Symptom perception theory, self-regulation theory, and theories on self-management emphasize the reality of subjective views of patients regarding their symptoms and the methods they employ in their management (Creer, 2000a,b; Pennebaker, 1982). The complex cascade of illness cognitions, symptom perception, self-management behaviors, and outcomes in medical, psychological, and social domains constitutes a major area for research and clinical care for behavioral scientists who work with patients with respiratory disorders.

Despite the high prevalence of respiratory disorders, the number of behavioral scientists working in this field is relatively small compared with the number of behavioral scientists involved with cardiovascular disorders and oncology. Figure 1.1 depicts the cumulative number of papers published in *Health Psychology* on cardiovascular disorders, cancer, asthma, and COPD in the period 1990–99. Two observations can be made when studying this figure. First, behavioral scientists who are active in the area of respiratory disorders apparently prefer publishing their papers in medical journals and, secondly, they are simply overwhelmed by the number of colleagues in the cardiology and oncology fields.

In this introductory chapter, I will briefly review how psychologists and other behavioral scientists have viewed asthma and COPD in the past century. I will then discuss some research topics for future behavioral research on patients with respiratory disorders, as well as the conditions necessary for this research to occur.

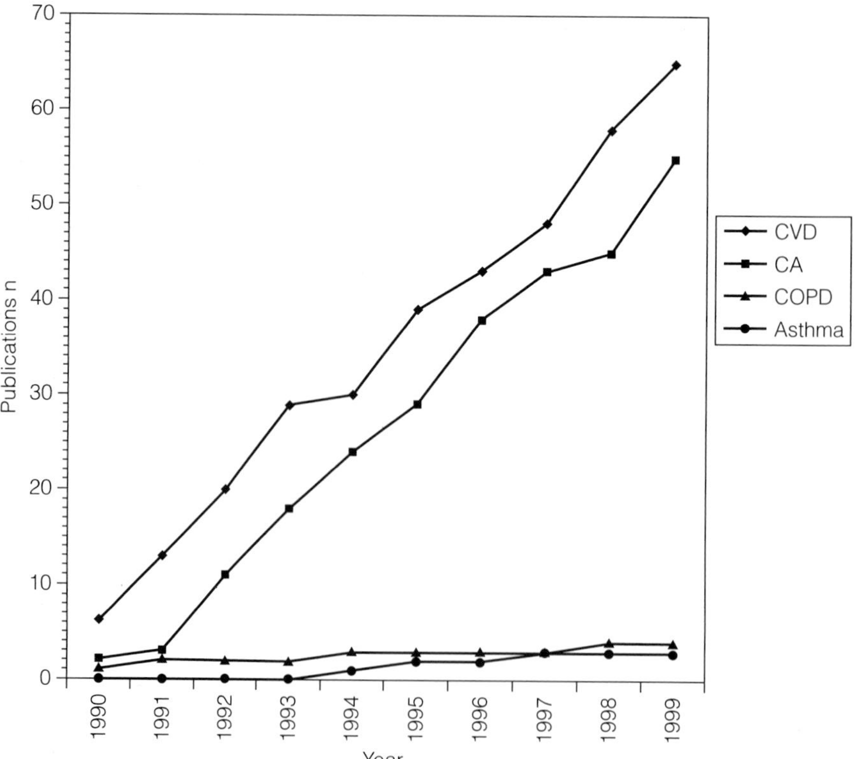

Figure 1.1

Papers on cardiovascular disease (CVD), cancer (CA), chronic obstructive pulmonary disease (COPD), and asthma published in *Health Psychology*, 1990–1999.

Asthma

'It's very frightening, I can't speak, I can't move.
I'm just like a statue, frozen stiff with fear.
You're gasping for air, and you feel as if
you're suffocating . . . it's just very, very frightening
you get into such a panic that you don't know
what's happening to you really,
it's terrible'

(Williams, 1993, p. 13)

Over the past century, three major theoretical approaches in psychological research on patients with asthma can be delineated. I will briefly outline these approaches to illustrate the changing foci in behavioral research on patients with asthma; the approaches concern psychoanalytic theory, behavioral approaches, and self-management.

Psychoanalytic Theories

Between World War I and World War II, psychoanalytic theories on various diseases were proposed and widely disseminated. At the same time, impressive medical successes that increased our understanding of the causes of bacterial diseases and how to treat them profoundly influenced the framework within which researchers viewed the relationship between psychological factors and disease processes. This was particularly important with asthma. As Knapp (1963, p. 235) remarked, these investigators 'often follow an implicit model of the germ theory and tried to find in one or another facet of the syndrome, a *bacillus asthmaticus psychosomaticus*'.

Dunbar (1935), in her *Emotions and Bodily Changes*, extensively reviewed the psychoanalytic and psychosomatic literature on somatic disorders. The review emphasized what were described as considerable similarities in the personality structure and behavior patterns of individuals with a certain bodily disease, and suggested these personality characteristics were causally related to diseases of specific organ systems. In a later publication, Dunbar (1938, p. 55) outlined specific similarities in personality, behavior, family background, and early experiences of three patients with asthma.

> *The element of separation from the mother was important ... the demand for love coexisting with a fear of love and revolt against it seemed to keep all three patients in a constant state of vibration between activity and passivity, between love and hate. They feared both love and loss of love; all spoke of fear being held too tight – 'smothered with kisses' – as well as of fear of sexual activity and of separation and rejection.*

According to Dunbar, patients with asthma not only had similar personality profiles but also these profiles were causally related to specific diseases. For example, personality profile A was said to lead to asthma, profile B to diabetes mellitus, and so on.

Another psychoanalytic theory of asthma had Franz Alexander, a contemporary of Dunbar, as its foremost proponent. Alexander and his coworkers at the Chicago Institute for Psychoanalysis proposed theories to account for different psychosomatic disorders. In addition, their research effort was devoted to accumulating evidence in support of their theoretical notions. In a series of publications, Alexander and his coworkers (1952, 1966, 1968) presented extensive theoretical and empirical information concerning the effects of emotional factors on the disease process. Based on these publications, an attempt will be made here to summarize Alexander's views on asthma.

The major underlying premise of the writings of Alexander and his colleagues is that continuous functional stress, arising out of everyday contacts with the environment, causes chronic disturbances in the organ systems of the individual. Built on Cannon's work on the autonomic nervous system, Alexander considered disturbance of vegetative functions to arise because either 'fight or flight' behavior or dependent help-seeking behavior is blocked. Whenever the overt expression of 'fight or flight' behavior is blocked, the resulting sustained excitation of the sympathetic nervous system leads to disturbances in the neuroendocrine system that ultimately leads to diseases such as hypertension or migraine headaches. On the other hand, when the wish of 'being taken care of' is blocked because of internal denial or external circumstances, increased parasympathetic activity mediated by the neuroendocrine system leads to diseases such as peptic ulcer or asthma.

When discussing the problem of specificity of emotional factors and somatic disturbances, Alexander (1952, p. 69) stated that 'it is not the presence of any one or more of these psychological factors (e.g., anxiety, repressed hostile and erotic impulses, frustration or dependent craving) that is specific, but the presence of the dynamic configuration in which they appear.' With regard to asthma specifically, Alexander (1952, p. 68) noted that 'attacks of asthma are correlated with an unconscious suppressed impulse to cry for the mother's help,' and that (Alexander 1952, pp. 133–134) 'the nuclear psychodynamic factor is a conflict centering in an excessive unresolved dependence upon the mother... it is the wish to be protected – to be encompassed by the mother or the maternal image.... Everything which threatens to separate the patient from the protective mother or her substitute is apt to precipitate an asthmatic attack.'

Alexander & Selesnick (1966) subsequently provided a revised set of conditions that must be present in order for an organic disease to occur: (a) a constitutional or acquired organ vulnerability; (b) a characteristic emotional–conflict pattern; and (c) a precipitating life event that leads to a breakdown of the patient's psychological defenses. With asthma, this 'summation of stimuli' gave Alexander the opportunity to incorporate the ever increasing knowledge on mechanisms between allergic stimuli and bronchoconstriction into his theory. These mechanisms supposedly constituted organ vulnerability.

In evaluating the theory in terms of its usefulness in explaining asthma, the conclusion is that that there is no substantial evidence for the existence of a specific nuclear conflict as hypothesized by Alexander. In addition, a number of criticisms can be raised about these beliefs. First, the patients studied were not representative of the general population of asthma patients because of the biased nature with which patients came to the attention of psychiatrists. A second criticism is that the nuclear conflict theory does not delineate mechanisms by which psychological and physiological factors are linked. Finally, rather than having a causal function, the dependency conflicts may very well arise as a consequence of having asthma.

Despite the lack of empirical evidence supporting psychoanalytic views on patients with asthma, many of these beliefs still survive. When mothers are asked to describe the causes of their child's asthma, some will reply, with some embarrassment, that they themselves may have caused their child's asthma because of faults in their rearing of the child. Other myths persist with respect to asthma. Recently, I was asked to review a manuscript for a high-impact journal in behavioral sciences. The manuscript described how family physicians in Germany viewed patients with asthma. One of the respondents remarked that patients with asthma are angry at those without asthma because the latter use up the air which is meant for patients (see Wahlström et al., 2001, p. 510).

Unscientific, or even anti-scientific views, about psychological factors and asthma will probably never disappear. The reason is found in the very nature of asthma itself. Gergen & Mitchell (Chapter 2) provide a comprehensive review of the risk factors for asthma. However, it is often difficult, if not impossible, to delineate the specific stimulus or stimuli that precipitate a given attack. There are a number of reasons for this state, including the presence of multiple stimuli, the additive effect of precipitating stimuli, and the fact that an attack may not occur for some time after the triggering stimulus has occurred (i.e., late onset asthma). For this reason, patients and those around them are prone to assume there is a correlation between an asthma exacerbation and events that occur concurrently with the onset of the attack even though no cause–effect relationship exists. By the same token, it is difficult to show causality between a treatment and the end of an attack. The reason? The fact that asthma can reverse either spontaneously or with treatment. As long as attacks may remit spontaneously, it is impossible to definitively prove a cause–effect relationship in determining why an episode was aborted (Creer, 1982).

Learning Theory

With the relatively successful applications of learning theory principles to mental health problems (e.g., phobias, social skills deficits, etc.), behavior therapists examined the effectiveness of applying learning principles to patients with somatic disorders. Creer (1979) presented an overview of the applications of behavior therapeutic approaches to patients with asthma and COPD. Relaxation training, systematic desensitization, biofeedback, and time-out from positive reinforcement were some of the techniques used in studies on these patients.

As many patients with asthma report physiological or psychological arousal as a trigger of an asthma attack, it seemed logical to examine the effects of relaxation training techniques on asthma symptoms. In 1978, Knapp & Wells reviewed the topic and concluded that relaxation therapy can produce statistically significant improvement in the respiratory functioning of asthma patients. An empirical study by Alexander *et al.* (1979, p. 33) with excellent design and outcome measures, concluded however, that

> *the most optimistic appraisal of the status of relaxation as a symptomatic therapy in asthma is that the effect may be very small indeed, if in fact it is reliable at all, even when present at full strength; and that, in any case, it is of little or no clinical significance even if real.*

The review in 1982 by Richter and Dahme supported this cautious summary.

One of the best studies in which systematic desensitization (SD) was employed in children with asthma was carried out by Miklich *et al.* (1977, p. 291). Pulmonary function, severity of medication, and frequency of symptoms were unaffected by the intervention. The authors conclude that 'we are in agreement, that, even at best, SD appears to have no more than an ancillary role in the management of asthma.' Similar rather disappointing conclusions have been drawn regarding biofeedback (Kotses & Glaus, 1981).

A focus of early studies on relaxation and behavior therapy for asthma patients was on asthma per se; hence, pulmonary function was a major outcome measure. As noted by Miklich *et al.* (1977), systematic desensitization was only effective as an adjunctive treatment for asthma with given patients in certain situations. As noted in the chapter by Mesters, Creer, and Gerards (Chapter 6), this does not mean that relaxation does not play a prominent role in the management and control of asthma. Instead of focusing on pulmonary function as an outcome variable, however, behavioral scientists have shifted their perspective so that relaxation is now considered as a significant factor if a patient is to manage asthma exacerbations as directed. In other words, patients must relax if they are to perform the sequential self-management steps outlined in their asthma action plan. In addition, as Creer (1979) pointed out, only by relaxing can patients be treated effectively by medical personnel and avoid the possibility of panicking, a behavior that both exacerbates ongoing attacks and is contagious to those around patients, including health care personnel. When considered in this manner, the teaching of relaxation, sometimes coupled with systematic desensitization, is a much more effective, efficient, and helpful tool to assist patients in dealing with asthma in their daily lives.

Behavioral techniques have increasingly been shown to be of value in the management of asthma and COPD. They are useful across all facets of treatment for allowing patients (a) to prevent exacerbations through medication compliance; (b) to avoid exacerbations of their conditions through the avoidance of triggers such as overexertion or smoking; (c) to control exacerbations efficiently and effectively; and (d) to develop the confidence and expectations that their actions make what is often the major contribution to controlling a chronic respiratory condition. All the procedures that permit patients to make optimal use of these techniques are often considered under the umbrella of self-management.

Self-Management

Self-management, self-regulation, self-control, self-directed behavior, and self-help are terms that are often considered as synonymous (Creer & Holroyd, 1997; Creer, 2000a,b). Basically, these terms refer to the following processes: (a) goal selection; (b) information collection; (c) information processing and evaluation; (d) decision making; (e) action; and (f) self-reaction (Creer & Holroyd, 1997). Chapter 6 is devoted to this topic. However, it can be said that self-management has emerged as a set of techniques that allows patients to become partners with health care personnel in the control and management of their condition, particularly asthma and COPD. As Mesters, Creer, and Gerards note (Chapter 6), we are only beginning to understand the potential of self-management in controlling asthma, COPD, and other chronic illness. As our knowledge of these procedures grows, it will shape the development of future programs and, hopefully, permit us to increase the control over chronic disorders.

I will end this discussion by describing three topics that may at first seem to be unrelated. The topics refer to fascinating parts of the behavioral research tradition on emotional and cognitive responses of patients with asthma. As will be argued, these components may, when all is said and done, be related to one another to some extent.

The first topic concerns the work by Kinsman and colleagues (summarized in Kinsman *et al.*, 1982, p. 435) on 'psychomaintenance of asthma,' which they define as 'the psychologic and behavioral perpetuation and exacerbation of physical illness.' Kinsman, the principal investigator of the research group, became fascinated by the wide variations in the psychological, behavioral, and physiological responses of individual military personnel as they were trained to parachute out of an airplane. An identical stimulus – actual parachute jumping – produced great variations in responses among subjects. Kinsman applied these findings to hospitalized patients with asthma by studying their emotional responses to severe episodes of shortness of breath and to their attitudes to being asthma patients. The research group identified two personality characteristics ('panic–fear symptomatology' and 'panic–fear personality') and a set of attitudes (e.g., stigma, optimism). These factors were found to be predictive of three aspects of medical outcome, irrespective of 'objective' measures of asthma severity: length of hospitalization, rates of rehospitalization, and severity of medication prescribed at discharge.

While the findings by Kinsman and his colleagues were not translated into intervention studies, other investigators replicated their findings – e.g., in Finland by Teiramaa, 1978; in France by Baron *et al.*, 1986; and in the Netherlands by Kaptein, 1982. Currently, Rietveld is using the concept of panic–fear symptomatology in his research on symptom perception in asthma (Rietveld, pers. comm., 2000).

The second topic concerns a recent study which falls within the scope of 'self-disclosure' (Smyth *et al.*, 1999). Self-disclosure, particularly talking or writing about stressful situations, leads to changes in immune function, well-being, and the use of health care resources (Pennebaker, 1995; Smyth, 1998). In the Smyth *et al.* (1999) study, patients with asthma were randomly assigned to an experimental or control condition. In the experimental condition, patients were asked to spend 20 min per day for 3 consecutive days in writing about the most stressful event that they ever encountered. In the control condition, patients were asked to spend an equal amount of time in writing about their plans for the day. Pulmonary function (forced expiratory volume (FEV_1)) was assessed before and after the study, and at a follow-up of 4 months. Statistically significant and clinically relevant improvements in pulmonary function were observed in the self-disclosure condition.

These two topics, in my view, underline the statements made in the introductory paragraphs of this chapter: affective and cognitive responses by patients to an illness or disorder are important as (co-)determinants of medical outcome and physiological processes. The concept of illness perceptions—the third topic—is the central theoretical framework that seems relevant for these two areas (Petrie & Weinman, 1997). Research on illness perceptions shows how these perceptions impact on, for example, resumption of work in patients with a myocardial infarction (Petrie *et al.*, 1996), or on psychological and physiological functioning in patients with COPD (Scharloo *et al.*, 2000). Intervention studies where illness perceptions are being modified in a cognitive-behavioral therapeutic approach are underway (Petrie, pers. comm., 1999). Self-disclosure and illness perceptions are not miles apart, conceptually speaking, and the 'cognitive revolution in psychology' may produce beneficial effects for patients with asthma as well (Hawton *et al.*, 1989).

Chronic Obstructive Pulmonary Disease

> *'I have a terrible lack of energy. I get terribly, terribly tired and worn out very easily, . . . you're always short of energy . . . whether it's getting up in the morning, washing and dressing, anything, you get so damned tired and breathless'.*
>
> *(Williams, 1993, p. 65)*

Behavioral scientists embarked on conducting empirical studies about patients with COPD only 40 years ago. Webb & Lawton (1961) are credited with performing the initial study in this area. They examined 33 patients with emphysema and compared them with healthy controls, using a now obsolete test, to assess personality traits.

Patients with COPD and their families did not have to overcome the barrier of psychoanalytic or psychosomatic theories, as were promulgated about asthma by physicians, psychiatrists, behavioral scientists, or society. COPD was excluded in the theorizing of the proponents of psychosomatic views because, from the outset, it was recognized that COPD was a condition that was irreversible, regardless of treatment, and often resulted in the death of the patient. The rise in the prevalence of COPD over the past decades is a direct result of the increase in cigarette smoking. The most parsimonious explanation for the rise in behavioral research and treatments of the disorder over this period is directly linked to the increase in the incidence of smoking and, in turn, the number of patients with COPD. Whereas a search of the literature only a couple of decades ago would have yielded only a few references to the topics of behavior, psychology, and COPD, a MEDLINE search in the year 2000 found 765 references on the topics. The number of studies, particularly those that integrate behavioral elements into the overall management of COPD, is bound to increase in the future. One reason is that, as predicted Murray & Lopez (1997), COPD will be the third leading cause of death 20 years from now.

Much of the collaborative research on COPD that has occurred is summarized throughout this book, particularly by Kaplan and Ries (Chapter 4) and Reynolds (Chapter 12). For this reason, only three areas of research on behavioral aspects of COPD will be briefly reviewed in order to illustrate the contributions of behavioral scientists to the overall management of COPD. These topics explore psychosocial consequences of COPD, quality of life, and self-management of the disorder.

Psychosocial Consequences of COPD

Behavioral scientists involved with patients with a chronic physical disorder have traditionally studied the consequences of these disorders on psychological and social functioning. Although the observations by Agle & Baum (1977) on various psychological aspects of patients with COPD were published some 25 years ago, they still make for fascinating reading. The authors outlined various psychological responses to the symptoms of COPD, including anxiety, depression, body preoccupation, alcoholism, paranoia, sexual dysfunction, and various defense mechanisms. Methods used to assess these consequences, such as selection of patients and sample size, can be criticized by current behavioral research standards. However, the clinical observations made by the authors have often been corroborated in behavioral studies on COPD patients (see, for example, Van Ede *et al.*, 1999 for a systematic review of the prevalence of depression in patients with COPD).

A second phase in empirical work on psychological aspects of COPD was reflected in the research of Kinsman and colleagues (Kinsman *et al.*, 1983). This group of psychologists, working at the National Jewish Hospital in Denver, Colorado, asked patients with chronic bronchitis and emphysema to rate the frequency of COPD symptoms. Results indicated that 10 symptom categories could be distinguished, with 'dyspnea' and 'fatigue' rated as the most frequent symptoms, and 'peripheral/sensory complaints' and 'alienation' as less-frequent reported symptoms.

In reviewing their research, it is evident that Kinsman and his colleagues planned to embark on a research line similar to the one they had followed in conducting asthma research in the 10 years prior to their initial studies on COPD. They demonstrated substantial differences in individual responses to COPD, and the relative lack of association between those responses and various indicators of 'objective' severity of the respiratory disorder. Their study, in what could have become a research line of psychomaintenance of COPD, was their last investigation. Soon after they published their findings, a significant conflict between psychologists, on the one hand, and physicians and administrators, on the other, terminated a line of research which no doubt would have been highly interesting and clinically useful. A more recent study (Ashutosh *et al.*, 1997), for example, focused on prognostic factors from a behavioral point of view in patients with COPD, and found psychological factors to be predictive of survival at 4 year follow-up, irrespective of objective measures of severity of COPD.

Quality of Life

As outlined in the chapter by Hyland (Chapter 9) and Kaplan and Ries (Chapter 4), quality of life (QOL) is a concept with a solid foundation in the area of behavioral research on respiratory disorders (Maillé *et al.*, 1996; McSweeny & Creer, 1995). A few years ago, I published a paper on the number of empirical studies on quality of life in COPD (Kaptein *et al.*, 1997). In Fig. 1.2 an update of the figure in that paper is given. A MEDLINE search on 'quality of life & lung diseases, obstructive' from 1975–1999 is the basis for the graph shown in Fig. 1.2 (included are only empirical papers in English; abstracts, editorials, and reviews are excluded). The figure illustrates the impressive increase in empirical work on quality of life in patients with COPD (see also *www.atsqol.org*).

Some 15 years ago, I was asked to participate in a multicenter randomized controlled trial on various medication regimens for patients with COPD. Quality of life was defined as 'secondary endpoint'; pulmonary function, as might be expected, was the primary endpoint. Validated, disease-specific QOL measures did not exist at that time. We compiled a test battery with instruments for assessing anxiety, depression, stigma, and activities of daily living as components (Kaptein *et al.*, 1993). At present, researchers in the area of QOL and COPD have at their disposal a substantial number of valid and reliable QOL measures (see Chapter 9).

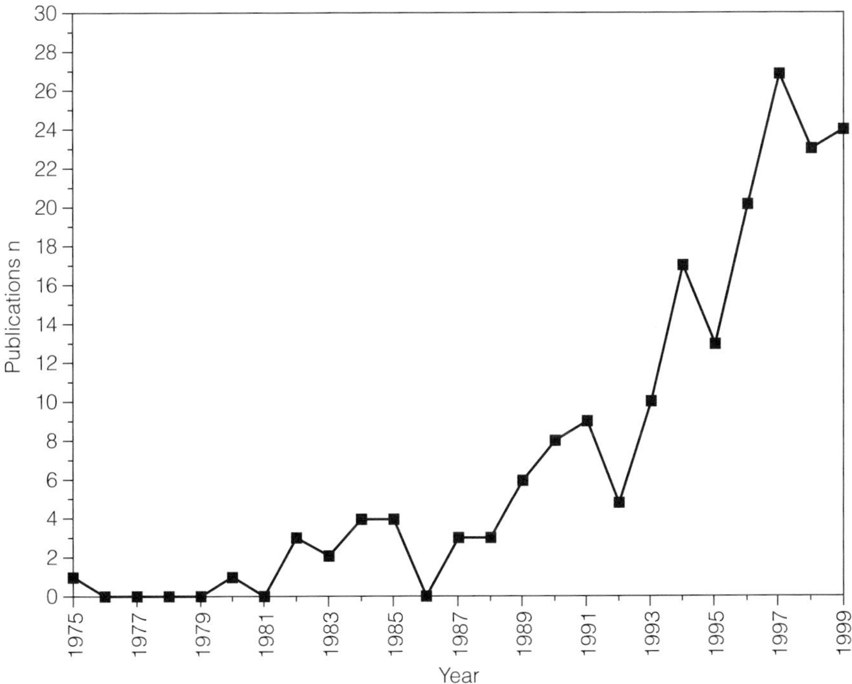

Figure 1.2

Lung disease (obstructive) and quality of life (MEDLINE 1975–1999).

Even in the highest impact journals in respiratory medicine, defining QOL as a primary endpoint is in vogue; this is particularly the case when QOL is considered within the perspective of discussions on outcome assessment in pulmonary medicine (Rubenfeld *et al.*, 1999).

Behavioral scientists have come a long way. As recently discussed by Wood-Dauphinee (1999), the challenges that still remain pertain to developing a more solid theoretical basis for quality of life research, and incorporating quality of life into clinical care.

The consequences of COPD on neuropsychological functioning of patients is a distinct area of research. In this book, Bender and Milgrom discuss the neuropsychological aspects of asthma in great detail (Chapter 7). Recent studies on the effects of hypoxia and hypercarbia on neuropsychological measures in COPD patients corroborate earlier research (e.g., Grant *et al.*, 1987): memory dysfunction and attentional deficits appear to be significantly more prevalent in COPD patients than in people of similar age without COPD (Antonelli Incalzi *et al.*, 1997; Stuss *et al.*, 1997). In quality of life research, neuropsychological functioning is rarely included as a separate domain. It could be argued, however, that neuropsychological measures could be part of QOL assessment in patients with a severe grade of COPD.

Self-Management and Pulmonary Rehabilitation

The history of behavioral research on patients with COPD may be relatively short, particularly when compared with behavioral research on patients with cardiovascular disease or cancer. Psychologists conducting research with COPD started by studying personality characteristics of patients with COPD (e.g., Webb & Lawton, 1961), and explored areas such as depression (van Ede *et al.*, 1999), sexuality (Kaptein *et al.*, 1991), and dyspnea (Mahler & Harver, 1996). Quality of life, despite its vagueness as a theoretical construct, is currently one of the dominant topics of research by behavioral scientists who work with COPD patients.

Behavioral interventions in patients with COPD have concentrated on four topics: smoking cessation, psychotherapy, self-management, and pulmonary rehabilitation programs. For the first topic, smoking cessation, see Chapter 12 by Reynolds and Chapter 4 by Kaplan and Ries. Early reports on psychotherapeutic management of patients with COPD are moving when read some 20 years later. Rosser *et al.* (1983), for example, used a randomized controlled trial design to study the effects of psychotherapy (both an analytic group and a supportive group were studied), nurse group intervention, and usual care on psychological and physiological measures. More recently Eiser *et al.* (1997) applied a similar approach in examining the effects of group psychotherapy with a cognitive–behavioral accent on anxiety, exercise tolerance, dyspnea, and quality of life. Results indicate that the psychotherapy condition produced a sustained improvement in exercise tolerance, without any changes in the other outcome measures.

Apart from questions raised about the effectiveness of psychotherapy with any patient group, COPD patients deserve better. Teaching patients self-managing skills in a cognitive–behavioral approach appears to be a more effective and cost-effective way to proceed. The chapter by Kaplan and Ries (Chapter 4) illustrates this statement. In a review of behavioral interventions in patients with COPD, 10 studies were identified with a randomized controlled design (Kaptein, 1997). Based on these studies, it can be concluded that cognitive–behavioral interventions, aimed at improving self-management skills of patients with COPD, result in favorable effects on outcome measures in the psychological domain (e.g., self-efficacy, quality of life, scores on scales that assess functional status) (Kaptein & Dekker, 2000). The study of Atkins *et al.* (1984) must still be considered as the classic study in this area.

Behavioral scientists are routinely involved in pulmonary rehabilitation programs. Recent meta-analyses (Lacasse *et al.*, 1996; Cambach *et al.*, 1999) indicated that pulmonary rehabilitation favorably impacts on psychological measures (e.g., depression), functional status (e.g., activities of daily living), and quality of life. Meta-analyses of the impact of behavioral interventions in patients with cardiovascular disease and cancer go a step further. Linden *et al.* (1996) and Meyer & Mark (1995) provide evidence that behavioral interventions in these patient categories may even be associated with prolonging survival. The survival curves in the paper by Ries *et al.* (1995) on the effects of psychosocial intervention in COPD patients seem to indicate a similar trend. However, Kaplan warned against being too optimistic regarding this trend (Kaplan, pers. comm., Toronto, May 2000).

Clearly, much more behavioral research on patients with COPD is required. Fundamental issues (e.g., sexuality, patients' partners, smoking cessation, etc.) need more attention. Theoretical issues should also be a focus of future research. Descriptive and experimental studies by psychologists with COPD patients will become stronger if a clear and solid theoretical perspective is adopted. Finally, behavioral scientists must be inventive and creative in ascertaining what would be adequate funding for their research.

Conclusions

I have never failed to be impressed by the impact of respiratory disorders on the daily lives of afflicted patients and their families. Equally impressive, however, is the amazing resilience of most patients in coping with their respiratory problems. Patients, pulmonary physicians, and behavioral scientists can further benefit patients and their families through mutual understanding and research collaboration. Cognitive–behavioral interventions for patients with asthma or COPD is potentially a promising area of research and clinical care. International consensus on assessment instruments specific for asthma and COPD will further help the cause of behavioral research in patients with respiratory disorders. It is a challenge for senior researchers in the area of behavioral research on patients with respiratory disorders to stimulate young behavioral scientists to enthusiastically conduct creative research on the fascinating subject of asthma and COPD. This book is intended to help them.

References

Agle, D.P. & Baum, G.L. (1977). Psychological aspects of chronic obstructive pulmonary disease. *Medical Clinics of North America*, 61, 749–758.

Alexander, F. (1952). *Psychosomatic medicine: its principles and applications*. London: Allen and Unwin.

Alexander, F. & Selesnick, S.T. (1966). *The history of psychiatry*. New York: Harper and Row, 1966.

Alexander, F., French, T.M. & Pollock, G.H. (1968). *Psychosomatic specificity*. Chicago: University of Chicago Press.

Alexander, A.B., Cropp, G.J.A. & Chai, H. (1979). Effects of relaxation training on pulmonary mechanics in children with asthma. *Journal of Applied Behavioral Analysis*, 12, 27–35.

Antonelli Incalzi, R., Gemma, A., Marra, C., Capparella, O., Fuso, L. & Carbonin, P. (1997). Verbal memory impairment in COPD. *Chest*, 112, 1506–1513.

Ashutosh, K., Haldipur, C. & Boucher, M.L. (1997). Clinical and personality profiles and survival in patients with COPD. *Chest*, 111, 95–98.

Atkins, C.J., Kaplan, R.M., Timms, R.M., Reinsch, S. & Lofback, K. (1984). Behavioral exercise programs in the management of chronic obstructive pulmonary disease. *Journal of Consulting and Clinical Psychology*, 52, 591–603.

Baron, C., Lamarre, A., Veilleux, P., Ducharme, G., Spier, S. & Lapierre, J-G. (1986). Psychomaintenance of childhood asthma: a study of 34 children. *Journal of Asthma*, 23, 69–79.

Bucknall, C.E., Slack, R., Godley, C.C., Mackay, T.W. & Wright, S.C. (1999). Scottish confidential inquiry into asthma deaths (SCIAD), 1994–6. *Thorax*, 54, 978–984.

Burr, M.L., Davies, B.H., Hoare, A., *et al.* (1999). A confidential inquiry into asthma deaths in Wales. *Thorax*, 54, 985–989.

Cambach, W., Wagenaar, R.C., Koelman, T.W., van Keimpema, T. & Kemper, H.C.G. (1999). The long-term effects of pulmonary rehabilitation in patients with asthma and chronic obstructive pulmonary disease: a research synthesis. *Archives of Physical and Medical Rehabilitation*, 80, 103–111.

Creer, T.L. (1979). *Asthma therapy: a behavioral health care system for respiratory disorders*. New York: Springer.

Creer, T.L. (1982). Asthma. *Journal of Consulting and Clinical Psychology*, 50, 912–921.

Creer, T.L. (2000a). Self-management of chronic diseases. In: M. Boekaerts, P.R. Pintrich & M. Zeidner (Eds), *Self-regulation: theory, research, applications*, (pp. 601–629). Orlando, FL: Academic Press.

Creer, T.L. (2000b). Self-management and the control of chronic pediatric illness. In: D. Drotar (Ed.), *Compliance in pediatric populations* (pp. 95–129). Mahwah, NJ: Lawrence Erlbaum Associates.

Creer, T.L. & Holroyd, K.H. (1997). Self-management. In: A. Baum, S. Newman, J.

Weinman, R. West & C. McManus (Eds), *Cambridge handbook of psychology, health and medicine* (pp. 255–258). Cambridge: Cambridge University Press.

Devine, E.C. (1996). Meta-analysis of the effects of psycho-educational care in adults with asthma. *Research in Nursing and Health*, 19, 367–376.

Devine, E.C. & Pearcy, J. (1996). Meta-analysis of the effects of psychoeducational care in adults with chronic obstructive pulmonary disease. *Patient Education and Counselling*, 29, 167–178.

Dunbar, F. (1935). *Emotions and bodily changes*. New York: Columbia University Press.

Dunbar, F. (1938). Psychoanalytic notes relating to syndromes of asthma and hay fever. *The Psychoanalytic Quarterly*, 7, 25–68.

Eiser, N., West, C., Evans, S., Jeffers, A. & Quirk, F. (1997). Effects of psychotherapy in moderately severe COPD: a pilot study. *European Respiratory Journal*, 10, 1581–1584.

Grant, I., Prigatano, G.P., Heaton, R.K., McSweeny, A.J., Wright, E.C. & Adams, K.M. (1987). Progressive neuropsychologic impairment and hypoxemia. *Archives of General Psychiatry*, 44, 999–1006.

Hawton, K., Salkovskis, P.M., Kirk, J. & Clark, D.M. (Eds) (1989). *Cognitive behaviour therapy for psychiatric problems*. Oxford: Oxford University Press.

Horowitz, H.W. (1996). Night attack. *The Lancet*, 348, 252.

Kaptein, A.A. (1982). Psychological correlates of length of hospitalization and rehospitalization in patients with acute, severe asthma. *Social Science and Medicine*, 16, 725–729.

Kaptein, A.A. (1997). Behavioural interventions in COPD: a pause for breath. *European Respiratory Review*, 7, 88–91.

Kaptein, A.A. & Dekker, F.W. (2000). Psychosocial support. *European Respiratory Monograph*, 13, 58–69.

Kaptein, A.A., Hooghiemstra, P., Wagenaar, J.P.M. & Wagenaar-Stoop, W.M.Th. (1991). Sexuality in patients with COPD. *American Review of Respiratory Disease*, 143, A676 [abstract].

Kaptein, A.A., Brand, P.L.P., Dekker, F.W., Kerstjens, H.A.M., Postma, D.S., Sluiter, H.J. & the Dutch CNSLD Study Group (1993). Quality-of-life in a long-term multicentre trial in chronic nonspecific lung disease: assessment at baseline. *European Respiratory Journal*, 6, 1479–1484.

Kinsman, R.A., Dirks, J.F. & Jones, N.F. (1982). Psychomaintenance of chronic physical illness. In: T. Millon, C. Green & R. Meagher (Eds), *Handbook of clinical health psychology* (pp. 435–466). New York: Plenum Press.

Kinsman, R.A., Fernandez, E., Schocket, M., Dirks, J.F. & Covino, N.A. (1983). Multidimensional analysis of the symptoms of chronic bronchitis and emphysema. *Journal of Behavioral Medicine*, 6, 339–357.

Kleinman, A. (1988). *The illness narratives*. New York: Basic Books.

Knapp, P.H. (1963). The asthmatic child and the psychosomatic problem of asthma: toward a general theory. In: H.I. Scheer (Ed.), *The asthmatic child* (pp. 234–255). New York: Harper & Row.

Knapp, T.J. & Wells, L.A. (1978). Behavior therapy for asthma: a review. *Behaviour Research and Therapy*, 16, 103–115.

Kotses, H. & Glaus, K.D. (1981). Applications of biofeedback to the treatment of asthma: a critical review. *Biofeedback and Selfregulation*, 6, 573–593.

Lacasse, Y., Guyatt, G.H., King, D., Cook, D.J. & Goldstein, R.S. (1996). Meta-analysis of respiratory rehabilitation in chronic obstructive pulmonary disease. *The Lancet*, 348, 1115–1119.

Leventhal, H., Benyami, Y., Brownlee, S., *et al.* (1997). Illness representations: theoretical foundations. In: K.J. Petrie & J.A. Weinman (Eds), *Perceptions of health and illness* (pp. 19–45). Amsterdam: Harwood Academic Publishers.

Linden, W., Stossel, C. & Maurice, J. (1996). Psychosocial interventions for patients with coronary artery disease. *Archives of Internal Medicine*, 156, 745–752.

McSweeny, A.J. & Creer, T.L. (1995). Health-related quality-of-life assessment in medical care. *Disease-a-Month*, 41, 1–72.

Mahler, D.A. & Harver, A. (1996). Dyspnea. In: A.P. Fishman (Ed.), *Pulmonary rehabilitation* (pp. 97–116). New York: Marcel Dekker.

Maillé, A.R., Kaptein, A.A., de Haes, J.C.J.M. & Everaerd, W.Th.A.M. (1996). Assessing quality of life in chronic nonspecific lung disease. A review of empirical studies published between 1980 and 1994. *Quality of Life Research*, 5, 287–301.

Meyer, T.J. & Mark, M.M. (1995). Effects of psychosocial interventions with adult cancer patients: a meta-analysis of randomized experiments. *Health Psychology*, 14, 101–108.

Miklich, D.R., Renne, C.M., Creer, T.L., *et al.* (1977). The clinical utility of behavior therapy as an adjunctive treatment for asthma. *Journal of Allergy and Clinical Immunology*, 60, 285–294.

Murray, C.J.L. & Lopez, A.D. (1997). Mortality by cause for eight regions of the world: Global burden of disease study. *The Lancet*, 349, 1269–1276.

Pennebaker, J.W. (1982). *The psychology of physical symptoms*. New York: Springer.

Pennebaker, J.W. (Ed.) (1995). *Emotion, disclosure, & health*. Washington DC: APA.

Petrie, K.J. & Weinman, J.A. (Eds) (1997). *Perceptions of health & illness*. Amsterdam: Harwood Academic Publishers.

Petrie, K.J., Weinman, J., Sharpe, N. & Buckley, J. (1996). Role of patients' view of their illness in predicting return to work and functioning after myocardial infarction: longitudinal study. *British Medical Journal*, 312, 1191–1194.

Richter, R. & Dahme, B. (1982). Bronchial asthma in adults: there is little evidence for the effectiveness of behavioural therapy and relaxation. *Journal of Psychosomatic Research*, 26, 533–540.

Ries, A.L., Kaplan, R.M., Limberg, T.M. & Prewitt, L.M. (1995). Effects of pulmonary rehabilitation on physiologic and psychosocial outcomes in patients with chronic obstructive pulmonary disease. *Annals of Internal Medicine*, 122, 823–832.

Rosser, R., Denford, J., Heslop, A., *et al.* (1983). Breathlessness and psychiatric morbidity in chronic bronchitis and emphysema: a study of psychotherapeutic management. *Psychological Medicine*, 13, 93–110.

Rubenfeld, G.D., Angus, D.C., Pinsky, M.R., Randall Curtis, J., Connors, A.F., Bernard, G.R. (1999). Outcomes research in critical care. *American Journal of Respiratory and Critical Care Medicine*, 160, 358–367.

Scharloo, M., Kaptein, A.A., Weinman, J.A., Willems, L.N.A. & Rooijmans, H.G.M. (2000). Physical and psychological correlates of functioning in patients with chronic obstructive pulmonary disease. *Journal of Asthma*, 37, 17–29.

Smyth, J.M. (1998). Written emotional expression: effect sizes, outcome types, and moderating variables. *Journal of Consulting and Clinical Psychology*, 66, 174–184.

Smyth, J.M., Stone, A.A., Hurewitz, A. & Kaell, A. (1999). Effects of writing about stressful experiences on symptom reduction in patients with asthma or rheumatoid arthritis. *Journal of the American Medical Association*, 281, 1304–1309.

Stuss, D.T., Peterkin, I., Guzman, D.A., Guzman, C. & Troyer, A.K. (1997). Chronic obstructive pulmonary disease: effects of hypoxia on neurological and neuropsychological measures. *Journal of Clinical and Experimental Neuropsychology*, 19, 515–524.

Teiramaa, E. (1978). Psychic disturbances and duration of asthma. *Journal of Psychosomatic Research*, 22, 401–408.

van Ede, L., Ijzermans, C.J. & Brouwer, H.J. (1999). Prevalence of depression in patients with chronic obstructive pulmonary disease: a systematic review. *Thorax*, 54, 688–692.

Wahlström, R., Lagerløv, P., Stålsby Lundborg C., Veninga, C.C.M., Hummers-Pradier, E., Dahlgren, L.O., Denig P., & the DEP group. (2001). Variations in general practitioners' views of asthma management in four European countries. *Social Science and Medicine* 53, 507–518.

Webb, M.W. & Lawton, A.H. (1961). Basic personality traits characteristic of patients with primary obstructive pulmonary emphysema. *Journal of the American Geriatrics Society*, 9, 590–610.

Williams, S.J. (1993). *Chronic respiratory illness*. London: Routledge.

Wood-Dauphinee, S. (1999). Assessing quality of life in clinical research: from where have we come and where are we going? *Journal of Clinical Epidemiology*, 52, 355–363.

2
Epidemiology of asthma

Peter J. Gergen and Herman E. Mitchell

Editors' note—*Peter Gergen and Herman Mitchell have performed an unusually thorough review in describing the epidemiology of asthma. They provide insights into the disorder, ranging from the evolution of the definition of asthma to the increasing prevalence of the condition. In doing so, Peter and Herman have extended both our knowledge of asthma and the potential uses of epidemiological data by medical and behavioral scientists. The comprehensive review has occurred, in the words of Pearce et al. (1998, p. vii), 'within the context of major concerns about asthma mortality and the increasing burden of asthma morbidity, and major developments in the understanding and management of asthma'. Such a review is of inestimable value to all who work with asthma.*

As described by Gergen and Mitchell, epidemiological data on asthma have a number of uses, as is apparent in reading this chapter. An oft-overlooked value of epidemiological information, however, is its role as base rates for making clinical decisions (Garb, 1998). Garb pointed out that a shortcoming of clinical practice is a disregard or underuse of information about base rates. If base rates for a disorder vary either as a function of patient variables, such as race, social class, gender, or age, or as a function of other variables such as context or diagnoses by other clinicians, then Garb argued, these should have an effect on diagnosis.

There are also times when it is inappropriate to use epidemiological data as a base rate: for example, when thorough physical testing and examination data confirms the diagnosis of asthma in someone with no family history of asthma or allergies. In this case, the clinician would base the diagnosis on other information and, correctly, ignore epidemiological data as a base rate. Base rates are most helpful when the case history is ambiguous and when base rates are very high or very low (Garb, 1998). It is then, when epidemiological data such as that summarized by Peter and Herman can make a major contribution to the diagnostic process. Including epidemiological information in the equation for diagnosing asthma should result in more accurate diagnoses of the condition and, in turn, provide a more accurate perspective of the increasing impact of asthma in the world.

Introduction

The epidemiology of asthma may appear confusing and contradictory to the casual observer. The lack of a gold standard for identifying asthma and the multitude of factors involved in the pathogenesis contribute to this confusion. Fundamental questions remain about the nature of asthma. Does the recurrent airway obstruction which we call asthma represent a single disease entity or a heterogeneous group of diseases which have a common final pathway? What role does allergy play in asthma? In the 1940s, Rackemann (1947) suggested there were at least two distinct subgroups – extrinsic asthmatics, who tend to start earlier in life (before age 30 years) and have other associated allergic manifestations, and intrinsic asthmatics, who tend to have onset of their disease later in life (after age 40 years) and do not have associated allergic manifestations. Burrows *et al.* (1989) reported that asthma at all ages is related to allergy. This chapter provides an overview of asthma epidemiology. It is hoped that the reader will look upon this area of research as a challenge and an excellent opportunity where important contributions can be made. There are many questions to be answered and a great deal of solid research that helps to point the way.

There have been many attempts to define asthma. Most early definitions of asthma have dealt with the physiological manifestation of the disease, i.e., recurrent airway obstruction. These definitions emphasized the role of bronchial muscular contraction, which was felt to play a dominant role in the airway obstruction. In accordance with this approach, the mainstay of treatment focused on relieving the muscle contraction by a variety of drugs, such as beta-agonists. In recent years the role of inflammation has received increasing attention. The current definition of asthma, as set forth by the National Asthma Education and Prevention Program's (NAEPP) Expert Panel Report 2 (National Institutes of Health, 1997), prominently features the inflammatory aspects of asthma:

> *Asthma is a chronic inflammatory disorder of the airways in which many cells and cellular elements play a role, in particular, mast cells, eosinophils, T lymphocytes, macrophages, neutrophils, and epithelial cells. In susceptible individuals, this inflammation causes recurrent episodes of wheezing, breathlessness, chest tightness, and coughing, particularly at night or in the early morning. These episodes are usually associated with widespread but variable airflow obstruction that is often reversible either spontaneously or with treatment. The inflammation also causes an associated increase in the existing bronchial hyperresponsiveness to a variety of stimuli.*
> *(National Institutes of Health, 1997, p. 8)*

Accordingly, the treatment recommendations from this Expert Panel have shifted in focus to a greater emphasis on anti-inflammatory treatment.

While the Expert Panel's definition of asthma emphasizes airway inflammation, it does not readily lend itself to use in clinical or epidemiologic studies. Gross (1980) suggested that, given this problem, each study should not simply use the term asthma but include a detailed definition of what is meant by asthma. Epidemiologic studies have taken a number of approaches to operationalizing asthma: a reported diagnosis with or without a doctor's confirmation; the report of certain symptoms, the presence of bronchoreactivity in response to a number of tests, such as methacholine or exercise; and any combination of the above. To study active asthmatics, researchers have required that symptoms occur within a defined period of time, usually 12 months, or that the study participants are currently taking asthma medications.

Each of these approaches has its strengths and weaknesses. Using a diagnosis of asthma with or without a physician's confirmation presumes an individual has been correctly evaluated, assigned the diagnostic label, and reported the diagnosis when asked. Population studies have shown a large amount of active asthma is undiagnosed in both children (Speight *et al.*, 1983) and adults (Banerjee *et al.*, 1987). Asthma that is no longer active tends to be forgotten. The National Child Development Study investigated asthma prevalence in a birth cohort interviewed at 7, 11, and 16 years of age. At age 16, 11.6% of patients reported asthma or wheezy bronchitis (AW) during their lifetime but, when all three interviews were evaluated, a total of 24.7% had reported AW in at least one of the interviews (Anderson *et al.*, 1986).

Similar sets of symptoms may not result in being assigned the same diagnosis. In a longitudinal study of respiratory disease in Tucson, Arizona, it was noted that among older subjects with wheeze, dyspnea, and shortness of breath, males tended to receive the diagnosis of emphysema while females tended to receive the diagnosis of asthma or chronic bronchitis (Dodge *et al.*, 1986). Similar problems occur among racial or ethnic groups. In a study of 9–11-year-old schoolchildren in Philadelphia, the prevalence of chronic wheezing was found to be similar between the racial or ethnic groups while the assignment of a diagnosis to chronic wheeze was related to race, with African-American children more likely to receive the diagnosis of asthma (Cunningham *et al.*, 1996). In New Zealand, all asthma deaths identified by death certificate during a 2-year period were evaluated by an expert panel based on a review of the clinical data. Under the age of 35 the accuracy of the death certificate for asthma being the certified cause of death was approximately 98%, but the accuracy dropped off with age and reached 39% at 70+ years of age (Sears *et al.*, 1986b).

The use of symptoms avoids the problem of diagnostic labeling while introducing other problems. Wheeze is the most common symptom of asthma (Lee *et al.*, 1983). However not all asthmatics wheeze. A cough-variant asthma has been reported among children where the predominant feature is a cough that responds to bronchodilator therapy (Corrao *et al.*, 1979; Cloutier & Loughlin, 1981; Johnson & Osborn, 1991). Bronchoreactivity, as measured by response to exercise or histamine, has been proposed as a gold standard for asthma. Population studies, however, have shown that this measure does not have a high degree of sensitivity and specificity (Sears *et al.*, 1986a; Pattemore *et al.*, 1990). In one school-based study among 7–10-year-old children in New Zealand, 41% of the children with bronchoreactivity had no current asthma symptoms while 42% of children with the diagnosis of asthma and current symptoms did not have bronchoreactivity (Pattemore *et al.*, 1990). A recent international consensus conference on asthma recommended that bronchoreactivity not be used as a criterion for the diagnosis of asthma among children (Warner *et al.*, 1998).

It has been shown by test–retest studies that the symptoms of asthma can be reliably reported (Mitchell & Miles, 1983). However, the prevalence of asthma can vary by the source of the report. Fathers have been noted to under report their children's asthma symptoms compared with mothers' reports (Schenker *et al.*, 1983). It has previously been assumed that one had to ask the parents to get accurate information on childhood asthma. However, a study by Guyatt *et al.* (1997) looked at symptoms, quality of life, and pulmonary functions and found that after age 11 little additional information was obtained by questioning the parents than that given by the child.

Burden

In the United States during 1996, there were an estimated 14.6 million people with asthma, 4.4 million of whom were less than 18 years old (Adams, Hendershot & Marano, 1999). Among children less than 18 years of age, asthma is the third most prevalent chronic disease after respiratory allergies and recurrent ear infections, and is responsible for approximately 10.1 million days lost from school (Taylor & Newacheck, 1992). During 1996, asthma was the first list diagnosis in 474,000 hospitalizations (Graves & Kuzak, 1998) and 5667 deaths (Anon., 1996a). In 1995, there were approximately 12.2 million visits to physician offices, outpatient departments, and emergency rooms (ER) for asthma (Schappert, 1997). Separate cost of illness studies have estimated the total economic cost of asthma in the United States during the early 1990s to be approximately $6 billion dollars a year (Weiss *et al.*, 1992; Smith *et al.*, 1997).

Prevalence

The prevalence of asthma is highly dependent on the definition chosen. The prevalence of asthma varied almost three-fold, from 3.6% to 9.5%, when various combinations of physician diagnosis and wheezing were used to define asthma among children 3–17 years of age who participated in the second National Health and Nutrition Examination Survey (NHANES II), 1976–80 (Gergen *et al.*, 1988).

Despite this dependence on definition, certain patterns appear consistently in the age distribution of asthma. Most childhood asthma begins before age 5 years (Gergen *et al.*, 1988b). A review of medical records of the Mayo Clinic found the highest incidence of asthma occurred in the first year of life, with rates falling throughout childhood and reaching their lowest levels among adults (Yunginger *et al.*, 1992) During childhood more males develop asthma, while during adolescence the prevalence in females surpasses males. After adolescence males and females have equivalent rates when a broad range of ages is examined (Turkeltaub & Gergen, 1991; Adams & Marano, 1995).

Other demographic characteristics have a less consistent relationship with asthma prevalence because of the definitional problems involved both with asthma and the particular demographic factor. Differences in asthma prevalence between African-American and whites depends upon both the age group and the particular study. The NHANES II reported higher rates in African-Americans at all ages (Gergen *et al.*, 1988; Turkeltaub & Gergen, 1991); the 1994 National Health Interview Study (NHIS) reported little to no difference in adults (Adams & Marano, 1995), while the 1981 and 1988 Child Health Supplement (CHS) of the NHIS reported more asthma in African-American children under age 18 years (Weitzman *et al.*, 1992). Hispanic children were reported to have the same asthma prevalence as non-Hispanic children in the 1981 and 1988 CHS, data from the Hispanic HANES and NHANES II using a different definition for Hispanics reported wide discrepancies in prevalence; Mexican American children in the Southwest reported some of the lowest rates of asthma in the United States while Puerto Rican children living on the East Coast of the United States reported some of the highest rates of asthma in the United States (Carter-Pokras & Gergen, 1993). Asthma prevalence has been reported to increase with poverty (Turkeltaub & Gergen, 1991; Adams & Marano, 1995), although not consistently (Gergen *et al.*, 1988; Adams, Hendershot, & Marano, 1996). The NHIS has shown that the prevalence of asthma increased in urban areas (Adams & Marano, 1995), although more focused studies have shown the prevalence of asthma can be just as high in nonurban areas of the United States, such as Los Alamos, New Mexico (Sporik *et al.*, 1995) as the Bronx in New York City (Crain *et al.*, 1994).

An understanding of the changing nature of asthma with age comes from a series of longitudinal cohort studies. Wheezing in the first several years of life appears to be transient in nature. Between 50 and 60% of children who wheeze at age 3 years will no longer report wheezing at 6 years of age (Brooke *et al.*, 1995; Martinez *et al.*, 1995b). Many asthmatics lose their symptoms as they grow older. In a 16-year follow-up of 6–14-year-old asthmatics evaluated at a hospital outpatient department,

57% were no longer wheezing at follow-up (Gerritsen *et al.*, 1989). In a 20-year follow-up of asthmatics less than 12 years of age recruited from a general practice in England, 28% reported no symptoms at the time of follow-up and 24% reported minimal symptoms (Blair, 1977). In a 33-year follow-up of children whose asthma began before age 7 years, only 50% were still wheezing by age 7 years, 18% at 11 years, and 10% at 16 and 23 years. However, wheezing increased to 27% at age 33 years (Strachan *et al.*, 1996). Others have reported a similar recurrence of wheezing in adulthood (Martin *et al.*, 1980; Kelly *et al.*, 1987). Among those who continue to wheeze, the severity of the wheezing in general tends to decrease as the individuals become adults (Martin *et al.*, 1980; Kelly *et al.*, 1987). A variety of factors have been associated with the persistence of asthma – early onset, severity, coexisting atopy such as eczema, allergic rhinitis, family history of atopy, and lower pulmonary function tests (Blair, 1977; Gerritsen *et al.*, 1989; Aberg & Engstrom, 1990; Strachan *et al.*, 1996).

International studies seem to indicate that asthma is lowest in developing countries and highest in Australia and New Zealand (Dowse *et al.*, 1985a; Woolcock, 1986; Yemaneberhan *et al.*, 1997). Comparisons of reported asthma prevalence among countries is hindered by a number of methodologic differences, such as the questions used to identify asthma, the age groups studied, and sampling techniques. Nonetheless, even when studies employ identical data collection techniques, international differences persist. In a study of schoolchildren 12 years of age in New Zealand, Wales, South Africa, and Sweden that involved both questionnaire and exercise challenge, a lifetime history of asthma was reported by 16.8% in New Zealand, 12% in Wales, 11.5% in South Africa, and 4% in Sweden. A similar pattern was found with the exercise challenge to define asthma (Burr *et al.*, 1994). An ongoing international effort to measure the reported prevalence of childhood asthma worldwide using a standardized questionnaire, International Study of Asthma and Allergies in Childhood (ISAAC), reports major differences in the prevalence of asthma worldwide with the lowest rates in the less developed parts of the world (ISAAC Steering Committee, 1998).

The prevalence of diagnosed asthma has been reported to be increasing worldwide during the 1980s and 1990s (Robertson *et al.*, 1991; Weitzman *et al.*, 1992; Anderson *et al.*, 1994). Much of this increase may be driven by an increase in the diagnosis of mild asthmatics who previously were undiagnosed as having asthma (Weitzman *et al.*, 1992; Anderson *et al.*, 1994). A critical review of the literature reporting the increase in asthma prevalence concluded that it is impossible to determine if the reported increase in prevalence is real due to the potential for increased labeling of previously unrecognized asthma, the changing meaning of the words used to describe the symptoms of asthma, such as wheeze, and the lack of objective measures for asthma (Magnus & Jaakkola,

1997). However, one of the few studies that used both questionnaire and objective data (exercise provocation testing) reported asthma had increased between 1973 and 1988 in Britain (Burr *et al.*, 1989).

Health Care Utilization

Asthma hospitalizations are highest among young children (especially those under age 5 years), with young males having higher rates than young females; adult females have higher rates than adult males, with the rates being higher in the inner cities and among the poor and minorities. (Gergen & Weiss, 1990; Carr *et al.*, 1992; Skolbeloff *et al.*, 1992; Taylor & Newacheck, 1992; Gottlieb *et al.*, 1995). The majority of asthma hospitalizations occur early in life – approximately 37% of all asthma hospitalizations occur among children less than 15 years of age – and over 65% occur among individuals less than 45 years of age. However, the hospitalization rate increases again for individuals over age 65 years. Readmission for asthma is not infrequent after an initial asthma hospitalization. Among Canadian children with asthma, the 6-month probability for rehospitalization was 20% for 0–4 year olds and 11.7% for 5–17 year olds (To *et al.*, 1996). Asthma hospitalizations have been reported to be rising in the United States (Gergen & Weiss, 1990) as they have been in the rest of the world (Mitchell, 1985). The rise is greatest in youngest children and among African-Americans. This increase does not appear to be due only to a rise in the readmission rate (Anderson *et al.*, 1980; Hisnanick *et al.*, 1994).

Poverty is an important factor in asthma hospitalizations, most likely through lack of access to medical care (Wissow *et al.*, 1988; Billings *et al.*, 1993). In a study of asthma hospitalizations among children 1–19 years of age in Maryland, differences in the rates between whites and African-American children all but disappeared when an ecological adjustment for poverty was included (Wissow *et al.*, 1988). However, poverty does not guarantee a high rate of asthma. Hisnanick *et al.* (1994) reported that both the level of and increase in asthma hospitalizations among American Indians and Alaskan Natives (AI/AN) was similar to whites, and much lower than African-Americans even though AI/AN have one of the highest levels of poverty in the United States. More open access to medical care through Indian Health Service facilities may play a role in keeping hospitalizations low among AI/AN.

Mortality

In contrast to hospitalizations, asthma mortality occurs mostly among the old – approximately 69% of all deaths from asthma in the United States occur after 54 years of age. In the United States, African-Americans have approximately twice the death rate from asthma as whites (Anon., 1994). However, depending on the age group studied, this discrepancy can increase to as much as six times (Anon, 1996b). Geographic-based studies have identified inner-city areas with high levels of minorities and poverty as areas with high levels of asthma mortality (Carr *et al.*, 1992; Lang & Polansky, 1994). Asthma mortality varies throughout the world, with the United States having a relatively low rate of asthma mortality, and the highest rates being noted in New Zealand, Germany, and Norway (Sears, 1991).

Asthma mortality is a multifaceted, multicausal event. Concern has been raised about excessive treatment with beta-agonists contributing to the increase in asthma morbidity and mortality (Sears *et al.*, 1990). Yet a meta-analysis found little to no relationship between beta-agonist use and mortality (Mullen *et al.*, 1993). In New Zealand, a long acting beta-agonist, fenoterol, has been implicated in the high level of asthma mortality (Grainger *et al.*, 1991). Identification and awareness of the problems associated with fenoterol has reduced the levels of asthma mortality, but the New Zealand rates still remain among the highest in the world (Pearce *et al.*, 1995). Local studies in the United States have implicated psychosocial factors and undertreatment in cases of asthma mortality (Strunk *et al.*, 1985; Birkhead *et al.*, 1989). A decreased sensitivity to the severity of the airway obstruction during an asthma attack may predispose some asthmatics to near-fatal and fatal outcomes (Kikuchi *et al.*, 1994).

Although asthma mortality is generally felt to be a result of prolonged, severe, uncontrolled asthma, a retrospective review of asthma deaths among individuals aged 20 years or less in Australia found that 33% were judged to have a history of mild asthma, while only 36% were judged to have severe asthma, and 32% had no previous hospitalizations for asthma (Robertson *et al.*, 1992). Although much emphasis is placed on mortality, the life expectancy of the average asthmatic is not shortened by the disease. A community-based study in Rochester, Minnesota, found asthmatics had the same life expectancy as residents without asthma, the only exception was asthmatics with diagnosis after age 35 years and with other concomitant lung disease where survival was jeopardized (Silverstein *et al.*, 1994).

Mortality due to asthma is not a recent phenomena. Speizer & Doll (1968) evaluated asthma mortality between 1867 through 1967 among people 5–34 years of age in England and Wales, and found the mortality rate was remarkably stable through 1962. Since the 1960s two epidemics of asthma mortality have occurred. During the 1960s, asthma mortality was found to be increasing in a number of countries around the world; mortality from asthma subsequently decreased during the 1970s. The increase during the 1960s has been associated with high doses of bronchodilators (Inman & Adelstein, 1969), but not all agree with this explanation (Gandevia, 1973). The second epidemic of asthma deaths began in the late 1970s and has continued through the 1990s (Sears, 1991), although there have been reports that the rate of increase is leveling off in the United States (Sly & O'Donnell, 1997) and falling in some countries such as New Zealand (Pearce *et al.*, 1995).

Inner Cities

As previously noted, inner-city areas have high levels of asthma morbidity and mortality (Carr *et al.*, 1992; Lang & Polansky, 1994; Gotlieb *et al.*, 1995). To help better understand the high rates of asthma in the inner city, the National Cooperative Inner-City Asthma Study (NCICAS) 1991–1996 was conducted. The first phase of the NCICAS study evaluated and followed for 1 year more than 1500 children (ages 5–9 years) with asthma living in eight inner-city areas in the eastern United States (Kattan *et al.*, 1997; Mitchell *et al.*, 1997). The NCICAS project reported high levels of morbidity of both symptoms and health care utilization. On average, the children reported 3–3.5 days of wheeze per 2-week period; approximately 66% had one or more unscheduled visits for asthma and 17% were hospitalized for asthma over the course of the year. While many risk factors for asthma were reported to be present among these children, no single asthma risk factor predominated. Environmental factors such as environmental tobacco smoke (ETS) and allergens, especially cockroaches, were observed to be at high levels in inner-city homes. Problems with access to care existed despite the majority of children having insurance; adherence problems and family disruptions contributed to the difficulty of managing the children's asthma. The findings of the NCICAS project suggest that a broad-based multifaceted intervention will be required to reduce asthma in the inner city.

Severity

Asthma severity is usually defined by any number of criteria: presence of symptoms; pulmonary functions (forced expiratory volume in one second (FEV_1) or peak flow); medication use, especially of beta-agonists; health care utilization (ER visits or hospitalizations); quality of life; or even death. However, the relationship among these various factors is not at all straightforward. Asthma mortality does not appear to occur predominately in severe asthmatics (Robertson *et al.*, 1992). Asthma symptoms recorded by means of a daily diary had little to no correlation to peak expiratory flow rate (PEFR) and albuterol use recorded during the same period (Apter *et al.*, 1994). Interventions can change medical use patterns such as decreasing ER usage without changing other manifestations of asthma, such as waking at night, beta-agonist use, or self-ratings of asthma severity (Cowie *et al.*, 1997). One reason for these discrepancies may be that these measures more accurately reflect asthma control than does severity (Cockcroft & Swystun, 1996). Asthma control can be influenced by a number of factors, including the quality of medical care received and the adherence of the patient to that care. Unfortunately, there is no method available to measure the underlying severity of asthma. Cockcroft & Swystun (1996) proposed that asthma severity would be better defined by the quantity and type of medication needed to keep the asthmatic under good control rather than the previously mentioned measures. However, this approach can be confounded by other factors, such as environmental control, which may reduce the need for asthma-controlling medications.

Role of Medical Care

Access to, and receipt of, appropriate care can make a substantial difference in the type and amount of health care utilized by an asthmatic. A retrospective chart review of children hospitalized for asthma in three cities in the United States with markedly different levels of asthma hospitalizations found the children in the city with the highest hospitalization rates appeared to have the least adequate primary care for their asthma (Homer *et al.*, 1996). Although the vast majority of children in the inner cities have access to care through Medicaid and similar programs, more than half of these families have reported significant difficulty in actually getting medications, making appointments, and getting to their physician's office or clinic (Crain *et al.*, 1998). In a managed care setting, the use of a written asthma management plan has been shown to be associated with reduced hospitalizations and ER visits (Lieu *et al.*, 1997).

Appropriate use of medications can decrease asthma morbidity and improve the quality of life of an asthmatic. Numerous reports have been produced by expert panels in the United States (Expert Panel 2 Report, 1997) and the world (Warner *et al.*, 1998) in an attempt to define what appropriate asthma therapy should be. Despite the concerns about overuse of certain medicines being associated with asthma mortality, the major problem appears to be underrecognition and under, or inadequate, treatment of asthma by both the doctor and the patient, especially among poor children (Kattan *et al.*, 1997; Eggleston *et al.*, 1998).

The type of treatment a child receives for asthma can be influenced by the site at which treatment is received and by who delivers the treatment. In a study in the United States of children aged 1–6 years hospitalized for asthma in Boston, children who received their primary care from hospital-based clinics or neighborhood health centers were receiving less optimal medication than those receiving care from private practitioners after adjustment for a variety of socioeconomic and medical factors (Finkelstein *et al.*, 1995). Studies comparing outcomes of asthmatics treated by specialists and nonspecialists have reported better outcomes in asthmatics treated by the specialist (Engel *et al.*, 1989; Zeiger *et al.*, 1991). When examined in detail, the important difference between specialist care and primary care appears to be a greater emphasis on asthma education, taking of inhaled steroids, and the use of ancillary devices such as spacers and peak flow meters among specialists. As the majority of care for asthma in the United States is provided by primary care givers, more emphasis must be paid to train primary care doctors to treat asthma properly (Weiss *et al.*, 1992).

Heredity versus Environment

Genetics plays an important role in asthma. For many years, it has been reported that individuals with asthma have a higher probability of having a parent or sibling with asthma than those without asthma (Van Arsdell & Motulsky, 1959; Sibbald *et al.*, 1980). The risk of asthma in children has been reported to increase as the number of parents with asthma increases (Sibbald & Turner-Warwick, 1979). Although a variety of mechanisms for inheritance have been suggested, including a dominant, recessive, or a polygenic system with incomplete penetrance, no one mechanism of inheritance has been agreed upon (Van Arsdell & Motulsky, 1959; Edfors-Lubs, 1971; Kjellman, 1977). As molecular genetic techniques have been developed, specific alleles have been identified for immunoglobulin E (IgE) (Cookson *et al.*, 1992) and bronchoreactivity (Postma *et al.*, 1995). A genomic-wide search for genes associated with asthma is underway and a variety of candidate genes have been identified (Anon, 1997). Further work is needed to determine the importance of the genes identified.

Environmental influences also appear to play a role in the development of asthma. Migrant populations tend to develop asthma at the levels of their adopted lands rather than their country of origin. A study of children living on Tokelau, an island in the Pacific Ocean, and children of Tokelauan origin living in New Zealand found that the Tokelauan children living in New Zealand had about double the prevalence of asthma as the Tokelauan children living in Tokelau. This was true even when the children were new immigrants to New Zealand (Waite *et al.*, 1980). Exposure to high levels of house dust mite has been shown in a longitudinal study of children from birth to 11 years of age to be associated with an increased in the development of asthma (Sporik *et al.*, 1990).

Twin studies have long been used to determine the relative importance of environment and heredity on disease development. Varying results have been reported from twin studies on asthma from a heritability estimate of 35.6% in a study of 13,888 Finnish twin pairs aged 18–70+ years. Surprisingly, when examined by gender, the heritability estimate was 67.8% for females and 0% for males (Nieminen *et al.*, 1991). In contrast, a report on 5864 Norwegian twins studied at 18–25 years of age reported a 75% heritability estimate (Harris *et al.*, 1997). No separate estimates were given by gender.

Correlates of Asthma

Atopy, as defined by IgE or allergen skin testing, is highly related to asthma (Gergen *et al.*, 1988; Zimmerman *et al.*, 1988; Burrows *et al.*, 1989; Kalliel *et al.*, 1989). The link between allergy skin test reactivity and asthma is not direct, as the level of skin test reactivity drops rapidly after the age of 40; by age 60, it reaches one-third the level found in patients during their 20s (Gergen *et al.*, 1987). This age trend is not found in the prevalence of asthma. In very old asthmatic patients (>70 years of age), allergen skin tests can be very infrequent (Braman *et al.*, 1991). Increasing levels of atopy, as defined by number of positive allergen skin tests, has been related to the severity of asthma in children (Zimmerman *et al.*, 1988) but not in adults (Inouye *et al.*, 1985).

Not all allergens seem to be related to asthma occurrence. In a longitudinal study of children from birth to age 13, only allergen skin test reactivity to dust mite and cat were associated with the development of asthma in New Zealand (Sears *et al.*, 1989). In a nationally representative sample of 6–24 year olds in the United States, house dust and Alternaria were associated with asthma (Gergen & Turkeltaub, 1992). Grass pollen was not associated with asthma in either study. Sensitivity to Alternaria was also implicated in attacks of respiratory arrest in young asthmatics in Minnesota (O'Hollaren *et al.*, 1991). Cat allergen has been implicated as a risk for children who have been hospitalized for asthma (Sarpong & Karrison, 1997).

The amount of allergen to which an individual is exposed also appears to play a role in the development and severity of asthma. A longitudinal study of English children up to 11 years old found increased levels of house dust mite associated with the development of asthma (Sporik *et al.*, 1990). Exposure to increasing amounts of a specific allergen, such as dust mites or cockroaches, has been associated with increasing levels of asthma severity (Chan-Yeung *et al.*, 1995; Rosenstreich *et al.*, 1997).

Other forms of atopy, such as infantile eczema and hayfever, have been associated with asthma (Duffy *et al.*, 1990; Anderson *et al.*, 1992; Jenkins *et al.*, 1993). Environmental factors such as dampness and molds have been associated with increased levels of asthma (Schenker *et al.*, 1983; Platt *et al.*, 1989). Soybean dust from unloading of ships has been associated with outbreaks of asthma in several port cities around the world (Anto *et al.*, 1989; White *et al.*, 1997).

Outdoor air pollution can affect respiratory health, causing both an increase in respiratory symptoms and a decrease in lung function (Goren & Hellmann, 1988; Schmitzberger *et al.*, 1993). Exposure to nitrogen dioxide, sulfur dioxide, ozone, particulates, and acid aerosols has been associated with increases in respiratory symptoms, decreases in spirometric functions, and increases in asthma ER visits and hospitalizations (Pope, 1989; Neas *et al.*, 1995; Romiue *et al.*, 1995; Jarvis *et al.*, 1996). Although specific pollutants have been studied in isolation, air pollution is not usually caused by a single agent, and the interaction of these pollutants has been shown to be important in asthma. Pre-exposure to ozone has been shown to increase bronchial reactivity to sulfur dioxide (Koenig *et al.*, 1990); simultaneous exposure to sulfur dioxide and nitrogen dioxide appears to be more effective in increasing bronchial reactivity to allergen exposure than exposure to either pollutant individually (Devalia *et al.*, 1994).

Outdoor air pollution does not appear to play an important role in the increase in asthma in the United States, since pollutant levels have been decreasing during the time of the increase. Between 1987 and 1996, the ambient concentrations of a number of pollutants decreased – nitrogen dioxide by 10%, ozone by 15%, and sulfur dioxide by 37% – and between 1988 and 1996, ambient particulate matter (PM10) decreased 25% (Anon, 1998).

Environmental Tobacco Smoke

Research regarding the role of ETS in asthma has not been consistent. Some researchers have found ETS exposure to be associated with an approximate doubling of the prevalence of asthma in children (Gortmaker *et al.*, 1982; Weitzman *et al.*, 1990). However, other studies linking ETS to the development of asthma have found less consistent results. In Arizona, ETS exposure was only associated with the development of asthma if mothers had less than 12 years of education but not among the children of more highly educated women (Martinez *et al.*, 1992). In Canada, only children with atopic dermatitis exposed to ETS developed asthma, while others exposed to ETS did not (Murray & Morrison, 1990). Longitudinal studies conducted in New Zealand and Norway have not found ETS to be associated with the development of asthma (Horwood *et al.*, 1985; Lilljeqvist *et al.*, 1997).

A similar lack of consistency is observed in research on the relationship between ETS exposure and asthma severity. The 1981 Child Health Supplement (CHS) of the NHIS reported ETS was associated with the greater use of 'physician-prescribed' asthma medication in the prior 2 weeks (Weitzman *et al.*, 1990), while no association was seen later in the NHANES III (Gergen *et al.*, 1998). Reduced pulmonary function and more reported acute exacerbations were found to be related to ETS exposure among asthmatics attending an allergy clinic (Chilmonczyk *et al.*, 1993). Among low-income urban children in New York City with asthma (average age 9 years old), passive smoking was associated with ER visits for asthma but not with hospitalizations or abnormalities in pulmonary function (Evans *et al.*, 1987). The effects of ETS on severity varied with age among asthmatics evaluated at a Canadian allergy clinic: in the youngest group (1–6 years old), no significant effect was found with exposure to smoke; in the middle age group (7–11 years old), the children of smokers had an increase in their asthma score; and in the oldest group (12–17 years old), the asthma symptom score was increased and the pulmonary functions were decreased in those children exposed to smoke (Murray & Morrison, 1989). In a recent report on 22 children (mean age 5 years old) followed for 1 month after being hospitalized for asthma, children living with a smoker reported 1.9 fewer days of daytime symptoms than those not living with a smoker ($p < 0.05$); however, no statistically significant difference was found in the mean number of nights of symptoms (Abulhosn *et al.*, 1997). Other studies looking at changes in ETS exposure did not find corresponding changes in acute attacks of asthma (Ehrlich *et al.*, 1992; Ogborn *et al.*, 1994).

One might argue that cigarette smoking does not appear to be playing an important role in the increase in asthma in the United States, since it has been decreasing during the time of the well-documented asthma increase. Between 1979 through 1994, the percent of active smokers dropped from 33.5% to 25.5% among individuals 18 or more years of age (Fingerhut & Warner, 1997).

Infections

Respiratory infections play an important role in asthma, and have been recognized as one of the most important triggers for asthma attacks in both children and adults (Minor *et al.*, 1974, 1976; Johnston *et al.*, 1995). Untreated infections of the respiratory tract such as sinusitis can make asthma more difficult to control (Rachelefsky & Spector, 1990). Infections such as chlamydia or respiratory syncytial virus (RSV) have been reported to be associated with the development of asthma by some, but not all, researchers (Pullan & Hey, 1982; Welliver *et al.*, 1986; Hahn *et al.*, 1991). The role respiratory infections play in the development of asthma and atopy is controversial (Frick *et al.*, 1979; Sporik *et al.*, 1990). It has been suggested that early infections may program lymphocytes into certain subsets, increasing the likelihood for the development of asthma (Martinez *et al.*, 1995a). Other researchers have suggested that certain early infections may actually have a protective effect against asthma development (Shirakawa *et al.*, 1997).

Birth and Family Factors

Birth factors seem to play a role in asthma. The prevalence of asthma has been found to be greater in premature infants followed until late childhood and adolescents (Chan *et al.*, 1989; Frischer *et al.*, 1992; Kitchen *et al.*, 1992; McCormick *et al.*, 1992; von Mutius *et al.*, 1993). This effect seems independent of the lung damage suffered as a result of bronchopulmonary disease secondary to premature birth (Smyth *et al.*, 1981).

Birth order has been reported to be associated with asthma – second-born children having a lower prevalence of asthma (Tay *et al.*, 1982). Asthma has been reported to be inversely related to family size (Jarvis *et al.*, 1997), while infants born to younger mothers have been reported to have a higher prevalence of asthma (Infante-Rivard, 1995). Month of birth has also been associated with development of asthma (Anderson *et al.*, 1981; Aberg, 1989).

Diet

The role of diet is unclear. Studies that have examined the effect of breast-feeding on the development of asthma have also reported conflicting results (Horwood *et al.*, 1985; Jonsson *et al.*, 1987; Saarinen & Kajosaari, 1995). In an intervention study where the mother was placed on a low allergenic diet in the last trimester of the pregnancy and the infant and mother had a low allergenic diet, no protection against the development of asthma was seen (Zeiger *et al.*, 1989). Another intervention which controlled both diet and exposure to house dust mite found that asthma was reduced at 2 years of age in the intervention group but that the effect had disappeared by age 4 years (Hide *et al.*, 1996). Other research has suggested that sodium in the diet contributes to bronchial reactivity (Burney *et al.*, 1986).

Weather Conditions

Certain weather conditions such as humidity and temperature have been shown to be associated with increased ER visits and hospitalizations for asthma (Carey & Cordon, 1986; Jamason *et al.*, 1997). Asthma outbreaks have been associated with thunderstorms, possibly as a result of the increased levels of aeroallergens put into the air by the weather disturbances (Davidson *et al.*, 1996).

Seasonality

Asthma has been shown to have a strong seasonal component that appears to vary by the age group and outcome measured. Asthma attacks, hospitalizations, and ER visits are highest in the fall and winter and lowest in the summer, especially in younger individuals (Khot *et al.*, 1984; Luyt *et al.*, 1994; Kljakovic, 1996). In the United States, both hospitalizations and mortality appear to be highest during the winter months for individuals over age 65 years, while for individuals under age 35 years hospitalizations peak in the fall and asthma mortality appears to be higher during the summer. Among individuals 35–64 years of age, hospitalizations peak in the winter; no seasonal trend was noted for mortality (Weiss, 1990). Many factors have been proposed for this seasonal variation, but it appears to be respiratory infections that are driving the fall and winter peaks.

Disease of Modern Civilization?

It has been speculated that the observed increase in asthma is associated with the advent of modern civilization. A number of studies have reported on populations in which the Western lifestyle has been recently introduced and/or the presence of asthma was noted to have appeared in that area in the last 10 years or so. Work from New Guinea found that the prevalence of asthma increased after the natives took up the habit of sleeping with blankets, which increased their exposure to dust mite allergen (Dowse *et al.*, 1985b). Comparison of urban (Western lifestyle) and rural areas in Ethiopia showed much higher levels of asthma associated with the urban areas where more modern living conditions prevail. Yet, despite this observed difference in asthma, the amount of allergen skin test reactivity was similar between urban and rural areas. In fact, reactivity to dust mite was much higher in the rural areas (Yemaneberhan *et al.*, 1997). In both of these populations asthma occurred primarily in adults, not in children. A study of ethnic Chinese secondary school students in Westernized (Hong Kong; Kota Kinabalu, Borneo) and non-Westernized (San Bu, China) areas of Asia reported the prevalence of wheeze and asthma to be much lower in the non-Westernized area, but atopy (as defined by skin test reactivity) was equivalent across the areas (Leung & Ho, 1994). Concern has been raised that the reported low levels of asthma reflect a lack of awareness of the disease due to cultural taboos or limited ascertainment. A number of studies have attempted to employ objective measures to circumvent this problem. A study of peak flow changes after exercise challenge among 7–9-year-old schoolchildren in Zimbabwe found a much lower prevalence of positive challenges in the non-Westernized rural area than in the Westernized urban areas (Keeley *et al.*, 1991). A similar finding was reported looking at Xhosa children in South Africa (Van Niekerk *et al.*, 1979).

Conclusion and Future Directions

As this review has shown, the epidemiology of asthma is full of conflicting, often confusing results. Clearly, there is the lack of a gold standard for the diagnosis of asthma, methodologic inconsistencies in the various studies, and the possibility that what we call asthma is not really a single disease at all, but rather a collection of related diseases with similar manifestations, but different causes. Large-scale epidemiologic studies, such as NCICAS (Kattan *et al.*, 1997; Mitchell *et al.*, 1997), have provided strong evidence that asthma is a multicausal disease with no one factor being identified as the main cause or risk associated with asthma symptoms and severity. In the future, asthma research must focus on identifying individuals who are susceptible to the development of asthma and environmental factors that convert this susceptibility to a reality. It is not clear that questionnaire-based assessments of asthma will accomplish this; yet unmade discoveries in the genetics of asthma and/or atopy may give us this ability. Additionally, it is a major challenge for asthma research to disentangle true etiologic factors from the mere correlates of the disease. This will only be accomplished by a greater emphasis on longitudinal studies and controlled, randomized clinical trials rather than the more common cross-sectional approach that dominates the field. Only by such methodologies, which permit causal determinations, will we be able to understand the importance of specific risk factors in the development and continuation of asthma. Until such time that the disease of asthma is better understood, when reading the asthma literature, one must be constantly aware of how the authors are defining asthma, the study methodology, the groups they are investigating, and the outcomes upon which they are basing their conclusions.

References

Aberg, N. (1989). Birth season variation in asthma and allergic rhinitis. *Clinical and Experimental Allergy*, 19, 643–648.

Aberg, N. & Engstrom, I. (1990). Natural history of allergic disease in children. *Acta Paediatrica Scandinavica*, 79, 206–211.

Abulhosn, R.S., Morray, B.H., Llewellyn, C.E. & Redding, G.J. (1997). Passive smoke exposure impairs recovery after hospitalization for acute asthma. *Archives of Pediatric and Adolescent Medicine*, 151, 135–139.

Adams, P.F. & Marano, M.A. (1995). Current estimates from the National Health Interview Survey, 1994. *National Center for Health Statistics. Vital Health Statistics*, 10, 193.

Adams, P.F., Hendershot, G.E., & Marano, M.A. (1999). Current estimates from the National Health Interview Survey, 1996. *National Center for Health Statistics. Vital Health Statistics,* 10, 200.

Anderson, H.R., Bailey, P. & West, S. (1980). Trends in the hospital care of acute childhood asthma 1970–8: a regional study. *British Medical Journal*, 281, 1191–1194.

Anderson, H.R., Bailey, P.A. & Bland, J.M. (1981). The effect of birth month on asthma, eczema, hayfever, respiratory symptoms, lung function, and hospital admissions for asthma. *International Journal of Epidemiology*, 10, 45–51.

Anderson, H.R., Bland, J.M., Patel, S. & Peckham, C. (1986). The natural history of asthma in childhood. *Journal of Epidemiology and Community Health*, 40, 121–129.

Anderson, H.R., Pottier, A.C. & Strachan, D.P. (1992). Asthma from birth to age 23 – incidence and relation to prior and concurrent atopic disease. *Thorax*, 47, 537–542.

Anderson, H.R., Butland, B.K. & Strachan, D.P. (1994). Trends in prevalence and severity of childhood asthma. *British Medical Journal*, 308, 1600–1604.

Anon. (1994). *U.S. vital statistics, mortality*. U.S. Government, Washington, DC.

Anon. (1996a). *U.S. vital statistics, mortality*. U.S. Government, Washington, DC.

Anon. (1996b). Asthma Mortality and hospitalization among children and young adults – United States, 1980–1993. *Morbidity and Mortality Weekly Report*, 45, 350–353.

Anon. (1997). A genome-wide search for asthma susceptibility loci in ethnically diverse populations. The Collaborative Study on the Genetics of Asthma (CSGA). *Nature Genetics*, 15, 389–392.

Anon. (1998). *National air quality and emissions trends report,* 1996 (EPA-454/R-97–013).

Research Triangle Park, NC 27711: U.S. Environmental Protection Agency, Office of Air Quality Planning and Standards.

Anto, J.M., Sunyer, J., Rodriguez-Roisin, R., Suarez-Cervera, M., Vazquez, L. & The Toxicoepidemiological Committee. (1989). Community outbreaks of asthma associated with inhalation of soybean dust. *New England Journal of Medicine*, 320, 1097–1102.

Apter, A.J., ZuWallack, R.L. & Clive, J. (1994). Common measures of asthma severity lack association for describing its clinical course. *Journal of Allergy and Clinical Immunology*, 94, 732–737.

Banerjee, D.K., Lee, G.S., Malik, S.K. & Daly, S. (1987). Underdiagnosis of asthma in the elderly. *British Journal of Diseases of the Chest*, 81, 23–29.

Billings, J., Zeitel, L., Lukomnik, J., Carey, T.S., Blank, A.E. & Newman, L. (1993). Impact of socioeconomic status on hospital use in New York City. Data Watch. *Health Affairs*, Spring, 162–173.

Birkhead, G., Attaway, N.J., Strunk, R.C., Townsend, M.C. & Teutsch, S. (1989). Investigation of a cluster of deaths of adolescents from asthma: evidence implicating inadequate treatment and poor patient adherence to medications. *Journal of Allergy and Clinical Immunology*, 84, 484–491.

Blair, H. (1977). Natural history of childhood asthma. *Archives of Disease in Childhood*, 52, 613–619.

Braman, S.S., Kaemmerlen, J.T. & Davis, S.M. (1991). Asthma in the elderly. A comparison between patients with recently acquired and long-standing disease. *American Review of Respiratory Disease*, 143, 336–340.

Brooke, A.M., Lambert, P.C., Burton, P.R., Clarke, C., Luyt, D.K. & Simpson, H. (1995). The natural history of respiratory symptoms in preschool children. *American Journal of Respiratory and Critical Care Medicine*, 152, 1872–1878.

Burney, P.G., Britton, J.R., Chinn, S., *et al.*. (1986). Response to inhaled histamine and 24 hour sodium excretion. *British Medical Journal (Clinical Research Edition)*, 292, 1483–1486.

Burr, M.L., Butland, B.K., King, S. & Vaughan-Williams, E. (1989). Changes in asthma prevalence: two surveys 15 years apart. *Archives of Disease in Childhood*, 64, 1452–1456.

Burr, M.L., Limb, E.S., Andrae, S., Barry, D.M. & Nagel, F. (1994). Childhood asthma in four countries – a comparative survey. *International Journal of Epidemiology*, 23, 341–347.

Burrows, B., Martinez, F.D., Halonen, M., Barbee, R.A. & Cline, M.G. (1989). Association of asthma with serum IgE levels and skin-test reactivity to allergens. *New England Journal of Medicine*, 320, 271–277.

Carey, M.J. & Cordon, I. (1986). Asthma and climatic conditions: experience from Bermuda, an isolated island community. *British Medical Journal (Clinical Research Edition)*, 293, 843–844.

Carr, W., Zeitel, L. & Weiss, K. (1992). Variations in asthma hospitalization and deaths in New York City. *American Journal of Public Health*, 82, 59–65.

Carter-Pokras, O.D. & Gergen, P.J. (1993). Reported asthma among Puerto Rican, Mexican-American, and Cuban children, 1982 through 1984. *American Journal of Public Health*, 83, 580–582.

Chan, K.N., Elliman, A., Bryan, E. & Silverman, M. (1989). Respiratory symptoms in children of low birth weight. *Archives of Disease in Childhood*, 64, 1294–1304.

Chan-Yeung, M., Manfreda, J., Dimich-Ward, H., *et al.* (1995). Mite and cat allergen levels in homes and severity of asthma. *American Journal of Respiratory and Critical Care Medicine*, 152(*6 Pt 1)*, 1805–1811.

Chilmonczyk, B.A., Salmun, L.M., Megathlin, K.N., *et al.* (1993). Association between exposure to environmental tobacco smoke and exacerbations of asthma in children. *New England Journal of Medicine*, 328, 1665–1669.

Cloutier, M.M. & Loughlin, G.M. (1981). Chronic cough in children: a manifestation of airway hyperactivity. *Pediatrics*, 67, 6–12.

Cockcroft, D.W. & Swystun, V.A. (1996). Asthma control vs asthma severity. *Journal of Allergy and Clinical Immunology*, 98, 1016–1018.

Cookson, W.O.C.M., Young, R.P., Sandford, A.J., *et al.* (1992). Maternal inheritance of atopic IgE responsiveness on chromosome 11q. *The Lancet*, 340, 381–384.

Corrao, W.M., Braman, S.S. & Irwin, R.S. (1979). Chronic cough as the sole presenting manifestation of bronchial asthma. *New England Journal of Medicine*, 300, 633– 637.

Cowie, R.L., Revitt, S.G., Underwood, M.F. & Field, S.K. (1997). The effect of a peak flow-based action plan in the prevention of exacerbations of asthma. *Chest*, 112, 1534–1538.

Crain, E.F., Weiss, K.B., Bijur, P.E., Hersh, M., Westbrook, L. & Stein, R.E. (1994). An estimate of the prevalence of asthma and wheezing among inner-city children. *Pediatrics*, 94, 356–362.

Crain, E.F., Kercsmar, C., Weiss, K.B., Mitchell, H. & Lynn, H. (1998). Reported difficulties in access to quality care for children with asthma in the inner city. *Archives of Pediatric and Adolescent Medicine*, 152, 333–339.

Cunningham, J., Dockery, D.W. & Speizer, F.E. (1996). Race, asthma and persistent wheeze in Philadelphia schoolchildren. *American Journal of Public Health*, 86, 1406–1409.

Davidson, A.C., Emberlin, J., Cook, A.D. & Venables, K.M. (1996). A major outbreak of asthma associated with a thunderstorm: experience of accident and emergency departments and patients' characteristics. Thames Regions Accident and Emergency Trainees Association. *British Medical Journal*, 312, 601–604.

Devalia, J.L., Rusznak, C., Herdman, M.J., Trigg, C.J., Tarraf, H. & Davies, R.J. (1994). Effect of nitrogen dioxide and sulfur dioxide on airway response of mild asthmatic patients to allergen inhalation. *The Lancet*, 344, 1668–1671.

Dodge, R., Cline, M.G. & Burrows, B. (1986). Comparison of asthma, emphysema, and chronic bronchitis diagnoses in a general population sample. *American Journal of Respiratory Disease*, 133, 981–986.

Dowse, G.K., Smith, D., Turner, K.J. & Alpers, M.P. (1985a). Prevalence and features of asthma in a sample survey of urban Goroka, Papua New Guinea. *Clinical Allergy*, 15, 429–438.

Dowse, G.K., Turner, K.J., Stewart, G.A., Alpers, M.P. & Woolcock, A.J. (1985b). The association between Dermatophagoides mites and the increasing prevalence of asthma in village communities with the Papua New Guinea highlands. *Journal of Allergy and Clinical Immunology*, 75, 75–83.

Duffy, D.L., Martin, N.G., Battistutta, D., Hopper, J.L. & Mathews, J.D. (1990). Genetics of asthma and hay fever in Australian twins. *American Review of Respiratory Disease*, 142, 1351–1358.

Edfors-Lubs, M.L. (1971). Allergy in 7,000 twin pairs. *Acta Allergologica*, 26, 249–285.

Eggleston, P.A., Malveaux, F.J., Butz, A.M., *et al.* (1998). Medications used by children with asthma living in the inner city. *Pediatrics*, 101, 349–354.

Ehrlich, R., Kattan, M., Godbold, J., *et al.* (1992). Childhood asthma and passive smoking. Urinary cotinine as a biomarker of exposure. *American Review of Respiratory Disease*, 145, 594–599.

Engel, W., Freund, D.A., Stein, J.S. & Fletcher, R.H. (1989). The treatment of patients with asthma by specialists and generalists. *Medical Care*, 27, 306–312.

Evans, D., Levron, M.J., Feldman, C.H., *et al.* (1987). The impact of smoking on emergency room visits of urban children with asthma. *American Review of Respiratory Disease*, 135, 567–572.

Fingerhut, L.A. & Warner, M. (1997). *Injury chartbook.* Health, United States, 1996–97. Hyattsville, MD: National Center for Health Statistics.

Finkelstein, J.A., Brown, R.W., Schneider, L.C., *et al.* (1995). Quality of care for preschool children with asthma: the role of social factors and practice setting. *Pediatrics*, 95, 389–394.

Frick, O.L., German, D.F. & Mills, J. (1979). Development of allergy in children I. Association with virus infections. *Journal of Allergy and Clinical Immunology*, 63, 228–241.

Frischer, T., Kuehr, J., Meinert, R., *et al.* (1992). Relationship between low-birth weight and respiratory symptoms in a cohort of primary school children. *Acta Paediatrica Scandinavica*, 81, 1040–1041.

Gandevia, B. (1973). Pressurized sympathomimetic aerosols and their lack of relationship to asthma mortality in Australia. *Medical Journal of Australia*, 1, 273–277.

Garb, H.N. (1998). *Studying the clinician. Judgment research and psychological assessment.* Washington, DC: American Psychological Association.

Gergen, P.J. & Turkeltaub, P.C. (1992). The association of individual allergen reactivity with respiratory disease in a national sample: data from the Second National Health and Nutrition Examination Survey, 1976–80 (NHANES II). *Journal of Allergy and Clinical Immunology*, 90, 579–588.

Gergen, P.J. & Weiss, K.B. (1990). Changing patterns of asthma hospitalization among children: 1979–1987. *Journal of the American Medical Association*, 264, 1688–1692.

Gergen, P.J., Turkeltaub, P.C. & Kovar, M.G. (1987). The prevalence of allergic skin test reactivity to eight common aeroallergens in the U.S. population: results from the Second National Health and Nutrition Examination Survey. *Journal of Allergy and Clinical Immunology*, 80, 669–679.

Gergen, P.J., Mullally, D.I. & Evans, R. III. (1988). National survey of prevalence of asthma among children in the United States, 1976 to 1980. *Pediatrics*, 81,1–7.

Gergen, P.J., Fowler, J.A., Maurer, K.R., Davis, W.W. & Overpeck, M.D. (1998). The burden of environmental tobacco smoke exposure on the respiratory health of children 2 months through 5 years of age in the United States: Third National Health and Nutrition Examination Survey, 1988–1994. *Pediatrics*, 101, e8.

Gerritsen, J., Koeter, G.H., Postma, D.S., Schouten, J.P. & Knol, K. (1989). Prognosis of asthma from childhood to adulthood. *American Review of Respiratory Disease*, 140, 1325–1330.

Goren, A.I. & Hellmann, S. (1988). Prevalence of respiratory symptoms and diseases in school children living in a polluted and in a low polluted of Israel. *Environmental Research*, 45, 28–37.

Gortmaker, S.L., Walker, D.K., Jacobs, F.H. & Ruch-Ross, H. (1982). Parental smoking and the risk of childhood asthma. *American Journal of Public Health*, 72, 574–579.

Gottlieb, D.J., Beiser, A.S. & O'Conner, G.T. (1995). Poverty, race and medication use are correlates of asthma hospitalization rates. A small area analysis in Boston. *Chest*, 108, 28–35.

Grainger, J., Woodman, K., Pearce, N., *et al.* (1991). Prescribed fenoterol and death from asthma in New Zealand, 1981–7: A further case-control study. *Thorax*, 46, 105–111.

Graves, E.J. & Kozak, L.J. (1998). Detailed diagnosis and procedures, National Hospital Discharge Survey, 1996. National Center for Health Statistics. *Vital Health Statistics*, 13, 138.

Gross, N.J. (1980). What is this thing called love? – Or, defining Asthma (Editorial). *American Review of Respiratory Disease*, 121, 203–204.

Guyatt, G.H., Juniper, E.F., Grifitth, L.E., Feeny, D.H. & Ferrie, P.J. (1997). Children and adult perceptions of childhood asthma. *Pediatrics*, 99, 165–168.

Hahn, D.L., Dodge, R.W. & Golubjatnikov, R. (1991). Association of *Chlamydia pneumoniae* (strain TWAR) infection with wheezing, asthmatic bronchitis, and adult-onset asthma. *Journal of the American Medical Association*, 266, 225–230.

Harris, J.R., Magnus, P., Samuelsen, S.O. & Tambs, K. (1997). No evidence for effects of family environment on asthma. A retrospective study of Norwegian twins. *American Journal of Respiratory Critical Care Medicine*, 156, 43–49.

Hide, D.W., Matthews, S., Tariq, S. & Arshad, S.H. (1996). Allergen avoidance in infancy and allergy at 4 years of age. *Allergy*, 51, 89–93.

Hisnanick, J.J., Coddington, D.A. & Gergen, P.J. (1994). Trends in asthma-related admissions among American Indian and Alaskan Native children from 1979 to 1989. Universal health care in the face of poverty. *Archives of Pediatric and Adolescent Medicine*, 148, 357–363.

Homer, C.J., Szilagyi, P., Rodewald, L., *et al.* (1996). Does quality of care affect rates of hospitalization for childhood asthma? *Pediatrics*, 98, 18–23.

Horwood, L.J., Fergusson, D.M., Hons, B.A. & Shannon, F.T. (1985). Social and familial factors in the development of early childhood asthma. *Pediatrics*, 75, 859–868.

Infante-Rivard, C. (1995). Young maternal age: a risk factor for childhood asthma? *Epidemiology*, 6, 178–180.

Inman, W.H.M. & Adelstein, A.M. (1969). Rise and fall of asthma mortality in England and Wales in relation to use of pressurized aerosols. *The Lancet*, 2, 279–285.

Inouye, T., Tarlo, S., Broder, I., *et al.* (1985). Severity of asthma in skin test-negative and skin test-positive patients. *Journal of Allergy and Clinical Immunology*, 75, 313–319.

The International Study of Asthma and Allergies in Childhood (ISAAC) Steering Committee (1998). Worldwide variation in the prevalence of asthma symptoms – the International Study of Asthma and Allergies in Childhood (ISAAC). *European Respiratory Journal* 12: 315–335.

Jamason, P.F., Kalkstein, L.S. & Gergen, P.J. (1997). A synoptic evaluation of asthma hospital admissions in New York City. *American Journal of Respiratory and Critical Care Medicine*, 156, 1781–1788.

Jarvis, D., Chinn, S., Luczynska, C. & Burney, P. (1996). Association of respiratory symptoms and lung function in young adults with use of domestic gas appliances. *The Lancet*, 347, 426–431.

Jarvis, D., Chinn, S., Luczynska, C. & Burney, P. (1997). The association of family size with atopy and atopic disease. *Clinical and Experimental Allergy*, 27, 240–245.

Jenkins, M.A., Hopper, J.L., Flander, L.B., Carlin, J.B. & Giles, G.G. (1993). The associations between childhood asthma and atopy, and parental asthma, hay fever and smoking. *Paediatric and Perinatal Epidemiology*, 7, 67–76.

Johnson, D. & Osborn, L.M. (1991). Cough variant asthma: a review of the clinical literature. *Journal of Asthma*, 28, 85–90.

Johnston, S.L., Pattemore, P.K., Sanderson, G., *et al.* (1995). Community study of role of viral infections in exacerbations of asthma in 9–11 year old children. *British Medical Journal*, 310, 1225–1229.

Jonsson, J.A., Boe, J. & Berlin, E. (1987). The long-term prognosis of childhood asthma in a predominantly rural Swedish county. *Acta Paediatrica Scandinavica*, 76, 950–954.

Kalliel, J.N., Goldstein, B.M., Braman, S.S. & Settipane, G.A. (1989). High frequency of atopic asthma in a pulmonary clinic population. *Chest*, 96, 1336–1340.

Kattan, M., Mitchell, H., Eggleston, P., *et al.* (1997). Characteristics of inner-city children with asthma: the National Cooperative Inner-City Asthma study. *Pediatric Pulmonology*, 24, 253–262.

Keeley, D.J., Neill, P. & Gallivan, S. (1991). Comparison of the prevalence of reversible airways obstruction in rural and urban Zimbabwean children. *Thorax*, 44, 549–553.

Kelly, W.J.W., Hudson, I., Phelan, P.D., Pain, M.C.F. & Olinsky, A. (1987). Childhood asthma in adult life: a further study at 28 years of age. *British Medical Journal*, 294, 1059- 1062.

Khot, A., Burn, R., Evans, N., Lenney, C. & Lenney, W. (1984). Seasonal variation and time trends in childhood asthma in England and Wales. *British Medical Journal*, 289, 235–237.

Kikuchi, Y., Okabe, S., Tamura, G., *et al.* (1994). Chemosensitivity and perception of dyspnea in patients with a history of near-fatal asthma. *New England Journal of Medicine*, 330, 1329–1334.

Kitchen, W.H., Olinsky, A., Doyle, L.W., *et al.* (1992). Respiratory health and lung function in 8-year-old children of very low birth weight: a cohort study. *Pediatrics*, 89, 1151–1158.

Kjellman, N-I.M. (1977). Atopic disease in seven-year old children. Incidence in relation to family history. *Acta Paediatrica Scandinavica*, 66, 465–471.

Kljaovic, M. (1996). The pattern consultations for asthma in a general practice over 5 years. *New Zealand Medical Journal*, 109, 48–50.

Koenig, J.Q., Covert, D.S., Hanley, Q.S., van Belle, G. & Pierson, W.E. (1990). Prior exposure to ozone potentates subsequent response to sulfur dioxide in adolescent asthmatic subjects. *American Review of Respiratory Disease*, 141, 377–380.

Lang, D.M. & Polansky, M. (1994). Patterns of asthma mortality in Philadelphia from 1969–1991. *New England Journal of Medicine*, 331, 1542–1546.

Lee, D.A., Winslow, N.R., Speight, A.N.P. & Hey, E.N. (1983). Prevalence and spectrum of asthma in childhood. *British Medical Journal*, 286, 1256- 1258.

Leung, R. & Ho, P. (1994). Asthma, allergy, and atopy in three south-east Asian populations. *Thorax*, 49, 1205- 1210.

Lieu, T.A., Quesenberry, C.P., Jr., Capra, A.M., Sorel, M.E., Martin, K.E. & Mendoza, G.R. (1997). Outpatient management practices associated with reduced risk of pediatric asthma hospitalization and emergency department visits. *Pediatrics*, 100, 334–341.

Lilljeqvist, A-C., Faleide, A.O. & Watten, R.G. (1997). Low birthweight, environmental tobacco smoke, and air pollution: risk factors for childhood asthma? *Pediatric Asthma and Allergy*, 11, 95–102.

Luyt, D.K., Burton, P., Brooke, A.M. & Simpson, H. (1994). Wheeze in preschool children and its relation with doctor diagnosed asthma. *Archives of Disease in Childhood*, 71, 24–30.

McCormick, M.C., Brooks-Gunn, J., Workman-Daniels, K., Turner, J. & Peckham, G.J. (1992). The health and developmental status of very low-birth-weight children at school age. *Journal of the American Medical Association*, 267, 2204–2208.

Magnus, P. & Jaakkola, J.J. (1997). Secular trend in the occurrence of asthma among children and young adults: critical appraisal of repeated cross sectional surveys. *British Medical Journal*, 314, 1795–1799.

Martin, A.J., McLennan, L.A., Landau, L.I. & Phelan, P.D. (1980). The natural history of childhood asthma to adult life. *British Medical Journal*, 280, 1397- 1400.

Martinez, F.D., Cline, M. & Burrows, B. (1992). Increased incidence of asthma in children of smoking mothers. *Pediatrics*, 89, 21–26.

Martinez, F.D., Stern, D.A., Wright, A.L., Holberg, C.J., Taussig, L.M. & Halonen, M. (1995a). Association of interleukin-2 and interferon-gamma production by blood mononuclear cells in infancy with parental allergy skin tests and with subsequent development of atopy. *Journal of Allergy and Clinical Immunology*, 96, 652- 660.

Martinez, F.D., Wright, A.L., Taussig, L.M., Holberg, C.J., Halonen, M., Morgan, W.J. & The Group Health Associates, (1995b). Asthma and wheezing in the first six years of life. *New England Journal of Medicine*, 332, 133- 138.

Minor, T.E., Dick, E.C., DeMeo, A.N., Ouellette, J.J., Cohen, M. & Reed, C.E. (1974). Viruses as precipitants of asthmatic attacks in children. *Journal of the American Medical Association*, 227, 292–298.

Minor, T.E., Dick, E.C., Baker, J.W., Ouellette, J.J., Cohen, M. & Reed, C.E. (1976). Rhinovirus and influenza type A infections as precipitants of asthma. *American Review of* Respiratory Disease, 113, 149–153.

Mitchell, C. & Miles, J. (1983). Lower respiratory tract symptoms in Queensland schoolchildren. The questionnaire: its reliability and validity. *Australian and New Zealand Journal of Medicine*, 13, 264–269.

Mitchell, E.A. (1985). International trends in hospital admission rates for asthma. *Archives of Disease in Childhood*, 60, 376–378.

Mitchell, H., Senturia, Y., Gergen, P., *et al.* (1997). Design and methods of the National Cooperative Inner-City Asthma Study. *Pediatric Pulmonology*, 24, 237–252.

Mullen, M.L., Mullen, B. & Carey, M. (1993). The association between beta-agonist use and death from asthma. A meta-analytic integration of case-control studies. *Journal of the American Medical Association*, 270, 1842–1845.

Murray, A.B. & Morrison, B.J. (1989). Passive smoking by asthmatics: its greater effect on boys than on girls and on older than younger children. *Pediatrics*, 84, 451–459.

Murray, A.B. & Morrison, B.J. (1990). It is children with atopic dermatitis who develop asthma more frequently if the mother smokes. *Journal of Allergy and Clinical Immunology*, 86, 732–739.

National Institutes of Health (1997). *Expert panel report II, guidelines for the diagnosis and management of asthma* (publication 97–4051). Washington, DC: US Department of Health and Human Services.

Neas, L.M., Dockery, D.W., Koutrakis, P., Tollerud, D.J. & Speizer, F.E. (1995). The association of ambient air pollution with twice daily peak expiratory flow rate measurements in children. *American Journal of Epidemi- ology*, 141, 111–112.

Nieminen, M.M., Kaprio, J. & Koskenvuo, M. (1991). A population-based study of bronchial asthma in adult twin pairs. *Chest*, 100, 70–75.

O'Hollaren, M.T., Yunginger, J.W., Offord, K.P., *et al.* (1991). Exposure to an aeroallergen as a possible precipitating factor in respiratory arrest in young patients with asthma. *New England Journal of Medicine*, 324, 359- 363.

Ogborn, C.J., Duggan, A.K. & DeAngelis, C. (1994). Urinary cotinine as a measure of passive smoke exposure in asthmatic children. *Clinical Pediatrics*, 33, 220–226.

Pattemore, P.K., Asher, M.I., Harrison, A.C., Mitchell, E.A., Rea, H.H. & Stewart, A.W. (1990). The interrelationship among bronchial hyperresponsiveness, the diagnosis of asthma, and asthma symptoms. *American Review of Respiratory Disease*, 142, 549–554.

Pearce, N., Beasley, R., Burgess, C. & Crane, J. (1998). *Asthma epidemiology: principles and methods.* New York: Oxford University Press.

Pearce, N., Beasley, R., Crane, J., Burgess, C. & Jackson, R. (1995). End of the New Zealand asthma epidemic. *The Lancet*, 345, 41–44.

Platt, D.S., Martin, C.J., Hunt, S.M. & Lewis, C.W. (1989). Damp housing, mold growth, and sympathetic health state. *British Medical Journal*, 298, 1673–1678.

Pope, C.A. 3rd. (1989). Respiratory disease associated with community air pollution and a steel mill, Utah Valley. *American Journal of Public Health*, 79, 623–628.

Postma, D.S., Bleecker, E.R., Amelung, P.J., *et al.* (1995). Genetic susceptibility to asthma – bronchial hyperresponsiveness coinherited with a major gene for atopy. *New England Journal of Medicine*, 333, 894–900.

Pullan, C.R. & Hey, E.N. (1982). Wheezing, asthma, pulmonary dysfunction 10 years after infection with respiratory syncytial virus in infancy. *British Medical Journal*, 284, 1665–1669.

Rachelefsky, G.S. & Spector, S.L. (1990). Sinusitis and asthma. *Journal of Asthma*, 27, 1–3.

Rackemann, F.M. (1947). A working classification of asthma. *American Journal of Medicine*, 3, 601–606.

Robertson, C.F., Heycock, E., Bishop, J., Nolan, T., Olinsky, A. & Phelan, P.D. (1991). Prevalence of asthma in Melbourne schoolchildren: changes over 26 years. *British Medical Journal*, 302, 1116–1118.

Robertson, C.F., Rubinfeld, A.R. & Bowes, G. (1992). Pediatric asthma deaths in Victoria: the mild are at risk. *Pediatric Pulmonology*, 13, 95–100.

Romiue, I., Meneses, F., Sienra-Monge, J.J.L., *et al.* (1995). Effects of urban air pollutants on emergency visits for childhood asthma in Mexico City. *American Journal of Epidemiology*, 141, 546–553.

Rosenstreich, D.L., Eggleston, P., Kattan, M., *et al.* (1997). The role of cockroach allergy and exposure to cockroach allergen in causing morbidity among inner-city children with asthma. *New England Journal of Medicine*, 336, 1356–1363.

Saarinen, U.M. & Kajosaari, M. (1995). Breastfeeding as prophylaxis against atopic disease: prospective follow-up study until 17 years old. *The Lancet*, 346, 1065–1069.

Sarpong, S.B. & Karrison, T. (1997). Sensitization to indoor allergens and the risk for asthma hospitalization in children. *Annals of Allergy and Asthma Immunology*, 79, 455–459.

Schappert, S.M. (1997). Ambulatory care visits to physician offices, hospital outpatient departments and emergency rooms: United States, 1995. *National Center for Health Statistics. Vital Health Statistics*, 13, 129.

Schenker, M.B., Samet, J.M. & Speizer, F.E. (1983). Risk factors for childhood respiratory disease. The effects of host factors and home environmental exposures. *American Review of Respiratory Disease*, 128, 1038–1043.

Schmitzberger, R., Rhomberg, K., Buchele, H., *et al.* (1993). Effects of air pollution on the respiratory tract of children. *Pediatric Pulmonology*, 15, 68–74.

Sears, M.R. (1991). Worldwide trends in asthma mortality. *Bulletin of the Union for Tuberculosis and Lung Disease*, 66, 79–83.

Sears, M.R., Jones, D.T., Holdaway, M.D., *et al.* (1986a). Prevalence of bronchial reactivity to inhaled methacholine in New Zealand children. *Thorax*, 41, 283–289.

Sears, M.R., Rea, H.H., De Boer, G., *et al.* (1986b). Accuracy of certification of deaths due to asthma. A national study. *American Journal of Epidemiology*, 124, 1004–1011.

Sears, M.R., Herbison, G.P., Holdaway, M.D., Hewitt, C.J., Flannery, E.M. & Silva, P.A. (1989). The relative risks of sensitivity to grass pollen, house dust mite, and cat dander in the development of childhood asthma. *Clinical and Experimental Allergy*, 19, 419–424.

Sears, M.R., Taylor, D.R., Print, C.G., *et al.* (1990). Regular inhaled beta-agonist treatment in bronchial asthma. *The Lancet*, 336, 1391–1399.

Shirakawa, T., Enomoto, T., Shimazu, S-I. & Hopkin, J.M. (1997). The inverse association between tuberculin responses and atopic disorder. *Science*, 275, 77–79.

Sibbald, B. & Turner-Warwick, M. (1979). Factors influencing the prevalence of asthma among first degree relatives of extrinsic and intrinsic asthmatics. *Thorax*, 34, 332–337.

Sibbald, B., Horn, M.E., Brain, E.A. & Gregg, I. (1980). Genetic factors in childhood asthma. *Thorax*, 35, 671–674.

Silverstein, M.D., Reed, C.E., O'Connell, E.J., Melton, L.J., O'Fallon, W.M. & Yunginger, J.W. (1994). Long-term survival of a cohort of community residents with asthma. *New England Journal of Medicine*, 331, 1537–1541.

Skobeloff, E.M., Spivey, W.H., St. Clair, S.S. & Schofstall, J.M. (1992). The influence of age and sex on asthma admissions. *Journal of the American Medical Association*, 268, 3437–3440.

Sly, R.M. & O'Donnell, R. (1997). Stabilization of asthma mortality. *Annals of Allergy and Asthma Immunology*, 78, 347–354.

Smith, D.H., Malone, D.C., Lawson, K.A., Okamoto, L.J., Battista, C. & Saunders, W.B. (1997). A national estimate of the economic costs of asthma. *American Journal of Respiratory and Critical Care Medicine*, 156, 787–793.

Smyth, J.A., Tabachnik, E., Duncan, W.J., Reily, B.J. & Levison, H. (1981). Pulmonary function and bronchial hyperactivity in long-term survivors of bronchopulmonary dysplasia. *Pediatrics*, 68, 336–340.

Speight, A.N.P., Lee, D.A. & Hey, E.N. (1983). Underdiagnosis and undertreatment of asthma in childhood. *British Medical Journal*, 286, 1253– 1256.

Speizer, F.E. & Doll, R. (1968). A century of asthma deaths in young people. *British Medical Journal*, 3, 245– 246.

Sporik, R., Holgate, S.T., Platts-Mills, T.A.E. & Cogswell, J.J. (1990). Exposure to house-dust mite allergen (Der p I) and the development of asthma in childhood. *New England Journal of Medicine*, 323, 502–507.

Sporik, R., Ingram, J.M., Price, W., Sussman, J.H., Honsinger, R.W. & Platts-Mills, T.A. (1995). Association of asthma with serum IgE and skin test reactivity to allergens among children living in high altitude. Tickling the dragon's breath. *American Journal of Respiratory and Critical Care Medicine*, 151, 1388–1392.

Strachan, D.P., Butland, B.K. & Anderson, H.R. (1996). Incidence and prognosis of asthma and wheezing illness from early childhood to age 33 in a national British cohort. *British Medical Journal*, 312, 1195–1199.

Strunk, R.C., Mrazek, D.A., Wolfson-Fuhrmann, G.S. & LaBrecque, J.F. (1985). Physiologic and psychological characteristics associated with deaths due to asthma in childhood. A case-controlled study. *Journal of the American Medical Association*, 254, 1193– 1198.

Tay, J.S.H., Ngiam, T.E. & Yip, W.C.L. (1982). Birth order of children with bronchial asthma. *Journal of the Singapore Paediatric Society*, 24, 152–155.

Taylor, W.R. & Newacheck, P.W. (1992). Impact of childhood asthma on health. *Pediatrics*, 90, 657–662.

To, T., Dick, P., Feldman, W. & Hernandez, R. (1996). A cohort study on childhood asthma admissions and readmissions. *Pediatrics*, 98, 191–195.

Turkeltaub, P.C. & Gergen, P.J. (1991). Prevalence of upper and lower respiratory conditions in the U.S. population by social and environmental factors: Data from the second National Health and Nutrition Examination Survey, 1976–80 (NHANES II). *Annals of Allergy*, 67, 147–154.

Van Arsdell, P.P., Jr. & Motulsky, A.G. (1959). Frequency and heritability of asthma and allergic rhinitis in college students. *Acta Genet (Basel)*, 9, 101–114.

Van Niekerk, C.H., Weinberg, E.G., Shore, S.C., Hesse, H. de V. & Van Schalkwyk, D.J. (1979). Prevalence of asthma: a comparative study of urban and rural Xhosa children. *Clinical Allergy*, 9, 319–324.

von Mutius, E., Nicolai, T. & Martinez, F.D. (1993). Prematurely as a risk factor for asthma in preadolescent children. *Journal of Pediatrics*, 123, 223–229.

Waite, D.A., Eyles, E.F., Tonkin, S.L. & O'Donnell, T.V. (1980). Asthma prevalence in Tokelauan children in two environments. *Clinical Allergy*, 10, 71–75.

Warner, J.O., Naspitz, C.K. & Cropp, G.J.A. (1998). Third International Pediatric Consensus Statement on the Management of Childhood Asthma. *Pediatric Pulmonology*, 25, 1–17.

Weiss, K.B. (1990). Seasonal trends in US asthma hospitalizations and mortality. *Journal of the American Medical Association*, 263, 2323–2328.

Weiss, K.B., Gergen, P.J. & Hodgson, T.A. (1992). An economic evaluation of asthma in the United States. *New England Journal of Medicine*, 326, 862–866.

Weitzman, M., Gortmaker, S., Walker, D.K. & Sobol, A. (1990). Maternal smoking and childhood asthma. *Pediatrics*, 85, 505–511.

Weitzman, M., Gortmaker, S.L., Sobol, A.M. & Perrin, J.M. (1992). Recent trends in the prevalence and severity of childhood asthma. *Journal of the American Medical Association*, 268, 2673–2677.

Welliver, R.C., Sun, M., Rinaldo D. & Ogra, P.L. (1986). Predictive value of respiratory syncytial virus-specific IgE responses for recurrent wheezing following bronchiolitis. *Journal of Pediatrics*, 109, 776–780.

White, M.C., Etzel, R.A., Olson, D.R. & Goldstein, I.F. (1997). Reexamination of epidemic asthma in New Orleans, Louisiana, in relation to the presence of soy at the harbor. *American Journal of Epidemiology*, 145, 432–438.

Wissow, L.S., Gittelsohn, A.M., Szklo, M., Starfield, B. & Mussman, M. (1988). Poverty, race and hospitalization for childhood asthma. *American Journal of Public Health*, 78, 777–782.

Woolcock, A.J. (1986). Worldwide differences in asthma prevalence and mortality. Why is asthma mortality so low in the USA? *Chest*, 90, 40S–45S.

Yemaneberhan, H., Bekele, Z., Venn, A., Lewis, S., Parry, E. & Britton, J. (1997). Prevalence of wheeze and asthma and relation to atopy in urban and rural Ethiopia. *The Lancet*, 350, 85–90.

Yunginger, J.W., Reed, C.E., O'Connell, E.J., Melton III, L.J., O'Fallon, W.M. & Silverstein, M.D. (1992). A community-based study of the epidemiology of asthma I. incidence rates 1964–84. *American Journal of Respiratory Disease*, 146, 888–894.

Zeiger, R.S., Heller, S., Mellon, M.H., *et al.* (1989). Effect of a combined maternal and infant food-allergen avoidance on development of atopy in early infancy: a randomized study. *Journal of Allergy and Clinical Immunology*, 84, 72–89.

Zeiger, R.S., Heller, S., Mellon, M.H., Wald, J., Falkoff, R. & Schatz, M., (1991). Facilitated referral to asthma specialist reduces relapses in asthma emergency room visits. *Journal of Allergy and Clinical Immunology*, 87, 1160–1168.

Zimmerman, B., Feanny, S., Reisman, J., *et al.* (1988). Allergy in asthma I. The dose relationship of allergy to severity of childhood asthma. *Journal of Allergy and Clinical Immunology*, 81, 63–70.

3
A family asthma management approach to behavioral assessment and treatment in children with asthma

Mary D. Klinnert and Bruce G. Bender

Editors' note—*In the chapter that follows, Mary Klinnert and Bruce Bender make the point that asthma, particularly pediatric asthma, is not simply a problem faced by patients. Rather, they note, asthma is a chronic disorder that involves everyone who has regular contact with a patient, including health care providers, educators, peers, behavioral scientists, and in particular, members of the patient's family. If, as the African proverb claims, it 'takes a village to raise a child,' it takes the collaboration of everyone significant in a patient's life to help an individual manage and cope with asthma. With such support, it is hoped that the patient can learn and perform the self-initiated skills needed to control asthma. Success in the latter will result in an improved quality of life for the patient and for all involved with the individual, particularly the patient's family.*

Potential problems in asthma and their assessment are outlined by Klinnert and Bender. An array of techniques, they note, have evolved to define and assess these problems. The techniques are based upon empirical research, including major contributions by the authors. Delineation of the problems, in turn, permit the development and application of procedures for changing inappropriate behaviors or patterns of behavior. As emphasized by the title of their chapter, Klinnert and Bender suggest much of the effort in changing behavior should be directed at using a family approach to assess and treat children with asthma. By building on a patient's family, the authors have both extended our knowledge of behavioral and psychological techniques useful in the management of asthma, and described the challenge we face in applying the methodology to control asthma. It is an important contribution.

Introduction

Research over the past 10 years has led to a redefinition of asthma as a 'chronic inflammatory disorder of the airways' (National Institutes of Health, 1997). New guidelines for the assessment and treatment of asthma in adults and children necessarily focus on symptom measurement, environmental control, and medication management. Improving patient health care behavior also receives significant emphasis in these revised guidelines. They include education, techniques for improving treatment adherence, and a suggestion about appropriate referral for mental health services. Patient education should be a continuous process, and one that is integrated into a 'partnership' between patient and health caregiver. Adherence may be enhanced through improved communication, sensitivity to the patient's perceptions and concerns, and the promotion of involvement of other family members. While not a central focus of the guidelines, psychological assessment and treatment are recommended when other efforts from the health care provider do not lead to improved outcomes and 'when stress seems to unduly interfere with daily asthma management' (National Institutes of Health, 1997).

The goal of this chapter is to develop a comprehensive portrayal of the circumstances among children with asthma that merit psychological assessment and treatment with respect to the impact of psychological dysfunction on asthma management. Principles and methods of assessing psychological barriers to asthma management are presented. A treatment approach is described that involves a team of professionals working closely with families with a focus on changing problematic behaviors that specifically impede asthma management.

Psychological Functioning and Nonadherence

Pharmacotherapy for asthma has improved significantly in the past decade, with consequent gains in our capacity to successfully manage asthma and prevent exacerbations of symptoms. Most asthma can be controlled without the need for hospitalization (Donahue *et al.*, 1997). Still, successful management of asthma requires a persistent effort on the part of the patients and their families. When families are unable to organize themselves to provide sufficient management of the child's asthma, and in particular, when anti-inflammatory medications are not taken as prescribed, disease control is seriously undermined. Many asthmatic patients take significantly less medication than is necessary; this finding has been established in adults (Spector *et al.*, 1986; Bailey *et al.*, 1990) and children (Baum & Creer, 1986; Coutts *et al.*, 1992). Furthermore, nonadherence occurs in numerous circumstances, regardless of whether medications are tablets (Christiannse *et al.*, 1989) or aerosolized medications (Spector *et al.*, 1986; Bender *et al.*, 1998). The degree of nonadherence can be dramatic. For example, subtherapeutic theophylline levels were found in 70% of outpatients treated at a children's hospital (Cox *et al.*, 1993). In a 90-day longitudinal study, eight children requiring urgent care visits resulting in oral steroid bursts (two of whom required subsequent hospitalization) had been markedly less adherent with a daily regimen of inhaled steroids than a group of 16 patients with stable symptom control (Milgrom *et al.*, 1995).

Inadequate health care behavior, poor symptom control, severe illness, and increased health care cost have been found in circumstances where psychological disturbance is present in the child or family (Strunk *et al.*, 1989; Bender & Klinnert, 1998; Klinnert *et al.*, 2000). Family dysfunction, and in particular family conflict, is a red flag signaling increased risk of nonadherence and, consequently, poorly controlled asthma (Wamboldt *et al.*, 1995). In a study of the families of 24 asthmatic children, underuse of aerosolized corticosteroids was associated with decreased communication and organization (Bender *et al.*, 1998). In other studies, high levels of family conflict were correlated with theophylline nonadherence (Christiannse *et al.*, 1989; Wamboldt *et al.*, 1995).

Reviews of the literature show that, in general, children with asthma do not have significantly more psychological problems than other children (Klinnert, 1997; Bender & Klinnert, 1998). However, among children with asthma, increases in psychological disturbance have been found to be associated with greater disease severity (Graham *et al.*, 1967; McNicol *et al.*, 1973; Bussing *et al.*, 1995; Klinnert *et al.*, 2000). There is reason to believe that increased asthma severity, which has been associated with greater psychological dysfunction in children, in reality often reflects asthma that is poorly controlled as a result of nonadherence (Norrish *et al.*, 1977; Klinnert, 1997; Bender & Klinnert, 1998). This is not to say that all children with severe, difficult-to-control asthma come from dysfunctional families or are seriously nonadherent. However, the frequency of adherence problems among severe, poorly controlled asthmatic patients is markedly increased (Bender & Klinnert, 1998). It appears that while asthma itself neither causes nor results from significant psychological dysfunction, when psychological disorders occur in conjunction with childhood asthma, psychological problems have a profound impact on the asthma through the adequacy of adherence or asthma management.

Family dysfunction and individual psychological disorders, at their extreme, increase the risk of asthma-related death. Using a stepwise discriminant analysis to evaluate the predictive role of 57 physiological and psychological variables, Strunk and colleagues examined the circumstances surrounding asthma death in 21 pediatric patients who later died from their asthma (Strunk *et al.*, 1985). The emerging asthma–death risk profile included families with histories of conflict between parents and their child and with medical staff; depressive symptoms in the child; family dysfunction, including parental psychopathology, intense marital conflict, or alcoholism; disregard of asthma symptoms; and deficient self-care and compliance. Results from other studies, generally based upon smaller samples, have similarly concluded that deaths from pediatric asthma are associated with denial of symptoms, poor asthma management including medication nonadherence, and increased psychological dysfunction (Fritz *et al.*, 1987; Kravis, 1987; Sly, 1988; Lanier, 1989).

It is no accident that pediatric asthma deaths have occurred primarily among adolescents. Because of their developmental status, adolescent asthmatics are particularly vulnerable to poor control of their disease (Randolph & Fraser, 1999). The primary developmental task of adolescence is the struggle to achieve autonomous functioning. The wish to make health care decisions on their own often precedes adolescents' capacity to make optimal decisions as well as to take preventive actions. During this time of transition to autonomous functioning, the safety net of parental supervision is often refused. Such struggles are normative behavior for well-adjusted adolescents, and the additional stress of having asthma has been shown to be associated with relatively poor social adjustment (Forero *et al.*, 1996). Adolescents whose parents were rated as being critical were found to have poorer medication compliance at admission to a national asthma referral center (Wamboldt *et al.*, 1995). High rates of psychiatric disorders have been found among adolescents with severe, out-of-control asthma (Wamboldt *et al.*, 1996). Adolescents from dysfunctional families or those with psychological problems appear to be especially vulnerable to denial of symptoms, poor medication adherence, and conflict with caregivers.

The relationship between psychological dysfunction and poor outcome has been increasingly well documented. However, information about what specific patterns of behavior lead to medical noncompliance, poorly controlled asthma, or in the worst case, death, has not been well documented. A traditional psychological evaluation may result in a diagnosis of a particular psychological disorder in the child, or may lead to improvement of family communicational difficulties, but is unlikely to lead to improved asthma management if the asthma management system is not the focus of the evaluation. The provision of psychological intervention to a disturbed child or a dysfunctional family that will result in better control of the asthma requires that the clinician determine the behaviors through which the psychological dysfunction is leading to increased asthma symptoms. Nonadherence with prescribed medications is a likely effect of psychological dysfunction. Still, given the complex systems of behavior required for good asthma care, nonadherence may take many forms. Various aspects of psychological functioning impact a family's ability to follow environmental recommendations, such as avoiding exposure to cigarette smoke or indoor allergens. Psychological functioning also affects how well a family monitors a child's symptoms and makes decisions about home management of symptoms and appropriate timing for involving the medical expertise of health care providers.

The impact of families' emotional functioning on children's asthma has long been recognized (Purcell *et al.*, 1969). However, the view of parents as home-based asthma managers is a more recent phenomenon. In the 1980s asthma education programs proliferated as a means of helping children to gain control over their illness (Creer *et al.*, 1988). Some of the asthma education programs put special emphasis on the role of parents in helping their children to manage their asthma or, in the case of younger children, teaching parents to be asthma managers (Wilson-Pessano & McNabb, 1985). The importance of working with the entire family to improve asthma management has also been emphasized in intensive inpatient programs with children with moderate to severe, out-of-control asthma (Strunk *et al.*, 1989; Weinstein *et al.*, 1992; Brazil *et al.*, 1997).

The processes involved in asthma management have been clarified through the theoretical approach of self-regulation (Clark & Zimmerman, 1990). Self-regulation theory provides a systematic means of assessing and teaching the various components of asthma management (Hindi-Alexander & Cropp, 1984; Wilson-Pessano & McNabb, 1985; Clark *et al.*, 1994). A number of intervention programs have based their outcome evaluation not only on increases in asthma knowledge but also on changes in asthma related self-regulation skills among both children and their parents (Taggart *et al.*, 1991; Clark *et al.*, 1994; Brazil *et al.*, 1997). A further development of self-regulation theory has defined the phases through which families progress in order to achieve self-regulation of the disease (Zimmerman *et al.*, 1999). Using a research interview, Zimmerman found support for four sequential phases that characterize families' management of asthma. Within this framework, 83% of the families assessed were 'precompliant' (i.e., were categorized as being at levels 1 or 2 of 4).

In addition to increased attention to the role of families in children's asthma management, there is now greater recognition that children and families are part of more extensive social systems. These systems include the physician, the alternative caregivers, the schoolteachers, and others (Kazak *et al.*, 1995). A number of assessment tools are available for evaluating the knowledge and self-management skills required for effective asthma management (Becker *et al.*, 1994). There is a need, however, for a systematic approach for assessing not only the individual child and family but also the social systems in which they are embedded. Further, there is a need for a systematic approach for assessing the problems that prevent families from benefiting from office-based or educational programs.

An interview methodology has been developed for assessing the multidimensional aspects of families' asthma management behavior, the Family Asthma Management System Scale (FAMSS; Klinnert *et al.*, 1997). The FAMSS includes interview guidelines for assessing the strengths and weaknesses of a family's asthma management system. The various dimensions and domains of behavior assessed by the FAMSS, described in Table 3.1, were derived conceptually from developmental psychopathology theory and research (Sroufe & Rutter, 1984), from a family systems approach to pediatric psychology (Kazak *et al.*, 1995), and from asthma self-management theory (Clark *et al.*, 1994). The FAMSS for

Table 3.1 Behavioral domains assessed in FAMSS interview

	Scale	Brief description of scale
I.	Family's perceived alliance with medical caregiver	Family has access to a medical caregiver; knows where to go and how to access the system; sees caregiver as knowledgeable and concerned; feels positively about care provided
II.	Collaborative relationship between family and medical caregiver	Communication between family and physician; family communicates symptom patterns; physician provides action plan; family follows home care plan; roles and boundaries are clear
III.	Knowledge of asthma and medications	Parents and child understand what asthma is, including chronicity, inflammation, hyperreactivity, triggers; they know different medications, their uses, and actions
IV.	Adherence with asthma medications	Family follows recommendations for medication usage; they have a system in place for preventive medications; they understand the indications for rescue medications, and use them appropriately
V.	Adequacy of care by alternative caregivers	Family communicates well with alternative caregivers; caregivers take responsibility for supervision when child is in their care, provide competent care
VI.	Adherence with environmental recommendations	Family follows recommendations for changes in environment; removes pets, practices dust control; helps child to avoid triggers and cigarette smoke
VII.	Knowledge and assessment of child's symptoms	Family is aware of various aspects of child's wheezing symptoms, including early warning signs, daily fluctuations, seasonal changes; use peak flow meter as directed; monitor response to rescue treatments

VIII. Appropriateness of action plan and emotional response to asthma symptoms	The family follows a coherent plan when exacerbations occur; they follow recommendations for home treatment, contact health care providers as directed; are aware of emotional response and management
IX. Balance of responsibility between parent and child	The child takes age-appropriate responsibility for managing those aspects of his asthma over which he has control; parent oversees appropriately
X. Parent–child interactions in arena of asthma care	Parents and child cooperate to monitor symptoms and take medications; child cooperates in an age-appropriate manner, and parent encourages increasing responsibility
XI. Parental resources	Parents have adequate intellectual, financial, and emotional resources; have capacity to trust and work with health care providers; and have adequate communication skills
XII. Balanced integration of asthma into family life	Concern and attention to asthma is balanced with other family and developmental needs; asthma is under control; child is progressing socially and academically

assessing families' functioning in each behavioral domain showed good inter-rater reliability, with excellent inter-rater reliability for the summary score. Internal consistency was also shown to be high (alpha = 0.91) (Klinnert *et al.*, 1997). The FAMSS summary score, together with an asthma severity score, jointly accounted for a significant proportion of the variance when predicting the functional severity of a group of children with mild to moderate asthma. Evidence for the concurrent validity of the subscales is being established. For example, the adherence subscale from the FAMSS interview, administered at admission, correlates highly and significantly ($r = 0.67$, $p < 0.0001$) with independent information about pediatric patients' functioning obtained by psychosocial clinicians during a several-week-long day treatment program at a tertiary referral center for asthma. The multidimensional nature of asthma management that is addressed in the FAMSS methodology provides a framework for discussing the assessment and treatment of behavioral problems among asthmatic children. We will demonstrate how, as each of the functional domains is explored and the specific behavioral deficits identified, the psychological disturbances which often underlie the failure of the system can be clarified, submitted to further evaluation, and treated.

It should be noted that this approach to assessing behavioral difficulties in children with asthma focuses primarily on the family, rather than on the individual child. This is not because the individual child's adjustment or self-management is seen as unimportant. Rather, it is because children develop physically and psychologically in the context of a family, whatever its composition. Under normal circumstances the child takes increasing responsibility for self-care with age. This developmental process is shaped by the attitudes and behaviors of the caregiver, who ultimately has responsibility for the child's safety and well-being. Thus, the psychological and material resources of the child's primary caregiver are of utmost importance, as is the quality of the relationship between the parent and the child with asthma. Although the caregiving system assumes particular importance for infants and younger children (Wilson *et al.*, 1993), there has been increasing recognition of the importance of the family system in asthma management for older children and adolescents (Wamboldt *et al.*, 1995).

Because the manner in which a family manages a child's asthma probably has the largest effect on symptom control, we recommend that the asthma management behaviors be the initial focus of a psychological consultation where the aim is to understand how 'stress is . . . interfering with daily asthma management' (National Institutes of Health, 1997). However, certain individual characteristics of children have been demonstrated to affect the controllability of their asthma, and should be considered as well. Depression among children with asthma has been viewed as a potentially 'lethal combination,' and a mechanism of vagal dysregulation has been described (Miller & Strunk, 1989). High levels of anxiety have been reported among some children and adolescents with asthma (Wamboldt *et al.*, 1996; Kashani *et al.*, 1988), and can have a debilitating effect on symptom control. In addition, some children with asthma are reported to have symptoms triggered by emotional upset, making it difficult to gain control of their asthma (Isenberg *et al.*, 1992; Vazquez & Buceta, 1993). There are instances where asthmatic and psychological symptoms become confused, and a psychological evaluation is required as part of the differential diagnosis (Baron & Marcotte, 1994). Finally, the secondary effects of having asthma, with psychological patterns such as stigmatization or physiological side effects of medication, or the family burden engendered by caring for the illness, may themselves interfere with asthma management and are deserving of evaluation and treatment. We will return to these behavioral difficulties after discussing an approach to evaluation of the family asthma management system.

Assessing the Family Asthma Management System

An integrated and comprehensive approach to psychological treatment for children with poorly controlled asthma must focus on the entire family system and on the entire range of behaviors required for effective asthma management. Adherence in asthma not only involves taking medications on time and in the appropriate manner but also working in partnership with a physician, having good environmental control of asthma triggers, and recognizing and treating asthma symptoms when they occur. The specific tasks to be accomplished for effective asthma management have been catalogued, and they are extensive (Wilson *et al.*, 1993). Because the required behaviors are complex and because families are so varied, individualized assessments of barriers that impede effective asthma management must precede the design of a treatment tailored to overcome those barriers.

Central to a family asthma management approach is a behaviorally focused assessment, conducted with the parents and asthmatic child together. This assessment includes an analysis of the family system and, in particular, the problem areas that serve as barriers to good asthma management. The assessment focuses on all aspects of the child's asthma, such as symptom patterns, triggers, monitoring of symptoms, medications prescribed, decision-making processes regarding administering medications, the relationship with the physician, and the distribution within the family of asthma-related tasks. The family's knowledge of asthma and management behaviors, their capacity to follow through with illness management procedures, and deficiencies undermining asthma control are determined. An exploration of the family's existing asthma management system uncovers impediments to more effective management. The family's current behavior deficits may be related to a lack of knowledge about asthma, counterproductive health beliefs or attitudes, organizational problems that prevent adherence, or interpersonal or relational difficulties. It is not uncommon to discover more systemic problems, such as parent–child interaction problems, spousal conflict, limited intellectual abilities, or financial limitations.

Referrals for Consultation

Referrals are appropriately made for psychological consultation when asthma management strategies known to be generally effective fail to result in reasonable control of asthma symptoms. What if despite the efforts of the primary clinician and support staff to educate a family, the provision of an action plan, and attempts to communicate effectively, the child's asthma remains out of control, which may be indicated by repeated emergency room (ER) visits or hospitalizations, or even by life-threatening events such as respiratory arrests or hypoxic seizures. Missing excessive amounts of school is a sure sign that asthma management efforts are failing.

The consulting psychologist who can be most helpful to the referring clinician is one who has extensive current knowledge of asthma and its medical treatment, as well as experience in working with families with asthma. Referral information should contain not only the behaviors and symptoms of concern but also information about the likely severity of the asthma, known allergies and other triggers, and the medication regimens that have met failure. This information is critical for the consultation, because the assessment focuses on the details of the family's asthma management system as a means of ferreting out barriers to effective implementation.

The FAMSS Interview

The primary strategy for assessing the family asthma management system is by means of a comprehensive, focused interview that can be completed in 1 hour. Although there are concerns among practitioners that people will not provide factual information about their health management behavior (Rand & Wise, 1994), the validity of self-report data has been shown to be variable, with a number of factors influencing reporting accuracy (Strecher *et al.*, 1989). Misreporting is greater under circumstances in which the demands are greater. The validity of responses is influenced by the relationship between the interviewer and the interviewee, what benefits will be accrued from answering in a particular manner, and the style in which questions are asked (Steele *et al.*, 1990). Thus, the possibility of obtaining accurate information will be increased in a sympathetic setting in which blaming or confrontation is avoided.

A semi-structured interview format is useful in its systematic review of specific behavioral domains that comprise the family asthma management system. At the same time, the open-ended format allows the family member the freedom to explain behavior, beliefs, and attitudes. The consultant probes until she has sufficient information to make a judgment about functioning in each domain. Unlike a self-report inventory, the parent's responses are not necessarily taken at face value. Rather, each piece of information is integrated into an overall picture by the consultant, so that a clinical judgment can be made about what is occurring in the home. This judgment relies on the consultant's knowledge of asthma, various asthma medications, preventive behaviors, and appropriate attack management strategies.

When the child with asthma is young, the interview can be effectively conducted with one or two caregivers in the absence of the affected child, although an opportunity to observe the parent–child interaction is helpful at some point. Older children and adolescents should be interviewed together with their caregivers. The consultant introduces the interview by indicating that managing asthma is a difficult task for families, and that they are going to talk about all of the different parts of it in order to understand how it works for this family.

The task of the interviewer is to gain as clear a picture as possible of various aspects of the family system for managing the asthma. Table 3.2 lists question areas of family asthma management in a natural progression that yields a wide range of specific information. Questions about the development of the child's asthma convey an understanding that there is a history to the illness, and an appreciation that the family has had to deal with the illness for some period of time. As well as providing factural information, the response will also provide a great deal of information on the family's emotional response to the illness, its meaning for the family, and the family's degree of acceptance of the illness. Parents can be asked directly what they understand about asthma and its treatment. Responses to this question inform the interviewer about the family's level of knowledge as well as their attitude about what they have learned or wish to learn. Finding out about the source of the parent's asthma knowledge provides information about the resources that have been tapped in the past, and the extent to which the medical caregiver has played a primary role in the family's asthma education. Subsequent topics to be covered include the caregiver's (and in the case of older children, the patient's) knowledge of the asthmatic child's triggers and symptom patterns, and knowledge and understanding of what medications have been prescribed and how they help the asthma. If asked in an open-ended and empathic fashion, responses to these questions may reveal poor symptom assessment and monitoring that impede early responses to symptoms, or a lack of understanding or acknowledgment of triggers. Questioning about medications may reveal knowledge deficits or blatant

Table 3.2 Areas of family asthma management to be assessed in a FAMSS interview

- Development of child's asthma and circumstances surrounding diagnosis
  - Course of the child's asthma since diagnosis
- Parent's understanding of the biological basis of asthma
  - Source of parent's understanding of asthma
- Child's symptom patterns within the past year
  - Type and severity of symptoms
  - Daily and seasonal patterns of symptoms
  - Early warning signs
  - Child's asthma triggers
- Parent's and child's response to asthma symptoms
  - Family member who first notices symptoms
  - Symptom management – use of medications, contacting physician
  - Parent's, child's emotional response to symptoms
  - Cooperation between parent and child to achieve symptom management
- Steps taken by parents to control environmental triggers
  - Presence or absence of pets in the home
  - Use of dust control procedures
  - Exposure to cigarette smoke
  - Efforts to prevent respiratory infections
- Use of asthma medications
  - Familiarity with type and dosage prescribed
  - Understanding of mechanisms of medication
  - Understanding of preventive vs rescue medications
  - System for administering regular medications
  - Circumstances under which medications are missed
- Family members' responsibility for asthma caretaking
  - Amount of responsibility taken by child vs parent
  - Involvement of other adults in asthma caretaking
- Relationship with physician treating asthma
  - Parent's view of physician's competence in treating asthma
  - Quality of communication with physician as reported by parent
  - Scheduled well checks vs sick visits only
  - Establishment of jointly developed action plan
  - Parent's report of physician's availability
- Effects of child's asthma on family
  - Child's adjustment to having asthma
  - Child's feelings about asthma
  - Effects of asthma on activities, school attendance

misunderstandings that preclude the appropriate use of medications. An assessment can be made as to whether the concept of prevention has meaning to the family members, or whether responding to symptoms using rescue medications or ER visits is consistent with the family's view of the disease.

The questions about what medications have been prescribed and when they are to be taken also reveal the family's perception of what the medical caregiver has recommended. Questioning about exactly what medications are taken, when they are used, and why they are taken at that time yields further information about how closely the family is adhering to medication recommendations. Probing about what prompts them to take the medication reveals information about whether scheduled medications are routinized as part of self-care, or whether they are generally taken following the occurrence of symptoms. It is useful to query regarding who remembers the medication and what cues serve as reminders. It is important to acknowledge with families that following medication schedules is a difficult task, and that most families have times when the medications are not taken. This approach reduces the shame or embarrassment that may lead to misrepresentation of adherence by the family. Rather, with a shared understanding with the family that non-adherence does occur, one can work with them to determine the times or circumstances under which adherence is most difficult.

Much information is gained as a result of questioning the family closely (but not judgmentally) regarding their medication-taking behavior. An estimate of adherence can be made, which itself is very useful for the primary clinician to understand why symptoms are not controlled. Equally important, the consultant can begin to make some inferences about the family's overall intentions and capacity for following through with recommendations. Information about the organization and routinization of family life, or lack thereof, will reveal important barriers to medication adherence. Knowledge, understanding, and attitudes toward giving the medications can be assessed throughout. However, the interviewer also learns about the physical and emotional availability of caregiving adults. Whether or not they have asthma, children require supervision 24 hours a day, a task that is optimally managed by more than one caregiver. Once it is determined who the caregivers are, more can be learned about the motivation and capability of both the primary and secondary caregivers.

The child's role in taking medications must be carefully assessed. The young child's response to being administered medication should be queried, and careful attention given to reports of lack of cooperation. The extent of the resistance, and the effect that such resistance has on the parent's efforts to administer further medication, should be assessed. For older children and adolescents, the critical issues for assessment are the age-appropriateness of the child's self-management and the ease with which the parent and child are negotiating increased independence in concert with ongoing supervision of medication adherence. When conflict about taking medications is present within the parent–child dyad, one can assess the pervasiveness of the conflict within the relationship.

It is very informative to ask a family member to describe exactly what happens when the child develops symptoms. Descriptions of who notices the symptoms reveals information about both the parent's and the child's symptom-monitoring habits. It also provides information about whether the child's perception and response to symptoms is developmentally appropriate, and whether the parental involvement is appropriate for the developmental level of the child. Inquiry can be made about peak flow meters – whether one was prescribed, whether and how it is utilized, and parent–child interactions related to its use. Once symptoms are noted, the family is asked what steps they usually take when asthma worsens. Responses will reveal a great deal about the effectiveness of the family's plan for managing asthma attacks. In this context, one can determine the manner in which decisions are made, including the extent to which an asthma action plan is utilized to manage exacerbations.

The family should be asked what recommendations regarding environmental control they remember hearing from their medical caregivers, how they feel about what they were told to do, and the completeness of their efforts to follow through. Whatever their medical caregiver's intended recommendations, the family's interpretation of the recommendations and their related efforts are paramount. Many parents will volunteer that they have made efforts in some areas: e.g., to eliminate dust mites. They should be asked specifically about pets in the home, because this topic presents major difficulties for many families. It is important to determine the owners of the pets, and the significance of the pets to the child with asthma, to siblings, or to the caregivers themselves. Parents may report having been told not to smoke around their children, and often they will present quite clearly where they stand. Under these circumstances it will be possible to determine their readiness for smoking cessation (Prochaska & DiClementi, 1983). Other parents will not acknowledge smoking unless they are asked explicitly, and so it is important to ask whether anyone in the household smokes cigarettes, and the amount of cigarette smoke to which the asthmatic child is exposed.

Throughout the interview, the family will have been providing information about their relationship with their medical care provider. Responses to being asked the source of their knowledge about asthma often reveal much about the adequacy of the education they have received in their health care setting. It will have become apparent whether they have an action plan and what they understand about calling the clinic for help. Similarly, the family's understanding of recommendations for environmental controls will have been probed. Nevertheless, it is helpful to ask explicitly about their access to and satisfaction with their health care provider, since the enhancement of this alliance is often an early intervention that can have far-reaching effects on the family's asthma management.

Behavioral Domains Assessed in the FAMSS Interview

By the completion of the interview, the consultant is able to make assessments in 12 interrelated domains of behavior, each of which must be functional for a family to effectively manage asthma (see Table 3.1). The areas represent domains of behavior specific to asthma management, yet almost all are conceptualized in terms of relationships and resources. The child with asthma is at the center of the system, and is cared for primarily by one or more adult caregivers. Most of the behaviors specific to asthma management, such as symptom assessment and medication adherence, take place within the parent–child relational system. Yet the asthma specific behaviors must be extended into both parents' and children's relationships with alternate caregivers (e.g., teachers, day care providers, grandparents). The supervision required by the child for asthma management, and hence the nature of the child–adult relationships, is dependent on the child's developmental level and individual capabilities for asthma self-care. Finally, the family interacts with the medical care providers, and the relational nature of these interactions is conveyed through the terms 'alliance' and 'collaborative relationship.'

Consistent with the asthma management approach, the consultant utilizes the information gained in the interview to evaluate the parent's and child's functioning in asthma-specific behavioral domains. In addition, there must be a first level or screening evaluation of both the child's and the parent's psychological functioning as it impacts on asthma management. Consideration must be given to the quality of the parent–child relationship, and the quality of the parent's relationship with alternate caregivers. Finally, the quality of the collaborative relationship between the health care provider and the child and parents must be evaluated. The manner in which family functioning in each of the areas is essential for asthma management is explained below. Family dynamics frequently associated with difficulties performing the functions are described, as are underlying problems that may limit the ability of family members to manage asthma effectively.

I. Alliance with Medical Caregiver

Treatment outcome studies have emphasized the importance of a positive working relationship between the patient and physician for achieving therapeutic gains (Kaplan *et al.*, 1983). To have an alliance with a medical care provider, it is obviously necessary for the family to know the name of a person or clinic who can medically evaluate and provide treatment guidance for a child with asthma. Speaking the same language or having access to adequate translation is a prerequisite for an alliance between a family and a health care provider. Parents feel allied with health care providers who listen to them, who respect their perspectives and efforts, and who appear to be genuinely concerned about the welfare of their child (Cramer & Spilker, 1991).

II. Collaborative Relationship with Medical Caregiver

Even though a family may feel very positively about their medical caregiver, this may not be sufficient to achieve effective joint management of the child's asthma. An effective collaborative relationship involves the provision of relevant medical information on the physician's part, and an accurate description of symptom patterns on the parent's part (Wilson *et al.*, 1993). It is important that the medical care provider has an opportunity to observe the child's symptoms during sick visits for clarification of diagnosis and symptom presentation. However, review of disease course and diagnostic test results and planning for ongoing management are effectively done during well visits. The construction of a written asthma action plan, covering steps for both prevention and exacerbation management, has now become the standard of care among physicians treating asthma (National Institutes of Health, 1997). Joint management is most effective when the roles and boundaries of the health care provider and the family are clear. This is facilitated by communicating to families a clear recommendation of how and to what extent they should pursue symptom management at home, and at what point they should call the health care provider.

III. Knowledge of Asthma

Asthma education has become the cornerstone of programs designed to improve asthma management. Increased knowledge has been shown to increase control and decrease morbidity due to asthma (Hindi-Alexander & Cropp, 1984; Clark *et al.*, 1986). However, the results of a meta-analysis of asthma education programs provided equivocal results regarding the association between increased education and decreased morbidity (Bernard-Bonnin *et al.*, 1995). As a result, there has been an increased awareness of the distinction between asthma knowledge and behavior that reduces asthma morbidity (Kolbe *et al.*, 1996; Cote *et al.*, 1997). Nevertheless, it is generally accepted that a minimum of knowledge about asthma is necessary, if not sufficient, for effective asthma management. In a study of the relationship between knowledge and behavior in asthmatic children, increasing asthma knowledge from 'little' to 'average' levels was correlated with behavior change, while further increases in asthma knowledge had little impact (Rubin *et al.*, 1989).

Parents need to understand basic anatomy of the airways and that asthma symptoms are reversible. The notion of chronicity and the role of inflammation seem to be prerequisite knowledge for appropriate use of anti-inflammatory medication. A working knowledge of the actions of medications that have been prescribed is another prerequisite. Parents can be expected to know the pattern of their own child's asthma symptoms, and the precipitants for wheezing episodes. When there is a lack of knowledge in any of these key areas, the consultant must begin to determine the underlying cause of the deficits. Such causes include, but are not limited to, inadequate education from health care providers, parent's intellectual limitations, or parent's motivational factors. Misinformation, abundantly available through the popular press, can lead to distortion of factual material and negative attitudes toward the medical model. A formulation of underlying problems will form the basis of a treatment plan, sometimes preceded by further specific evaluation.

IV. Medication Adherence

As noted above, failure to adhere with the medical care provider's recommendations for prescribed medication is often considered the primary reason for poorly controlled asthma (Rand & Wise, 1994). Therefore, for families in which a child has poorly controlled asthma it is useful to determine the proportion of medications that are actually taken. But while it is important to determine how much medication gets taken, it is equally important to understand the process by which medications end up in the child with asthma. To understand the medication delivery system for the regular (usually preventive) medications, it should be determined which person remembers that medications are to be taken and what cues that person uses as memory aids. Administering regular medications several times a day requires a high level of family organization (Bender & Klinnert, 1998). Families who do this successfully usually incorporate the medication times into family routines, such as mealtimes or bedtimes. Families without regularity in their schedules tend to have more difficulties with this.

The lack of family organization or routine can be exacerbated by numerous psychosocial problems, including spousal conflict or abuse, parental psychopathology, or parental substance abuse. Obviously, suspicion of underlying severe dysfunction will require further evaluation and possible treatment. If the primary caregiver is in charge of the medication delivery system, she either must be present all the time (a heavy burden for the most committed of parents) or there must be alternative caregivers who are well trained in following directions and making decisions, and with whom the primary caregiver is able to communicate effectively. If the child is in charge of the medication delivery system, the developmental appropriateness of the level of responsibility becomes pertinent.

The appropriate utilization of as-needed medications is even more complex, since it cannot rely on family routines. Rather, the child with asthma or the caregiver must perceive or notice the breakthrough asthma symptoms, have the medication available, know how to judge the severity and progression of symptoms, and know what symptoms dictate what treatment and under what conditions to call the physician. This is made more complex for school-age children, whose independent asthma self-care capacities come into play. The cooperation, commitment, and knowledge of alternative caregivers are also especially important with appropriate prn (as required) medication administration.

V. Alternative Caregivers

Medical care providers typically give directions and recommendations for a child's asthma care to the person who brings the child into the office or clinic. In a study of low-income African-American mothers of preschool-age children, 94% of the mothers identified themselves as having the primary responsibility for their children's asthma management (Brown *et al.*, 1996). However, 77% indicated that they received help with the asthma management from at least one other adult, whether grandmothers or fathers. While this sample may not be representative of the general population, the numbers regarding asthma care responsibilities and aid appear fairly typical. This study described how the involvement of family members adds complexity to the mother's task, since the helping adults may have different ideas about asthma management than those prescribed by the health care provider. The mothers also reported expending considerable energy in coordinating asthma management with caregivers outside the home. Adequate day care can be difficult to find, particularly for children with regular or severe exacerbations (Schultz *et al.*, 1994), and requires extensive communication with day care personnel. For school-age children, classroom and physical education teachers must be able and willing to monitor children's conditions, and the school must be prepared for prompt response to serious symptoms. Parents have reported that getting schoolteachers to learn about asthma and to cooperate with them was one of the biggest obstacles they had encountered (Brown *et al.*, 1996). When divorced couples are co-parenting, there is great potential for the differences that resulted in a divorce to be acted out in the management of a child's asthma. For example, in such cases, children may return from visitation with the noncustodial parent having not received any preventive medication for days. It is clear from these reports that effective asthma management requires the primary caregiver to be able to communicate and plan with numerous other caregivers. An effective system across settings is impeded when the caregiver is herself unclear about how to manage the asthma, when she has deficits in communication and relationship skills, or when she is unable to cope with the complexity of these requirements. Each of these areas is affected by parental psychiatric problems or intellectual limitations.

VI. Adherence with Environmental Recommendations

Exposure to indoor allergens and cigarette smoke contributes significantly to out-of-control asthma (Ehnert *et al.*, 1992). Follow-through with environmental recommendations from medical care providers is a good indication of the family's motivation to use available information to gain control over the asthma. A lack of understanding of what measures to take, or how environmental factors affect asthma, frequently underlies the failure of families to follow through. Other considerations for determining whether families have been nonadherent include feelings such as shame or associated financial burdens. Acknowledgment of the presence of cockroaches or rodents can be embarrassing, due to the implication of slovenliness, and lead to resentment, because elimination may be financially impossible. Procedures for the elimination of dust mites can also be financially draining, or represent a large housekeeping burden (e.g., removing carpet, washing bedding frequently in very hot water).

Recommendations to remove family pets from the home are often met with a great deal of resistance. Parents may be concerned about their child's attachment to the pet, and the importance to the child of having a pet like a 'normal' child. Sometimes the parents are strongly attached to the pets, and they must consider the relative importance to themselves of the pet versus the child's health. For emotionally needy children or adults, pets can serve as attachment objects imbued with great meaning. There may even be circumstances where it is ill-advised to remove a pet from a child who has nothing else in the world. In such instances the unavailability of secure and competent caregivers may be the most salient psychological issue. It should be clear from these examples that failure to 'get rid of the cat' may not be as simple as it seems. The manner in which families respond to this difficult issue reveals a great deal about individual and family psychological functioning and capacities for adaptive coping.

The presence of cigarette smoking in the home is an even more emotionally loaded problem. Most physicians will have inquired about smoke exposure and made a recommendation against it, but smoking parents often become extremely defensive. Being a cigarette smoker was found to characterize dropouts from an asthma management program (Fish *et al.*, 1996), and indeed the need to maintain this behavior may motivate some families to any avoid in-depth discussion of their asthma management system. It is wise to approach the topic without conveying the expectation that the smoker must quit. Most smokers have some history of trying to quit, and will relate the stressful circumstances that precipitated their resumption of smoking. It is important that the interviewer understand the social, psychological, and physiological reasons for maintenance of cigarette smoking, so that this difficult topic can be explored in an empathic manner. For evaluation purposes, the consultant should determine the smokers' readiness to quit (Prochaska & DiClementi, 1983), and their openness to discussing the effects of cigarette smoke exposure on their child with asthma. In some cases, nonsmoking parents may have difficulty protecting their asthmatic children from smoke, as when an extended family member continues to smoke in the child's presence. This situation provides an opportunity to evaluate the parent's assertiveness and personal resources to protect their child from asthma triggers.

VII. Symptom Knowledge and Assessment

To manage asthma effectively, it is essential that the caretaker recognize symptoms of breathing problems. This is especially true in caring for younger children who may not recognize their own symptoms or whose developing recognition of symptoms may be unreliable. Children develop the ability to notice that they are having breathing difficulties, and to tell their caregiver, at about 3–4 years of age (Brown *et al.*, 1996). Nevertheless, young children's motivation to attend to symptoms is variable, and their ability to notice early signs of breathing problems comes later. It falls to the caretaker to recognize impending breathing difficulties at the earliest possible time, in order to initiate treatment and make adjustments to prevent worsening symptoms. It is also important that the caretaker be attuned to patterns of daily functioning and seasonal variations, in order to maintain an accurate view of the course of a child's asthma.

As children get older and take on more responsibility for their asthma self-care, their perceptions of their breathing become increasingly important. Symptom perception studies have shown that there is marked variability in the accuracy with which children perceive their respiratory functioning (Fritz & Overholser, 1990). Thus, for older children whose symptom reports determine the use of prn medications or even emergency intervention, it is important to evaluate their ability to perceive symptoms accurately, in addition to their motivation to do so. Many medical care providers follow the Expert Panel guidelines and recommend daily use of peak flow meters for patients with moderate to severe asthma (National Institutes of Health, 1997). Peak flow meters are clearly a useful tool for children with poor symptom perception. Follow-through with utilization of a peak flow meter, and the quality of the parent–child interactions around such usage, represent one of the many behavioral systems within the family asthma management system that must function well to achieve well-controlled asthma.

VIII. Action Plan and Emotional Response

The quality of attack management skills is a central component of effective asthma management that becomes relevant when a child displays breathing difficulties. Appropriate behaviors include assessment of symptom severity, decision-making regarding medication administration, and prompt intervention. Following initial medications, symptoms must be monitored and decisions made regarding appropriate steps for further intervention, such as calling the medical care provider or taking the child for urgent care. Many factors influence the manner in which families manage asthma attacks. Caregivers may be slow to react adaptively because they are unaware of early or subtle signs of breathing difficulties, because they are uninformed about appropriate home management of symptoms, because they are lacking necessary medication or equipment, and so on. Under such circumstances, symptoms may worsen until urgent care is in fact required. Obviously, the high costs associated with ER care for asthma (Weiss *et al.*, 1992) would be much lower if families learned to intervene early with effective home management plans for asthma attacks.

The emotional response of the caregiver and of the asthmatic child to an exacerbation of symptoms is key to an effective response to symptoms. Appropriate concern without excessive anxiety is associated with effective care. Research with adults showed that anxiety levels that were either too high or too low were related to more hospitalizations (Kinsman *et al.*, 1982), and this pattern has also been shown to be true for children (Baron *et al.*, 1986). Low anxiety levels may be associated with a delay in treatment and, ultimately, with a need for more intensive treatment, as described above. In contrast, high anxiety may be related to overresponding to symptoms, and therefore to overutilization of medical treatment. Repeated use of ERs for asthma in children has been associated with parental attitudinal variables relating to appraisal of their child's asthma severity, management of asthma attacks, and parental worry (Wakefield *et al.*, 1997). The caregiver's emotional response is also transmitted to the child, who learns through emotional communication whether to be anxious and fearful about his condition (Klinnert *et al.*, 1983). This brings into question the adult's awareness of her own anxiety in response to the stress of the asthma exacerbation, and the adequacy of her coping strategies for managing internal distress.

IX. Balance of Responsibility

Optimally, children who grow up with asthma develop better awareness of their symptoms and take increasing responsibility for managing their own illnesses. This is a developmental process during which children learn about their breathing, and how to care for themselves by avoiding triggers and utilizing medication appropriately. As children learn more, their caregivers decrease the amount of surveillance and structure they provided earlier in the child's life. This can be seen as a shift in the balance of responsibility that occurs between parents and their asthmatic children during the course of normal development (Klinnert & LumLung, 1991). Guidelines are available for assessing the developmental appropriateness of responsibility taken by the child and the parent (Klinnert & LumLung, 1991). The expectations for specific asthma self-care tasks are determined by increasing developmental capabilities of the child, and are associated with the decreasing role of the parent.

Problems arise if children fail to learn self-care and caretakers continue to take full responsibility for their children's asthma. These children may appear as excessively dependent, and may be delayed in social and emotional development. Such dependency may be fueled by overly anxious caregivers who have difficulty allowing children to take responsibility for themselves and experiencing the negative consequences that may come from making mistakes.

In contrast, in some families young children are given far too much responsibility for monitoring their symptoms and taking their medications. In the National Cooperative Inner-City Asthma Study (NCICAS) of children's asthma management, about 5% of the children aged 6–9 reported that they were functioning as their own primary caretaker (Wade *et al.*, 1997). Given the developmental needs and limitations of growing children, either too much or too little involvement on the part of caregivers represents poor adjustment to the illness and a malfunctioning asthma management system.

X. Parent–Child Interaction

An asthmatic child's poor cooperation with the parent's management efforts often results in nonadherence with recommended medications or environmental controls. Parent–child conflict during asthma attacks mitigates against effective management by interfering with adherence on a day-to-day basis. Children may refuse to take medications, to use peak flow meters effectively, or to avoid triggers such as pets to which they are allergic. When a child resists a parent's attempts to administer medications, parents may initially increase the coerciveness of their attempts to get the child to take medications, but ultimately the aversiveness of the process may result in their giving up (Patterson, 1982).

Such conflict between parents and children is indicative of more pervasive problems that require assessment and treatment. The assessment addresses the quality of the relationship throughout the child's lifetime, and the duration of conflictual interactions. On the mild side, parent–child conflict can represent transitory difficulties in coping related to disease events or to unrelated life stresses. In contrast, problems with the attachment relationship are typically long-standing and have ramifications throughout the family's functioning. Attachment problems are reflected in the interaction with the child. Parents may be emotionally uninvolved, they may be affectively negative toward the child, or they may vacillate between these behavioral patterns. Children with insecure attachments to their parents have poorer coping skills in general, and have more negative interpersonal interactions (Bates *et al.*, 1985; Erikson *et al.*, 1985). Given the requisite components of the asthma management system described above, such family dysfunction would probably be related to poorly controlled asthma. Indeed, a study of preschoolers with severe, uncontrolled asthma revealed that significantly more of the children had insecure attachments to their mothers than would be expected within a group of normal preschoolers (Mrazek *et al.*, 1987). Among older children, parental negativity, or criticism, has been shown to increase with greater asthma severity (Hermanns *et al.*, 1989). Parental criticism has been related to medication noncompliance in a group of adolescents with severe, poorly controlled asthma (Wamboldt *et al.*, 1995).

Children who are difficult to control may be diagnosed as 'oppositional' or as having a 'conduct disorder' (American Psychiatric Association, 1994). These disorders, which most often occur in the context of parent–child problems, constitute significant problems for achieving asthma management. When children are out of control and refuse to follow the rules set for them by adults, they are unlikely to comply with recommendations for any specific self-management behaviors, whether made by their parents or their medical care provider. Children with 'attention deficit hyperactivity disorder' (ADHD) also display a behavioral pattern that complicates family asthma management. Thus, although ADHD is not more common among children with asthma than among normal children (Biederman *et al.*, 1994), when it occurs in conjunction with asthma it has the potential to impede effective asthma management and ultimately to lead to more poorly controlled asthma.

The assessment of the quality of interactions between parents and their children deserves particularly close attention within the asthma management system. The consistency with which family conflict and negative affective exchanges have been associated with poor asthma outcome is striking. Conflict, coerciveness, and criticism have been shown to be increased in families with severe, poorly controlled asthma (Mrazek *et al.*, 1985; Hermanns *et al.*, 1989; Wamboldt *et al.*, 1995). Asthma death in children has been shown to be associated with conflict among all parties of the system – child–parent, child–staff, and parent–staff conflict were all present in the cases of children who died from asthma as compared with case controls (Strunk *et al.*, 1985). Family dysfunction is mentioned repeatedly as a factor in asthma death (Fritz *et al.*, 1987), and excessive conflict and negativity may be the most pernicious as well as common form of family dysfunction.

XI. Parental Resources

Since parents or caretakers have primary responsibility for children with asthma, limitations in their resources can affect asthma management in the family. For example, poverty is often associated with poor access to health care, difficulty in obtaining prescribed medications, lack of transportation to medical care facilities, and inability to exert control over environmental precipitants (Huss *et al.*, 1994). Likewise, intellectual deficits on the part of caretakers impede an adequate understanding of asthma, medications and their mechanisms, and optimal judgment and decision making. Life stressors such as unemployment, housing inadequacy, or legal difficulties drain parents' psychological and material resources. In the face of overwhelming life stresses, taking measures to prevent a child's asthma exacerbations becomes a low priority.

Parental difficulties in forming or maintaining relationships can also seriously impede effective asthma management. This is seen most clearly when parents are unable to identify a medical care provider for their child whom they can trust, with whom they can jointly form an asthma management plan, and to whom they can appropriately turn for help. Psychiatric problems in parents of asthmatic children impede effective asthma management in numerous ways, such as lack of ability or motivation to organize family life, or the maintenance of interpersonal conflict. In the NCICAS study of asthma management among inner-city children, 50% of the caregivers were found to report psychological symptoms in themselves which were in the clinical range (Wade *et al.*, 1997). Although the relationship between parents' psychological symptoms and management of their children's asthma was not reported, it is likely that this amount of impairment is related to inadequate asthma management. Relationships between parents' psychological adjustment and parenting behavior have been well documented in child development research, and can be expected to show similar relationships when asthma management is the caretaking behavior of focus. For example, mothers suffering from depression have been shown to be more aversive towards their children (Dumas & Serketich, 1994), to give more critical descriptions of their children (Goodman *et al.*, 1994), and to be less effective in disciplining their children's behavior (Fox & Gelfand, 1994) compared with nondepressed mothers. It can be assumed that depressed mothers of children with asthma would have more difficulty in managing their children's asthma management behavior. Parents who have been found to be critical of their children are significantly more likely to suffer from psychiatric disorders than parents who do not make critical comments (Hibbs *et al.*, 1991). In a study of children with chronic illnesses including asthma, children with more functional limitations were found to have mothers with more psychiatric symptoms (Jessop *et al.*, 1988).

XII. Balanced Integration of Asthma into Family Life

Adjustment to an asthmatic condition in one or more members of the family involves giving attention to learning about asthma, establishing a management system including taking preventive measures, and dealing with exacerbations when they occur. Ideally, however, once the system is established and maintenance procedures are in place, attention to and concern about the asthma should not occupy the center of a family's life (Gonzalez *et al.*, 1989). When attention to asthma outweighs the objective requirements of the illness, there appears to be an overinvestment in the illness that does not bode well for the psychological adjustment of the family or its individual members. Alternatively, some families may deny the importance of asthma and fail to invest the time and energy required for establishing an effective asthma management system, resulting in undertreatment. Either of these patterns represents a poor integration of the asthma into the family.

Asthmatic children's peer relationships can be seen as an index of whether a child's asthma is well integrated into the child's sense of self and the family life. Problems with integration are indicated if a child's peer relationships are overly restricted due to asthma. If the asthma is as well controlled as possible, the family should be working with the child to develop and maintain developmentally appropriate peer relationships. Children who are embarrassed to use an inhaler in front of peers may need help in explaining their asthma and related medications. For example, a parent can help by making a class presentation about asthma. Children do at times experience teasing by peers about their asthma, but being teased is a normative childhood experience that provides an opportunity for children to learn to cope with such experiences. Blaming peer problems on asthma is often an indication that the asthma is not being integrated into the child's life in a healthy manner.

The Asthma Management Profile

Once a family's asthma management system has been characterized along each of the relevant dimensions, the strengths and weaknesses of the system become clear. Table 3.3 illustrates the results of a FAMSS evaluation with the family of a child whose asthma was out of control. It can be seen that the available information leads directly to a treatment plan. Before discussing treatment, however, we will review, in a limited fashion, behavioral and emotional problems that may be experienced by the individual child with asthma.

Secondary Effects of Asthma on Child Functioning

Although deficits in the family asthma management system are the most common reason for psychological consultation regarding children with asthma, there are occasions where the asthma management system is found to be functioning fairly well, but the child nevertheless experiences negative effects from the asthma. While children with asthma as a group may not be more prone to depression than other children (Klinnert, 1997), some children with asthma experience depression that appears to be unrelated to negative family circumstances (Gizynski & Shapiro, 1990). When depression includes hopelessness or self-destructive feelings, it has the potential for affecting medication adherence. Although this is one of the problems associated with depression among children with asthma, nonadherence is only one of the pathways to poor outcome among children with asthma. Depression among children with asthma has been

Table 3.3 Case illustration: FAMSS multidimensional assessment

David was an 8-year-old African-American male who was referred for psychological consultation because his asthma was out of control as indicated by his missing a significant amount of school through the previous fall months. David's asthma, which he had had since infancy, was triggered primarily by his severe allergies. David was an only child, and he lived with his mother and his stepfather. Both parents worked full time.

An interview regarding the family asthma management system revealed difficulties in many of the 12 areas. Of equal importance, the problems experienced by the family in each of the areas pointed toward specific areas of underlying psychological problems, in some cases requiring further evaluation, and ultimately to a treatment plan.

I. Alliance with medical caregiver. David's mother was strongly allied with her physician; she believed in his competence and trusted his opinion.

II. Collaborative relationship. David's mother liked their physician, and he had tried to help her gain control over her son's asthma. It was unclear whether she had been given an action plan; she was not approaching the management of the asthma in a systematic way. It was not clear that she would be able to do her part in monitoring and reporting symptoms accurately.

III. Knowledge of asthma. David's mother had some knowledge of asthma, including the role of environmental precipitants. However, she did not understand the role of inflammation and that inhaled steroids would be effective against inflammation only if taken twice every day as prescribed.

IV. Medication adherence. There were multiple reasons why David was not receiving his medications as prescribed. His mother had cut his inhaled steroids to once a day because she believed that side effects from the medication were causing him to be inattentive and uncooperative at school. Further, her work schedule prevented her from being available in the mornings to administer the medication.

V. Alternative caregivers. Because both the mother and stepfather had long and erratic work schedules, David had to be awakened at 4:00 a.m. and taken to a sitter. The sitters were irregular, with extended family sometimes serving in this role and paid sitters sometimes caring for David and sending him off to school. The sitters were unaware of his need for regular medication in the morning. At school, there was no school nurse to help David with his asthma. His teacher had a large classroom of children and found it burdensome to monitor David's symptoms and give him medication as needed. This caused his mother to be anxious about David's well-being at school and to take him home whenever he had symptoms.

VI. Environmental adherence. There were no pets in the home, and no one smoked cigarettes. Dust control measures had been taken.

VII. Symptom knowledge and assessment. David's mother was vague about the pattern of David's symptoms. This was in contrast with how clearly she spoke about his allergic symptoms, their precipitants, and effective treatment. David had been given a peak flow meter, but he used it sporadically and played games with it rather than utilizing the information it could provide.

VIII. Action plan and emotional response. David's mother did not have a clear plan for managing his symptoms. She would take him home from school and give him treatments, but sometimes would take him directly to the

Table 3.3 *contd*

doctor. Her decisions seemed to be prompted by her level of anxiety, rather than by working her way through a plan. She often became quite frightened by David's attacks, and she knew that he was very attuned to her fear.

IX. Balance of responsibility. David's mother admitted that David was not taking responsibility for his asthma as would be expected at his age. Although he did notice his symptoms, he did not show initiative in taking medications. His mother was very involved in monitoring his symptoms, and frequently brought him home from school to watch over him.

X. Parent–child interaction. David often fought with his mother about taking his medications, actively refusing a good deal of the time. At the same time the dyad was overinvolved, with David experiencing separation anxiety and his mother being anxious and guilty about her parenting with him.

XI. Parental resources. This family had adequate finances, including medical insurance. However, the mother's job required her to work swing shifts, and to work a great deal of overtime. This limited her time with her son, and made it difficult to have a regular schedule. The stepfather was unable to compensate for her absence, since he had a full time job and another part-time job. The mother's mental health was a serious problem in this case, since she suffered from anxiety and depression, which appeared to be related to how she was parented.

XII. Balanced integration. For this family, David's asthma had become the focus of their lives. David had missed significant amounts of school, which contributed to poor performance. His mother had missed excessive work and worried about the security of her job. David hated and feared his asthma, rather than taking it in stride and learning to live with it.

Supplementary evaluation. Because of his school difficulties and his excessive absences, David received cognitive testing, including a screen for learning disabilities, testing of his attentional capacities, and brief emotional testing. His intellectual ability was in the average range, he had no learning disabilities, and his attentional capacities, while diminished, did not indicate a child with attention deficit disorder. Testing supported the impression of significant anxiety and depression. David's academic delay was believed to be caused by his emotional problems and his school absence.

Treatment. The components of treatment included:
1. Informing the family regarding factors underlying David's behavior problems, and in particular that they were not caused by his asthma medications.
2. Educating the family regarding asthma, symptom assessment, effective use of medications, and behavioral approaches for managing David's self-management behavior.
3. Assisting the family and the physician in clarifying an asthma action plan.
4. Increasing the family's awareness of the need for supervision of David's asthma management, and problem-solving regarding parental availability.
5. Assisting the family in utilizing the county nurse to educate school personnel and ensure adequate supervision in the school setting.
6. Referring David and his parents for psychotherapy to address parent–child relationship problems as well as David's significant anxiety and depression, and to assess the mother's anxiety and depression.

described as a significant risk factor in childhood asthma death due to the increased cholinergic tone that characterizes depression and which can lead to an explosive parasympathetic outpouring, and death (Miller, 1987).

The breathlessness that is intrinsic to asthma symptoms can result in anxiety; the fear of dying is not uncommonly reported (Carrieri *et al.*, 1991). Family studies have shown that anxiety disorders are more common among children with allergies (Kagan *et al.*, 1991). Further, parents have consistently reported that their asthmatic children have increased internalizing problems, including anxiety (Hamlett *et al.*, 1992; MacLean *et al.*, 1992). As noted above, such anxiety can result in overresponding and overtreating asthma symptoms. Anxiety has been reported to serve as an emotional trigger for asthma exacerbations, and may worsen asthma symptoms when they occur (Vazquez & Buceta, 1993). But even if there is no discernible effect of anxiety on the asthma or its management, high anxiety is in itself a disorder deserving of evaluation and treatment.

Post-traumatic stress disorder can occur secondary to asthma, particularly among children with severe asthma who have experienced invasive procedures. Children who have required intubation have been described as demonstrating elements of post-traumatic stress (Gavin & Roesler, 1997). For younger children, hospitalizations which entail separation from parents or even repeated medical procedures have long been known to result in stress reactions (Garmezy, 1983). Asthma that appears to be intractable has been found to be associated with panic disorder (Baron & Marcotte, 1994). The patients apparently confuse their panic symptoms with asthma, and report symptoms that naturally are not controlled by their asthma medications.

Medication side effects may serve as a source of distress for children whose asthma is otherwise under control. While the psychological effects of theophylline are not as severe as once believed (Rachelefsky *et al.*, 1986), the caffeine-like effects of theophylline have been documented and include a slight trend towards more anxiety and hand tremor in treated versus untreated children. This may be accompanied by slightly increased attention and/or verbal memory (Bender *et al.*, 1991; Schlieper *et al.*, 1991; Bender & Milgrom, 1992). Classic antihistamines, such as diphenhydramine, have been found to cause drowsiness in some children (Vuurman *et al.*, 1993). Individual case studies have reported an association between sympathomimetics and a variety of unusual behaviors in children, including aggressiveness and visual hallucinations (Bender & Milgrom, 1995). Asthmatic children stabilized on high doses of corticosteroids (40–80 mg per day) can experience significant depression, anxiety, and impairment of long-term memory compared with children on low maintenance doses (2–20 mg per day) (Bender *et al.*, 1988). However, steroid-induced psychosis, which has been reported in adults, has not been documented in children. Of particular interest is the finding that children with a pre-existing history of emotional difficulties were more likely to become anxious and depressed while receiving high doses of prednisone than children without such histories (Bender *et al.*, 1991).

Treatment: A Family Asthma Management Approach

The evaluation of the family asthma management system and the identification of problem areas within the multidimensional system lead directly to the forms of psychosocial intervention required to gain improved control of symptoms. Interventions are conducted within the family context, because this is where the interactions comprising asthma management occur. This asthma-focused family therapy should be distinguished from traditional family therapy in its targeting of asthma management behaviors. Treatment should specifically address the deficits in the system that have been identified during the evaluation. Given the multidimensional nature of the asthma management system, treatment will by necessity be multidimensional.

As discussed, knowledge about asthma may not be sufficient for effective asthma management, but it is probably necessary. If it has been determined that a family is lacking in knowledge about asthma, this should be remedied. Asthma education classes may be useful, or clinic-based individualized instruction may be necessary (Wilson *et al.*, 1993). Special attention should be paid to the mastery of specific component skills, such as symptom perception or monitoring, training in the use of a peak flow meter, or good inhaler technique. The therapist can provide valuable input to the educators regarding the parents' or child's intellectual capacity or cognitive style, cultural biases or beliefs, or emotional experiences and orientation. At the same time the therapist can continue to evaluate the family's knowledge, while exploring a family's resistance to certain recommendations. The interplay between family factors and the education process is illustrated by a family who declares unwillingness to administer inhaled steroids. Exploration may reveal a lack of understanding of the inflammatory basis of chronic asthma or misconceptions about side effects of steroids. Individualized education may be sufficient to address the problem. However, fears about side effects of medication are often based not only on ignorance but also on previous emotionally complex experiences. An examination of the source of the fears is necessary to dispel them and clear the way for a more enlightened view.

Along with asthma knowledge, the relationship with the medical care provider must be addressed early on. As recognized in the *Expert Panel Report 2* (National Institutes of Health, 1997), the control of asthma is not possible without an effective collaborative relationship with the medical care provider. Families need to have an asthma action plan and to be clear about its meaning. Supporting and clarifying prescriptions, making recommendations, and establishing expectations is a useful and appropriate activity for the psychosocial clinician. Sources of misunderstanding can be identified and communications clarified. For example, a family may reveal their confusion about the circumstances under which they should treat attacks at home as opposed to calling their physician for guidance. Such a family would benefit from help in communicating with their physician and obtaining clarity regarding this component of their asthma management plan.

For some families, increased knowledge and clarification of recommendations and the action plan will improve control of asthma symptoms. The next level of intervention involves behavioral guidance for specific activities that must occur. For example, a family may require assistance in setting up a system for an adolescent to take inhaled steroids independently, but with parental supervision. Some parents desire help in removing pets from their home in a manner that is sensitive to the needs of all family members, as well as the pets. Decreasing the child's exposure to cigarette smoke may be facilitated at this level. With input from their physician, families may wish to clarify their plan for addressing symptom exacerbations. In this context, parents with good psychological resources may be able to examine their own anxiety in the face of their child's asthma attack, and find ways to manage it in the interest of optimal home management and modeling positive coping for the child.

While improving the routine medication system will commonly be a treatment goal, the therapist should continue to evaluate the underlying difficulties that impede an effective system. Insight and guidance may not be sufficient for the anxious parent described above, whose child's wheezing symptoms may meet with high anxiety, an overestimate of symptom severity, and inappropriate attack management. Exploration may reveal that the anxiety underlying the appropriate responses is related to a relative's death from asthma. In this case, it would be necessary to address the loss of the relative, while also educating regarding symptom assessment and rehearsing appropriate responses to symptoms. However, anxiety symptoms are sometimes not situation-specific, but are pervasive and debilitating. In such cases, it is helpful to identify the problem, including its relationship to asthma management, and to refer for psychiatric assessment and possible medical and psychotherapeutic management.

Families can be seriously in need of help in their communications with alternative caregivers. The provision of guidance, including educational materials, can be helpful. In this context, many parents need help in improving their communication skills. They may need to work on clarifying what it is they need or want done, becoming more assertive, or changing an aggressive style to one that is appropriately assertive. Interventions with alternative caregivers may involve not only family members but also members of the extended family or co-parenting ex-spouses. In working on communication skills, parents' personal problems such as poor self-esteem or excessive dependency needs may become apparent and require attention. If these problems are severe, they will undoubtedly be interfering with asthma management in a number of ways, and may require evaluation and treatment.

As asthma management knowledge and techniques improve, impediments caused by dysfunction in the family system become more apparent. Systemic family problems that impede asthma management include the physical unavailability of caregivers and lack of family routines or organization. Parents may need support in reconsidering work schedules that take them away from their children. Some families need feedback and guidance about the importance of family routine and structure, not only for asthma management but also for optimal overall child development. However, family disorganization may be symptomatic of marital problems or of parental psychiatric disorders. Evaluation and treatment of the disorder, whether in the medical setting or through referral, may be necessary before an improvement is seen in family functioning.

Interventions aimed at the parent–child relationship and at parenting problems will be appropriate in those cases with conflict related to tasks such as taking medications or measuring peak flows, or where the balance of responsibility for asthma care is developmentally inappropriate. Behavior modification techniques are extremely useful tools for the parents of infants and younger children. Besides learning the principles of reinforcement and time out, parents typically need help in defining the asthma self-care behaviors they should expect from their children. With adolescents, communication and clarification regarding expected behaviors on the part of the parent and the teenager, with some provision for age-appropriate supervision, can be very helpful for families with functional relationships. When parents of children of any age feel that the child is out of control and that poor asthma self-care is only one of a multitude of behavioral problems, diagnoses of oppositional behavior or conduct disorder must be considered. Evaluation and treatment of the child and the family will follow recommended interventions for this family pattern (Patterson, 1982).

The treatment of families in which the responsibility for the illness is unbalanced requires different forms of family therapy. For those where the child has too much responsibility for his asthma, there may be a lack of information about what is developmentally appropriate for the child. Often there are systemic family problems that involve the lack of physical or emotional availability of the parents. When necessary, the attachment relationship between the parent and the child can be addressed in parent–child therapy, or may require referral to professionals trained in this area. Family therapy is also appropriate for those families where the parent has taken responsibility for the asthma and the child is overly dependent. In these cases it is helpful to clarify developmentally appropriate expectations, and also to explore the fears and needs of each person in the dyad that have impeded the normal course of development. For these families, therapy should include all members of family, since there may be a shifting of roles throughout the family system that has supported the dysfunctional development of the child with asthma (Gustafsson *et al.*, 1986).

Finally, for many families with children with severe, poorly controlled asthma, overwhelming problems in living take precedence over attending to the specific needs of their asthmatic child. These families are often 'multiproblem' families with a variety of financial, social, and psychological needs. Intervention requires the involvement of mental health providers who can help to address the organizational and programmatic problems that face these families. With such families, behavioral contracting provides a focus on specific, manageable problems and an arena within which to address the family's motivation to change.

Despite the evaluation and treatment approach promoted here, where the focus is on the family system and asthma management, there are situations where individual therapy with the child with asthma is the treatment of choice. For example, children who suffer anxiety about their asthma despite good control and a supportive, resourceful family can benefit from relaxation therapy. Such therapy can have positive effects on the asthma itself. A carefully controlled study has shown that asthmatic children with emotional triggers showed symptom improvement following relaxation therapy, in contrast with non-emotionally triggered children (Vazquez & Buceta, 1993). Similarly, certain forms of depression in children and adolescents are effectively treated individually.

Conclusions and Future Directions

Innovative behavioral interventions are critically needed to alter the course of treatment for children with asthma. The need for these programs comes from the combined influence of increasing morbidity and mortality among inner-city children with asthma (Wade *et al.*, 1997) and changes in health care management which emphasize cost efficiency. Despite numerous programmatic efforts to decrease asthma morbidity, significant improvements have been difficult to document (Bernard-Bonnin *et al.*, 1995). We suggest that, for families of children with asthma who have failed to achieve disease management, whether working with a physician or through educational programs, an individualized assessment and treatment plan is in order. A systematic assessment of the psychological characteristics of the patient and the family, of the social system of which they are a part, and of the barriers which prevent appropriate management must precede the introduction of a planned intervention. The FAMSS framework focuses specifically on the family's asthma management system, and thereby provides a promising model for a collaborative, disease-focused behavioral intervention. Since treatment focuses on those aspects of the system that are found to be impeding disease management, specific treatment modules can then be developed to address the particular deficits of a family's asthma management system.

The FAMSS interview and treatment approach is currently being utilized in a number of clinical and research studies. In a tertiary care setting for severe, out-of-control asthma, the FAMSS is being administered at admission to assess the strengths and weaknesses of the asthma management system the family has had in place at home (Bratton *et al.*, 1999). In a study of asthma symptom perception, family asthma management assessed with the FAMSS will be combined with symptom perception to jointly predict asthma morbidity (Fritz *et al.*, 1996). Since the latter study is utilizing computerized metered dose inhalers to assess medication adherence, data will soon be available regarding agreement between the FAMSS medication adherence subscale and actual inhaler usage. The FAMSS assessment approach is also being utilized in a randomized, controlled preventive intervention study with infants from low-income families who are at high risk for developing asthma, to assess illness management before and after intervention. The interview format is particularly useful with these low-resource families who have variable management skills, and who are generally inexperienced with asthma and unexposed to asthma management information. Preliminary data from this study show that the environmental adherence subscale is significantly correlated with the house dust evidence of animal dander and infant urinary cotinine. Evidence is accumulating that this focused family interview provides valid information about various aspects of the asthma management system.

Ultimately, changing the behavior of patients with chronic illness and their families is an enormous challenge. The value of such programs is put to the test when the final endpoint is improvement of asthma symptoms accompanied by decreased school or work absence and health care costs. Randomized, controlled studies of these programs and instruments must therefore be conducted before agreement is reached about their ultimate contributions (Creer *et al.*, 1990).

Acknowledgment

The writing of this paper was supported by NIH grants #R18 AI41137 and #M01-RR00051. The authors express their sincere thanks to Dr Elizabeth McQuaid and Dr Donna Bratton for their helpful comments during the preparation of this manuscript.

References

American Psychiatric Association (1994). *Diagnostic and statistical manual of mental disorders*, 4th edn. Washington, DC: American Psychiatric Association, 1994.

Bailey, W., Richards, J., Brooks, C., Soong, S., Windsor, R., & Manzella, B. (1990). A randomized trial to improve self-management practices in adults with asthma. *Archives of Internal Medicine*, 150, 1664–1668.

Baron, C., & Marcotte, J.E. (1994). Role of panic attacks in the intractibility of asthma in children. *Pediatrics*, 94, 108–110.

Baron, C., Lamarre, A., Veilleux, P., Ducharme, G., Spier, S., & Lapierre, J. (1986). Psychomaintenance of childhood asthma: a study of 34 children. *Journal of Asthma*, 23, 69–79.

Bates, J.E., Maslin, C.A., & Frankel, K.A. (1985). Attachment security, mother–child interaction, and temperament as predictors of behavior– problem ratings at age three years, *Monographs of the Society for Research in Child Development*, 50, 167–193.

Baum, D. & Creer, T.L. (1986). Medication compliance in children with asthma. *Journal of Asthma*, 23, 49–59.

Becker, A., McGhan, S., Dolovich, J., Proudlock, M., & Mitchell, I. (1994). Essential ingredients for an ideal education program for children with asthma and their families. *Chest*, 106, 231S–234S.

Bender, B. & Klinnert, M.D. (1998). Psychological correlates of asthma severity and treatment outcome. In: H. Kotses & A. Harver (Eds), *Behavioral contributions to the management of asthma.* New York: Marcel Dekker.

Bender, B. & Milgrom, H. (1992). Theophylline-induced behavior change in children: an objective evaluation of parent's perceptions. *Journal of the American Medical Association*, 267, 2621–2624.

Bender, B. & Milgrom, H. (1995). Neuropsychiatric effects of medications for allergic diseases. *Journal of Allergy and Clinical Immunology*, 95, 523–528.

Bender, B., Lerner, J., & Kollasch, E. (1988). Mood and memory changes in asthmatic children receiving corticosteroids. *Journal of the American Academy of Child and Adolescent Psychiatry*, 6, 720–725.

Bender, B., Lerner, J., & Polland, J. (1991). Association between corticosteroids and psychologic change in hospitalized asthmatic children. *Annals of Allergy*, 66, 414–419.

Bender, B., Milgrom, H., Rand, C., & Ackerson, L. (1998). Psychological factors associated with medication nonadherence in asthmatic children. *Journal of Asthma*, 35, 347–353.

Bernard-Bonnin, A., Stachenko, S., Bonin, D., Charette, C., & Rousseau, E. (1995). Self management teaching programs and morbidity of pediatric asthma: a meta-analysis. *Journal of Allergy and Clinical Immunology*, 95, 34–41.

Biederman, J., Milberger, S., Faraone, S., Guite, J., & Warburton, R. (1994). Associations between childhood asthma and ADHD: issues of psychiatric comorbidity and familiality. *Journal of the American Academy of Child and Adolescent Psychiatry*, 33, 842–848.

Bratton, D., Gavin, L.A., Price, M., *et al.* (2000). Outcomes of a multidisciplinary day treatment program for children and adolescents with severe asthma: a two-year follow-up study. *Pediatric Pulmonology*, 1, 177–189.

Brazil, K., McLean, L., Abbey, D., & Musselman, C. (1997). The influence of health education on family management of childhood asthma. *Patient Education and Counseling*, 30, 107–118.

Brown, J.V., Avery, E., Mobley, C., Boccuti, L., & Golbach, T. (1996). Asthma management by preschool children and their families: a developmental framework. *Journal of Asthma*, 33, 299–311.

Bussing, R., Halfon, N., Binjamin, B., & Wells, K.B. (1995). Prevalence of behavior problems in US children with asthma. *Archives of Pediatric and Adolescent Medicine*, 149, 169–174.

Carrieri, V., Kieckhefer, G., Janson-Bjerklie, S., & Souza, J. (1991). The sensation of pulmonary dyspnea in school-age children. *Nursing Research*, 40, 81–85.

Christiannse, M.E., Lavigne, J.V., & Lerner, C.V. (1989). Psychosocial aspects of compliance in children and adolescents with asthma. *Developmental and Behavioral Pediatrics*, 10, 75–80.

Clark, N.M. & Zimmerman, B.J. (1990). A social cognitive view of self-regulated learning about health. *Health Education Research: Theory and Practice*, 5, 371–379.

Clark, N.M., Feldman, C., Evans, D., Levison, M., Wasilewski, Y., & Mellins, R. (1986). The impact of health education on frequency and cost of health care use by low income children with asthma. *Journal of Allergy and Clinical Immunology*, 78, 108–115.

Clark, N.M., Evans, D., Zimmerman, B.J., Levison, M.J., & Mellins, R.B. (1994). Patient and family management of asthma: theory-based techniques for the clinician. *Journal of Asthma*, 31, 427–435.

Cote, J., Cartier, A., Robichaud, P., *et al.* (1997). Influence on asthma morbidity of asthma education programs based on self-management plans following treatment optimization. *American Journal of Respiratory & Critical Care Medicine*, 155, 1509–1514.

Coutts, J., Gibson, N., & Paton, J. (1992). Measuring compliance with inhaled medication in asthma. *Archives of Diseases of Childhood*, 67, 332–333.

Cox, S., Webster, M., Ilett, K., & Walson, P. (1993). Audit of theophylline plasma level monitoring in a pediatric hospital. *Therapeutic Drug Monitor*, 15, 289–293.

Cramer, J. & Spilker, B. (1991). *Patient compliance in medical practice and clinical trials*. New York: Raven Press.

Creer, T.L., Backial, M., Burns, K.L., *et al.* (1988). Living with asthma. I. Genesis and development of a self-management program for childhood asthma. *Journal of Asthma*, 25, 335–362.

Creer, T.L., Wigal, J.K., Kotses, H., & Lewis, P. (1990). A critique of 19 self-management programs for childhood asthma: Part II. Comments regarding the scientific merit of the programs. *Pediatric Asthma, Allergy, and Immunology*, 4, 41–55.

Donahue, J.G., Weiss, S.T., Livingston, J.M., Goetsch, M.A., Greineder, D.K., & Platt, R. (1997). Inhaled steroids and the risk of hospitalization for asthma. *Journal of the American Medical Association*, 277, 887–891.

Dumas, J.E. & Serketich, W.J. (1994). Maternal depressive symptomatology and child maladjustment: a comparison of three process models. *Behavior Therapy*, 25, 161–181.

Ehnert, B., Lau-Schadendorf, S., Wever, A., Buettner, P., Schou, C., & Wahn, U. (1992). Reducing domestic exposure to dust mite allergen reduces bronchial hyperreactivity in sensitive children with asthma. *Journal of Allergy and Clinical Immunology*, 90, 135–138.

Erikson, M.F., Sroufe, L.A., & Egeland, B. (1985). The relationship between quality of attachment and behavior problems in preschool in a high-risk sample. *Monographs of the Society for Research in Child Development*, 50, 147–166.

Fish, L., Wilson, S.R., Latini, D.M., & Starr, N.J. (1996). An education program for parents of children with asthma: differences in attendance between smoking and non-smoking parents. *American Journal of Public Health*, 85, 246–248.

Forero, R., Bauman, A., Young, L., Booth, M., & Nutbeam, D. (1996). Asthma, health behaviors, social adjustment, and psychosomatic symptoms in adolescence. *Journal of Asthma*, 33, 157–164.

Fox, C.R. & Gelfand, D.M. (1994). Maternal depressed mood and stress as related to vigilance, self-efficacy, and mother–child interactions. *Early Development and Parenting*, 3, 82.1–82.11.

Fritz, G.K. & Overholser, J.D. (1990). Accuracy of symptom perception in childhood asthma. *Psychosomatic Medicine*, 11, 69–72.

Fritz, G.K., Rubinstein, S., & Lewiston, N.J. (1987). Psychological factors in fatal childhood asthma. *American Journal of Orthopsychiatry*, 57, 253–257.

Fritz, G.K., McQuaid, E.L., Spirito, A., & Klein, R.B. (1996). Symptom perception in pediatric asthma: relationship to functional morbidity and psychological factors. *Journal of the American Academy of Child and Adolescent Psychiatry*, 35, 1033–1041.

Garmezy, N. (1983). Stressors of childhood. In: N. Garmezy & M. Rutter (Eds), *Stress, coping, and development in children* (pp. 43–82). New York: McGraw-Hill.

Gavin, L. & Roesler, T. (1997). Post traumatic stress symptoms in children and families after intubation. *Pediatric Emergency Care*, 6, 222–224.

Gizynski, M. & Shapiro, V. (1990). Depression and childhood illness. *Child and Adolescent Social Work* 7, 179–197.

Gonzalez, S., Steinglass, P., & Reiss, D. (1989). Putting the illness in its place. *Family Process*, 28, 69–87.

Goodman, S.H., Adamson, L.B., Rinit, J., & Cole, S. (1994). Mothers' expressed attitudes: associations with maternal depression and children's self-esteem and psychopathology. *Journal of the American Academy of Child and Adolescent Psychiatry*, 33, 1265–1274.

Graham, P.J., Rutter, M., Yule, W., & Pless, I.B. (1967). Childhood asthma: a psychosomatic disorder? *British Journal of Preventative and Social Medicine*, 21, 78–85.

Gustafsson, P.A., Kjellman, N.I., & Cederbald, M. (1986). Family therapy in the treatment of severe childhood asthma. *Journal of Psychosomatic Research*, 30, 369–374.

Hamlett, K.W., Pelligrini, D.S., & Katz, K.S. (1992). Childhood chronic illness as a family stressor. *Journal of Pediatric Psychology*, 17, 33–47.

Hermanns, J., Florin, I., Dietrich, M., Rieger, C., & Hahlweg, K. (1989). Maternal criticism, mother–child interaction, and bronchial asthma. *Journal of Psychosomatic Research*, 33, 469–476.

Hibbs, E.D., Hamburger, S.D., Lenane, M., *et al.* (1991). Determinants of expressed emotion in families of disturbed and normal children. *Journal of Child Psychology and Psychiatry*, 32, 757–770.

Hindi-Alexander, M. & Cropp, G. (1984). Evaluation of a family asthma program. *Journal of Allergy and Clinical Immunology* 74, 505–510.

Huss, K., Rand, C., Butz, A., *et al.* (1994). Home environmental risk factors in urban minority asthmatic children. *Annals of Allergy*, 72, 173–177.

Isenberg, S.A., Lehrer, P.M. & Hochron, S. (1992). The effects of suggestion and emotional arousal on pulmonary function in asthma: a review and a hypothesis regarding vagal mediation. *Psychosomatic Medicine*, 54, 192–216.

Jessop, D., Riessman, C., & Stein, R. (1988). Chronic childhood illness and maternal mental health. *Journal of Developmental and Behavioral Pediatrics*, 9, 147–156.

Kagan, J., Snidman, N., Julia-Sellers, M., & Johnson, M.O. (1991). Temperament and allergic symptoms. *Psychosomatic Medicine*, 53, 332–340.

Kaplan, S., Greenfield, S., & Ware, J. (1983). Assessing the effects of physician–patient interactions on the outcomes of chronic disease. *Medical Care*, 27, S110–S127.

Kashani, J.H., Konig, P., Shepperd, J.A., Wilfley, D., & Morris, D.A. (1988). Psychopathology and self-concept in asthmatic children. *Journal of Pediatric Psychology*, 13, 509–520.

Kazak, A., Segal-Andrews, A., & Johnson, K. (1995). Pediatric psychology research and practice: a family/systems approach. In: M. Roberts (Ed.), *Handbook of pediatric psychology*. New York: Guilford Press.

Kinsman, R.A., Dirks, J.F., & Jones, N.F. (1982). Psychomaintenance of chronic physical illness. In: T. Millon & C.J. Green (Eds), *Handbook of clinical health psychology* (pp. 435–465). New York: Plenum Press.

Klinnert, M.D. (1997). The psychology of asthma in the school-age child. In: P.F. Kernberg & J.R. Bemporad (Eds), *Handbook of child and adolescent psychiatry. Volume 2. The grade school child: development and syndromes* (pp. 579–594). New York: John Wiley & Sons.

Klinnert, M.D., Campos, J., Sorce, J.F., Emde, R.N., & Svejda, M. (1983). *Emotions as behavior regulators: social referencing in infancy*, Vol. 2. New York: Academic Press.

Klinnert, M., & Lumlung (1991). Developmental guidelines for children's asthma self-care. Unpublished manuscript.

Klinnert, M., McQuaid, E., & Gavin, L. (1997). Assessing the family asthma management system. *Journal of Asthma*, 34, 77–88.

Klinnert, M., McQuaid, E., McCormick, D., Adinoff, A., & Bryant, N. (2000). A multimethod assessment of behavioral and emotional adjustment in children with asthma. *Journal of Pediatric Psychology*, 25, 35–40.

Kolbe, J., Vamos, M., Fergusson, W., Elkind, G., & Garrett, J. (1996). Differential influences on asthma self-management knowledge and self-management behavior in acute severe asthma. *Chest*, 110, 1463–1468.

Kravis, L. (1987). An analysis of fifteen childhood asthma fatalities. *Journal of Allergy and Clinical Immunology*, 80, 467–471.

Lanier, B. (1989). Who is dying of asthma and why? *Journal of Pediatrics*, 115, 838–840.

MacLean, W.E., Perrin, J.M., Gortmaker, S., & Pierre, C.B. (1992). Psychological adjustment of children with asthma: effects of illness severity and recent stressful life events. *Journal of Pediatric Psychology*, 17, 159–171.

McNicol, K.N., Williams, H.E., Allan, J., & McAndrew, I. (1973). Spectrum of asthma in children: III. psychological and social components. *British Medical Journal*, 4, 16–20.

Milgrom, H., Bender, B., Acherson, L., Bowry, P., Smith, B., & Rand, C. (1995). Children's compliance with inhaled asthma medications. *Journal of Allergy and Clinical Immunology* 95, 217.

Miller, B. (1987). Depression and asthma: a potentially lethal mixture. *Journal of Allergy and Clinical Immunology*, 80, 481–486.

Miller, B.D. & Strunk, R.C. (1989). Circumstances surrounding the deaths of children due to asthma. *American Journal of Diseases of Children*, 143, 1294–1299.

Mrazek, D., Anderson, I., & Strunk, R. (1985). Disturbed emotional development of severely asthmatic preschool children. In: Stevenson (Ed.), *Recent research in developmental psychopathology, Journal of Child Psychology and Psychiatry Book* (pp. 81–94). Oxford: Pergamon.

Mrazek, D., Casey, B., & Anderson, I. (1987). Insecure attachment in severely asthmatic preschool children: Is it a risk factor? *Journal of the American Academy of Child and Adolescent Psychiatry*, 26, 516–520.

National Institutes of Health (1997). *Highlights of the expert panel report 2: Guidelines for the diagnosis and management of asthma (2)*. Bethesda: National Institutes of Health; National Heart, Lung, and Blood Institute, 1997.

Norrish, M., Tooley, M., & Godfrey, S. (1977). Clinical, physiological, and psychological study of asthmatic children attending a hospital clinic. *Archives of Diseases of Childhood*, 52, 912–917.

Patterson, G.R. (1982). *Coercive family process*. Eugene, OR: Castalia.

Prochaska, J.O. & DiClementi, C.C. (1983). Stages and processes of self-change in smoking. *Journal of Consulting and Clinical Psychology*, 51, 390–395.

Purcell, K., Brady, K., Chai, H., *et al.* (1969). The effect on asthma in children of experimental separation from the family. *Psychosomatic Medicine*, 31, 144–164.

Rachelefsky, G., Wo, J., Adelson, J., *et al.* (1986), Behavior abnormalities and poor school performance due to oral theophylline use. *Pediatrics*, 78, 1133–1138.

Rand, C. & Wise, R. (1994). Measuring adherence to asthma medication regimens. *American Journal of Respiratory and Critical Care Medicine*, 149, S69–S76.

Randolph, C. & Fraser, B. (1999). Stressors and concerns in teen asthma. *Current Problems in Pediatrics*, 29, 82–93.

Rubin, D., Bauman, L., & Lauby, J. (1989). The relationship between knowledge and reported behavior in childhood asthma. *Developmental and Behavioral Pediatrics*, 10, 307–312.

Schlieper, A., Adcock, D., Beaudry, P., Feldman, W., & Leikin, L. (1991). Effect of therapeutic plasma concentrations of theophylline on behavior, cognitive processing, and affect in children with asthma. *Journal of Pediatrics*, 118, 449–455.

Schultz, R.M., Dye, J., Jolicoeur, L., Cafferty, T., & Watson, J. (1994). Quality-of-life factors for parents of children with asthma. *Journal of Asthma*, 31, 209–219.

Sly, R.M. (1988). Mortality from asthma, 1979–1984. *Journal of Allergy and Clinical Immunology*, 82, 705–717.

Spector, S., Kinsman, R., Mawhinney, H., *et al.* (1986). Compliance of patients with asthma on experimental aerosolized medication: implications for controlled clinical trials. *Journal of Allergy and Clinical Immunology*, 77, 65–70.

Sroufe, L.A. & Rutter, M. (1984). The domain of developmental psychopathology. *Child Development*, 55, 17–29.

Steele, D., Jackson, T. & Gutmann, M. (1990). Have you been taking your pills? The adherence-monitoring sequence in the medical interview. *Journal of Family Practice*, 30, 294.

Strecher, V., Becker, M., Clark, N., & Prasada-Rao, P. (1989). Using patients' descriptions of alcohol consumption, diet, medication compliance, and cigarette smoking: the validity of self-reports in research and practice. *Journal of General Internal Medicine*, 4, 160.

Strunk, R.C., Mrazek, D.A., Wolfson Fuhrmann, G.S., & LaBrecque, J.F. (1985). Physiological and psychological characteristics associated with deaths from asthma in childhood: a case-controlled study. *Journal of the American Medical Association*, 254, 1193–1198.

Strunk, R.C., Fukuhara, J.T., LaBrecque, J.F., & Mrazek, D.A. (1989). Outcome of long-term hospitalization for asthma in children. *Journal of Allergy and Clinical Immunology*, 83, 17–25.

Taggart, V., Zuckerman, A.E., Sly, M., *et al.* (1991). You can control asthma: evaluation of an asthma education program for hospitalized inner-city children. *Patient Education and Counseling*, 17, 35–47.

Vazquez, M.I. & Buceta, J.M. (1993). Effectiveness of self-management programmes and relaxation training in the treatment of bronchial asthma: relationships with trait anxiety and emotional attack triggers. *Journal of Psychosomatic Research*, 37, 71–81.

Vuurman, E., Veggel, B., Uiterwijk, M., Leutner, D., & O'Hanlon, J.F. (1993). Seasonal allergic rhinitis and antihistamine effects on children's learning. *Annals of Allergy*, 71, 121–126.

Wade, S., Weil, C., Holden, G., *et al.* (1997). Psychosocial characteristics of inner-city children with asthma: a description of the NCICAS psychosocial protocol. *Pediatric Pulmonology*, 24, 263–276.

Wakefield, M., Staugas, R., Ruffin, R., Campbell, D., Beilby, J., & McCaul, K. (1997). Risk factors for repeat attendance at hospital emergency departments among adults and children with asthma. *Australia and New Zealand Journal of Medicine*, 27, 277–284.

Wamboldt, F.S., Wamboldt, M.Z., Gavin, L.A., Roesler, T.A., & Brugman, S.M. (1995). Parental criticism and treatment of outcome in adolescents hospitalized for severe, chronic asthma. *Journal of Psychosomatic Research*, 39, 995–1005.

Wamboldt, M.Z., Weintraub, P., Krafchick, D., & Wamboldt, F.A. (1996). Psychiatric family history in adolescents with severe asthma. *Journal of the American Academy of Child and Adolescent Psychiatry*, 35, 1042–1049.

Weinstein, A.G., Faust, D.S., McKee, L., & Padman, R. (1992). Outcome of short-term hospitalization for children with severe asthma. *Journal of Allergy and Clinical Immunology*, 90, 66–75.

Weiss, K.B., Gergen, P.J., & Hodgson, T.A. (1992). An economic evaluation of asthma in the United States. *New England Journal of Medicine*, 326, 862–866.

Wilson, S.R., Mitchell, J.H., Rolnick, S., & Fish, L. (1993). Effective and ineffective management behaviors of parents of infants and young children with asthma. *Journal of Pediatric Psychology*, 18, 63–81.

Wilson-Pessano, S., & McNabb, W. (1985). The role of patient education in the management of childhood asthma. *Preventive Medicine*, 14, 670–687.

Zimmerman, B.J., Bonner, S., Evans, D., & Mellins, R.B. (1999). Self-regulating childhood asthma: a developmental model of family change. *Health Education and Behavior*, 26, 55–71.

4
Chronic obstructive pulmonary disease: Behavioral assessment and treatment

Robert M. Kaplan and Andrew L. Ries

Editors' note—*Chronic obstructive pulmonary disease (COPD) is a condition that has increased throughout the world as a direct function of the number of people who smoke cigarettes. While smoking rates have decreased in the United States and many European countries in recent years (World Health Organization, 1999), this trend is not observed in many other nations. China, for example, is the world's largest producer and consumer of cigarette products. A National Prevalence Survey of 120,298 Chinese people was conducted by Yang and his colleagues (1999). The survey revealed that 34.1% of the respondents smoked, an increase of 3.4% since 1984. Smoking was more prevalent among men (63%) than women (3.8%). While 70% of the smokers knew of the link between smoking and COPD, particularly bronchitis, only a minority recognized that lung cancer (36%) and heart disease (4%) were associated with smoking. Of the nonsmokers, 53.5% were exposed to environmental tobacco smoke at least 15 min each day on more than 1 day per week.*

Two pioneering investigators in the rehabilitation of COPD patients, Bob Kaplan and Andrew Ries, describe cutting-edge research on the condition. In particular, they focus on various approaches taken to reduce the impact of COPD on patients and their families. The task Bob and Andrew have faced has been difficult because of the need to persuade COPD patients to abandon long-time behaviors, particularly smoking, while convincing them to perform new behaviors, particularly regular exercise. In addition, medical and behavioral scientists who work with the disorder have had to overcome a strong skepticism among their colleagues as to the value of rehabilitation as a treatment for patients with COPD. Only a few years ago, the schism was highlighted by a debate on the merit of pulmonary rehabilitation as an effective treatment for COPD: Albert (1997) argued that it was not effective and Celli (1997) argued that it was.

Despite the barriers they've faced, Kaplan and Ries describe progress made in synthesizing medical and behavioral procedures to treat COPD. In doing so, they not only discuss progress in the management of COPD but also provide a glimpse of what promises to be an exciting area of research to both medical and behavioral scientists.

Introduction

The term chronic obstructive pulmonary disease (COPD) is used to describe a collection of chronic disabling lung diseases. The American Thoracic Society defines COPD as

> *a disease state characterized by the presence of air flow obstruction due to chronic bronchitis or emphysema. The air flow obstruction is generally progressive, may be accompanied by airway hyperreactivity and may be partially reversible*
>
> *(American Thoracic Society, 1995)*

Chronic bronchitis, emphysema, and chronic asthma are the three diseases that contribute to the diagnosis of COPD. These diseases are similar because they all are disorders of expiration associated with obstruction of air flow out of inflated lungs. Chronic bronchitis, emphysema, and asthma differ in the nature of the airway obstruction. However, it is most common for patients to have components of more than one of these diseases.

The Obstructive Lung Diseases

Until recently, the diagnosis of emphysema was anatomic and typically made at the time of autopsy. However, newer techniques in radiology have made it possible to separate emphysema from chronic bronchitis in living people. Emphysema is caused by the loss of elastic recoil of the lung parenchyma, resulting in overinflation of the lung. These changes are typically associated with destruction of the alveolar walls, which are the walls of the small air sacs in the lung that inflate and deflate during breathing. Emphysema is a chronic condition that develops over many years and is characterized by symptoms of progressive shortness of breath on activity. The disease process is largely irreversible, and results in considerable disability for affected individuals, with high morbidity and mortality.

The consequences of chronic bronchitis are similar. However, chronic bronchitis is defined as the presence of a chronic cough and sputum production that lasts at least 3 months in 2 consecutive years. This results in chronic inflammation of the bronchi, which are the cell linings of the breathing passages. In some patients, the airways became obstructed, making breathing difficult.

Asthma is a condition associated with a reversible airway narrowing that may occur in response to stimuli such as infection, allergy, cold air, or cigarette smoke. The narrowing of the airways may be caused by a spasm of smooth muscles, inflammation, or the oversecretion of mucus. Chronic asthma occurs when the narrowing persists over the course of time. Chronic asthma and bronchitis often coexist, resulting in a diagnosis of 'asthmatic bronchitis.'

What Causes COPD?

Most of the causes and consequences of COPD are behavioral. Cigarette smoking is clearly the major risk factor for the development of these diseases. It has been estimated that 90% of cases of COPD are directly attributable to the use of cigarettes (Austin, 1976; Higgins, 1989). Compared with people who do not smoke cigarettes, current smokers are 10 times more likely to develop COPD (Higgins, 1989). The risks are approximately equal for men and women. For many years it was assumed that COPD was a disease of men. However, in recent years, as women have gained in cigarette use, rates of COPD have been escalating for females (National Heart, Lung, and Blood Institute, 1996).

Genetic factors also play an important role in development of COPD. Even among cigarette smokers, only about 15–20% develop significant COPD. Some individuals may be genetically susceptible, leaving them at much greater risk if they are exposed to cigarette smoke or other irritants. There is still debate about whether or not second-hand smoke is a significant risk factor for COPD. However, there is evidence suggesting that environmental exposures such as air pollution and exposure to dusts and fumes in the workplace may exacerbate underlying lung disease and may increase the risks of developing COPD. In addition, frequent respiratory infections in childhood increase the risk of developing COPD later in life.

Public Health Impact

COPD is a major cause of death and disability in the United States. In 1995, it was estimated that 97,262 people in the United States died of COPD (National Center for Health Statistics, 1995). This represents an age-adjusted death rate of 21 per 100,000 in the population. COPD is the fourth most common cause of death in the United States. Recent estimates suggest that there are approximately 14 million cases of chronic bronchitis reported each year and 2 million cases of emphysema (Vital and Health Statistics, Series 10, #193, 1986). In contrast to heart diseases that have been declining as a cause of death, deaths resulting from COPD increased by 38% between 1979 and 1991. Also, because COPD is an insidious disease typically diagnosed only late in the course of illness, official health statistics underestimate the burden of disease in the population.

Worldwide, COPD has ranked lower as a cause of disease burden, because smoking has been more prevalent in the industrialized countries. However, an analysis completed by the World Bank and the World Health Organization ranked disease burden in disability-adjusted life years' (DALYs) lost. They reported that COPD ranked 12th of all causes in 1990. However, the report suggests that by the year 2020, COPD will be the fifth leading cause of death worldwide (Fig. 4.1). Although smok-

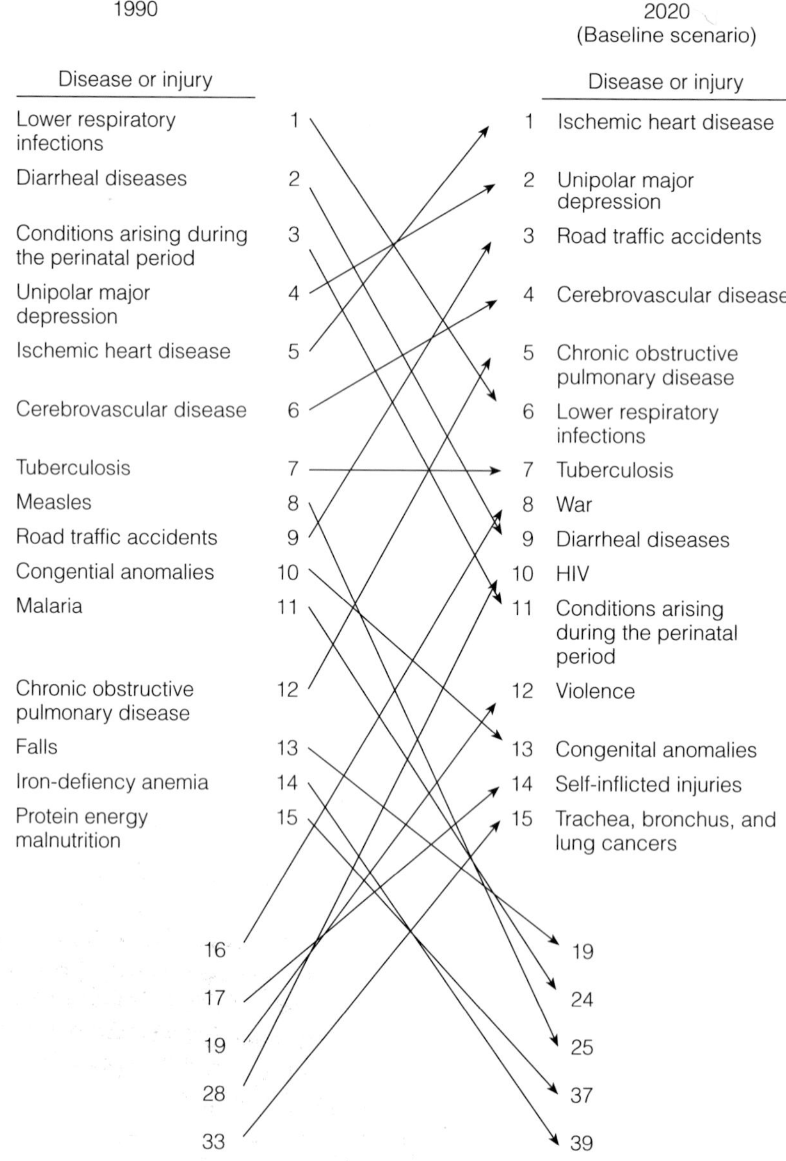

Figure 4.1

Disease burden estimated using disability-adjusted life years (DALYs), showing rank order of 15 major causes of death in the world, 1990–2020. (Reprinted with permission from Murray & Lopez, 1996.)

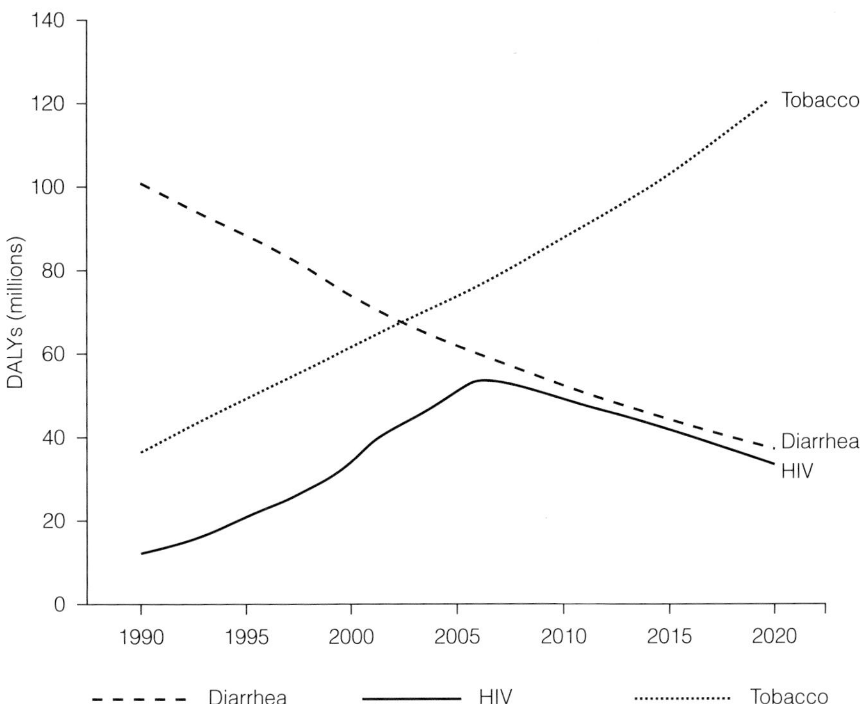

Figure 4.2

Disability adjusted life years (DALYs) for diarrhea, HIV, and tobacco use; projections for 1990–2020. (Reprinted with permission from Murray & Lopez, 1996.)

ing may have leveled off or declined in the industrialized countries, the worldwide trend is toward greater tobacco use. Figure 4.2 summarizes the WHO–World Bank estimates of DALYs lost to diarrheal disease, HIV, and tobacco between 1990 and 2020. Diarrheal disease is expected to decline steadily over this interval, while HIV is expected to peak in 2005. However, loss of life attributable to tobacco use is expected to increase steadily (Murray & Lopez, 1996).

Medical and Surgical Treatment

Medical management of COPD involves the use of medications to stabilize and/or improve airway function and symptoms, and strategies to minimize the consequences and prevent complications of the disease. Patients with COPD often use bronchodilator medicines to maximize airway size. In addition, some patients may use corticosteroids to reduce inflammation. Further, medications are sometimes used to control secretions, which is sometimes achieved by consumption of several glasses of fluid per day. Antibiotics are commonly used to control infections. Vaccinations against influenza and certain types of bacteria can prevent and reduce the risk of pneumonia. For patients with severe reductions in oxygen levels in their blood, continuous oxygen therapy has been shown to improve survival and reduce complications of the disease (Fishman, 1996).

Considerable evidence suggests that some patients may be genetically susceptible to the development of emphysema. Some of these individuals have an identified genetic abnormality that causes deficiency of a protective enzyme called α_1-antitrypsin. Recently, there has been experimentation with methods to replace the deficient protein in people affected by this condition. However, this treatment remains unproven, and the drug costs can exceed $25,000/year.

A recent development in the treatment of severe emphysema is lung volume reduction surgery (Cooper *et al.*, 1996; McKenna *et al.*, 1997). Patients with emphysema have areas of damaged lung that lose elasticity, become overinflated, and compress areas of better-functioning lung. Surgical techniques have been developed to remove these diseased sections from the lungs. However, evidence for the effectiveness of this surgery is still accumulating and the National Institutes of Health, in conjunction with the Health Care Finance Administration, is conducting a major clinical trial to evaluate the risks and benefits of these procedures.

In some patients with severe COPD, lung transplantation may be a therapeutic option. However, the expense and limited availability of donor organs means that transplantation can be made available for only a small fraction of eligible patients.

At present, medical and surgical interventions are limited because there is no cure for COPD. Behavioral interventions designed to improve functioning or to help patients cope with the illness retain an important role in contemporary care.

This chapter is divided into two major sections: the first section considers behavioral intervention and rehabilitation; the second section discusses behavioral assessments for patients with COPD.

Behavioral Intervention Studies

Kaptein (1997) reviewed randomized behavioral intervention studies involving patients with COPD: he found 15 published studies, among which 13 suggested some benefit of intervention. The outcome measures used in these studies vary considerably. Common outcome measures assess quality of life, knowledge, exercise duration, and mood. In this section intervention techniques are considered. In the next section psychosocial moderators of outcomes are reviewed.

Most behavioral intervention programs are part of comprehensive rehabilitation programs. These rehabilitation programs use multidisciplin teams to develop individualized programs aimed at restoring patients to their highest levels of functioning. A 1994 workshop at the US National Institutes of Health defined pulmonary rehabilitation as

> *a multi-dimensional continuum of services directed to persons with pulmonary disease and their families, usually by an interdisciplinary team of specialists with a goal of achieving and maintaining the individuals maximum level of independence and functioning in the community.*
>
> *(Fishman, 1996, pp. 8–9)*

Comprehensive rehabilitation programs typically include several components. Most of the programs perform individual assessments, and offer education, instruction in respiratory and chest physiotherapy, psychological and social support, and supervised exercise training. The programs differ in the extent to which they emphasize these different components (American Thoracic Society, 1987; Guyatt *et al.*, 1987).

Hodgkin *et al.* (1993) provided a long list of methods that have established value in rehabilitation programs. The benefits suggested include reduced respiratory symptoms, reduced anxiety and depression, enhanced ability to carry out activities of daily living, increased exercise ability, improved quality of life, reduction in hospital days, and prolonged life.

These claims are difficult to validate. However, a growing literature testifies to the benefits of pulmonary rehabilitation, as documented in a series of important textbooks on pulmonary rehabilitation (Hodgkin *et al.*, 1993; Bach, 1996; Fishman, 1996). Also, a recent evidence-based guideline document reviewing the published literature has been published and supports the scientific foundation of these programs (ACCP/AACVPR, 1997).

Figure 4.3 summarizes the relationship between disability and COPD. Rehabilitation programs attempt to attend to each of these levels. The top of the figure describes the domains of pathophysiology, impairment, functional limitation, disability, and societal limitation. The bottom of the figure relates these domains to aspects of COPD. For example, the pathophysiology of COPD is obstruction of the airways. The impairment is represented by symptoms such as breathlessness, cough, or psychological depression. Functional limitations include limited abilities to exercise and perform activities of daily living. The disability associated with COPD is reflected in limitations in constructive work, deterioration of social relationships, and loss of capability of engaging in many recreational activities. Finally, the social limitation might be the inability to gain or maintain employment, the inability to use stairs or access public facilities, and so on.

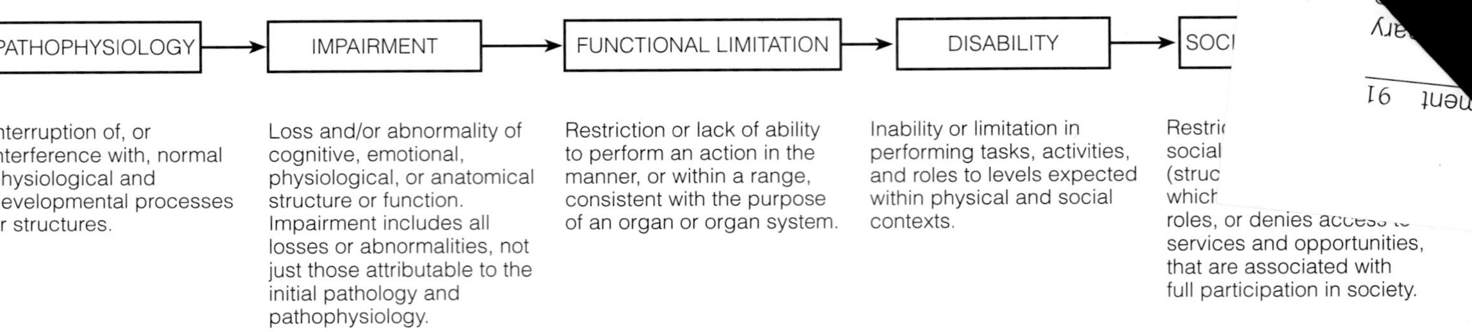

PATHOPHYSIOLOGY
IMPAIRMENT
FUNCTIONAL LIMITATION
DISABILITY
SOCI
Interruption of, or interference with, normal physiological and developmental processes or structures.
Loss and/or abnormality of cognitive, emotional, physiological, or anatomical structure or function. Impairment includes all losses or abnormalities, not just those attributable to the initial pathology and pathophysiology.
Restriction or lack of ability to perform an action in the manner, or within a range, consistent with the purpose of an organ or organ system.
Inability or limitation in performing tasks, activities, and roles to levels expected within physical and social contexts.
Restri
social
(struc
which
roles, or denies access
services and opportunities, that are associated with full participation in society.

Example: Chronic Obstructive Pulmonary Disease

Adult with chronic bronchitis and emphysema.	Shortness of breath upon limited activity; easy fatigability; malnutrition; depression.	Difficulties with activities of daily living, such as eating, dressing, personal hygiene; requires supplemental oxygen during sleep and activity.	Activities of daily life require extra time and assistance; cannot do work mechanic; cannot do hobbies and recreational activities; not independent with family and peers.	Difficulties in finding employment; lack of involvement in social activities; health insurer limits home care; limited access to recreational activies.

Figure 4.3

Relationship between disability and COPD. (Reprinted with permission from Fishman, 1996.)

History

Rehabilitation has always been part of medical care. However, developments in 18th century Europe may have set the stage for contemporary rehabilitation programs. With the French Revolution in 1789 came a declaration of rights of man and the citizen. The declaration proclaimed that unfortunate citizens should be supported by society and that society should make education available to everyone. Another 18th century development was the spread of tuberculosis during the industrial revolution; epidemic-proportion tuberculosis may have resulted from rapid urbanization. Treatments involved separating the infected individuals and relocating them to sanatoriums with clean, dry air. Relaxation was a part of the therapy in the sanitoria until the introduction of antibiotics changed the treatment of the disease (van den Broek, 1995).

San Diego Programs

Over the last few decades, we have conducted several studies to evaluate behavioral and rehabilitation interventions for patients with COPD. Our first experimental study was published in 1984. This was not an evaluation of comprehensive rehabilitation. Instead, the study focused on behavioral interventions designed to increase exercise. At the time, we were persuaded that exercise was the key component of rehabilitation for patients with COPD. A variety of earlier studies had shown benefits of exercise interventions in small or non-controlled studies (Bell & Jensen, 1977; McGavin *et al.*, 1977; Mertens *et al.*, 1978; Ambrosino *et al.*, 1981; Belman & Wasserman, 1981). Each of these studies demonstrated some benefit of physical activity, but the studies differed greatly in the percentage of patients followed for longer than 3 months and the methods of outcome assessment.

The issue addressed in our original study was not whether exercise benefits patients, but rather how to enhance regular physical activity among patients with COPD. Many patients with COPD experience shortness of breath and discomfort during physical activity. Thus, behavior modification and cognitive modification were used to train patients to cope with the discomfort associated with regular physical activity. The study randomly assigned 78 COPD patients to one of five experimental groups. Three of the five groups were given various behavioral interventions. One group received traditional behaviour modification that emphasized goal setting, analysis of reinforcers, and behavior contracts. A second group received cognitive modification and emphasized self-taught and positive self-statements. A third cognitive–behavior modification group received an intervention that used the technology of behavior modification to modify patient self-statements.

Each of these interventions was designed to enhance regular physical activity during everyday activities. Sessions were conducted in the patient's home and the interventions were designed to promote activity in the patient's usual home environment. The study included two control groups: one group received attention but did not have behaviorally based sessions; the second control received no treatment at all.

Patients in this study were evaluated at baseline, 3 months, 6 months, 12 months, and 18 months. Figure 4.4 shows changes in self-reported physical activity during the first three months for the five groups. The figure suggests that the cognitive–behavior modification and cognitive modification groups increased their physical activity significantly more than the behavior modification group or the control groups.

All the participants were given treadmill endurance tests by a technician blinded to the experimental conditions. Changes in self-reported

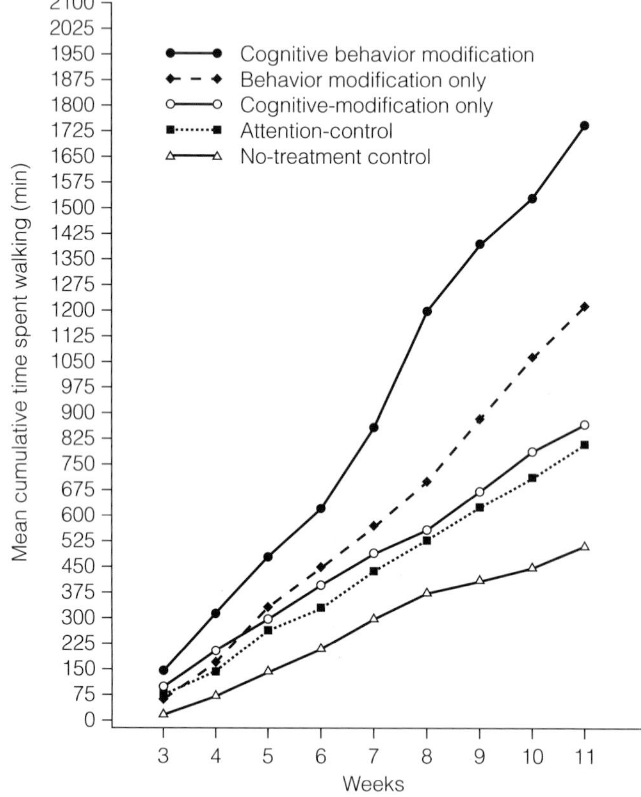

Figure 4.4

Cumulative self-reported walking in five groups. The three behavior modification groups exceed the two control groups. (Reprinted with permission from Atkins *et al.*, 1984.)

exercise were validated by improvements in laboratory exercise endurance tests taken 1 month following the end of treatment (Fig. 4.5).

In addition to changes in exercise endurance, we also measured quality of life outcomes using a general assessment procedure known as the quality of well-being scale (QWB). After 3 months, differences between the small treatment groups began to disappear. However, averaging over three experimental groups and two control groups, differences between treated and untreated patients remained. These are shown in Fig. 4.6. Those in treated groups declined slightly over the course of 18 months, while those randomly assigned to control conditions showed a significant reduction in the quality of life over 18 months.

The study also included an extensive battery of pulmonary function tests. Consistent with most other studies in the literature, pulmonary function did not improve or decline as a function of treatment (Atkins *et al.*, 1984).

Several noncontrolled studies have also supported the use of cognitive behavioral interventions. For example, Lisansky & Clough (1996) offered an 8-week cognitive behavioral self-help education program to eight patients with COPD. They found significant improvements for the

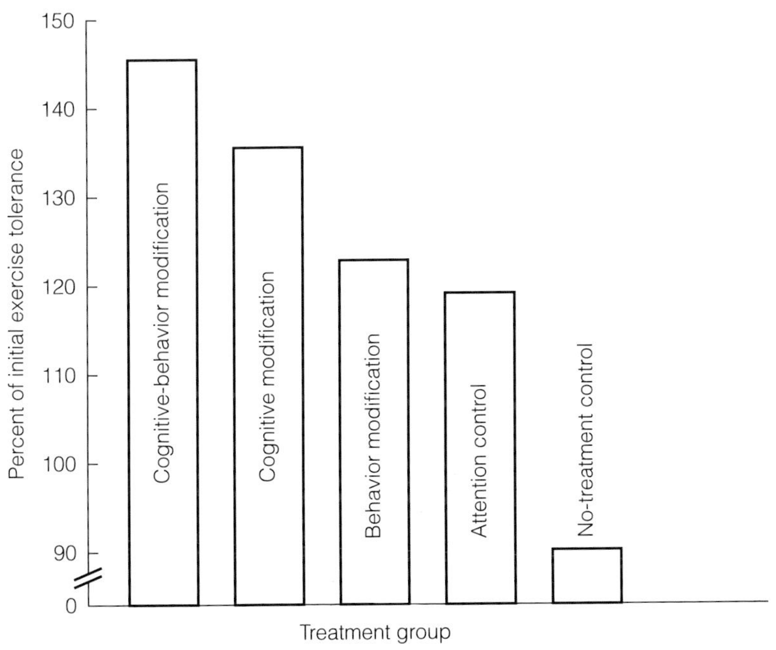

Figure 4.5

Percent of initial exercise endurance for five groups at 3 months. (From Atkins *et al.*, 1984.)

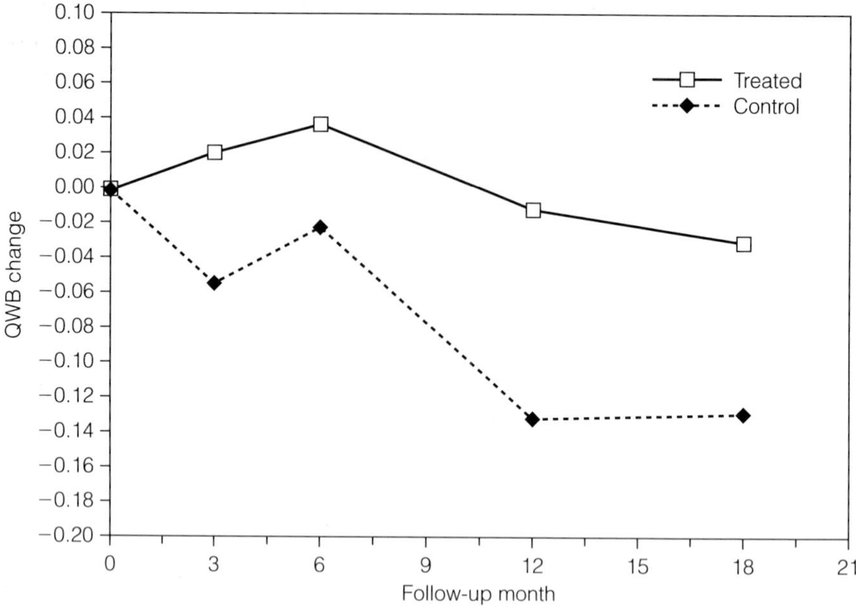

Figure 4.6

Change in quality of well-being (QWB) for three treatment groups (combined into 'treated' line) and two control groups (combined into 'control' line). (From Toevs *et al.*, 1984.)

psychosocial and total scores of the sickness impact profile. Eiser *et al.* (1997) compared cognitive behavioral psychotherapy to a control group that included lung function, testing, and walking. Their psychotherapy and controlled interventions lasted 6 weeks. Those who completed the behavioral program showed sustained improvement in exercise tolerance but did not improve on measures of anxiety or depression.

Because of the complexity of COPD, psychological intervention independent of a comprehensive program is usually not advisable. Typically, psychological and behavioral treatments are components of a comprehensive rehabilitation program. Pulmonary rehabilitation is now an established therapy for people with advanced COPD. A variety of studies have demonstrated that rehabilitation can alleviate symptoms, improve function, and reduce medical care costs (Toevs *et al.*, 1984; Bach, 1996; Fishman, 1996; ACCP/AACVPR, 1997). Pulmonary rehabilitation usually requires a multidisciplinary team of experts in behavioral science, respiratory and chest physiotherapy, medicine, and exercise science.

We have conducted several studies designed to evaluate outcomes of pulmonary rehabilitation. In one study, 119 outpatients with stable but advanced COPD were randomly assigned to pulmonary rehabilitation or to a control condition. The pulmonary rehabilitation program lasted 8 weeks and included twelve 4-hour sessions that integrated education, physical and respiratory care instruction, psychosocial support, and supervised exercise training. In addition, participants attended monthly reinforcing sessions for 1 year. The control group emphasized education alone. Control participants attended two 4-hour sessions that included videotapes, lectures, and discussions about lung diseases. However, those in the control group did not receive individualized instruction or training in exercise.

A variety of physiological and psychological measures were used to evaluate the program, including measures of lung function, maximum exercise tolerance and endurance, gas exchange, symptoms of perceived breathlessness, physical fatigue during exercise, shortness of breath, self-efficacy for walking, depression, medical care utilization, and quality of life. Prior to the intervention, the treatment and control groups were equivalent on a wide range of physiological and psychosocial measures. Following the treatment, those in the pulmonary rehabilitation program (compared with education controls) showed significant improvements in exercise endurance, maximum exercise tolerance, symptoms of perceived breathlessness, muscle fatigue during exercise, reported shortness of breath with daily activities, and self-efficacy for walking. Some of these benefits gradually declined over the course of 1–2 years. However, the benefits for perceived muscle fatigue and breathlessness persisted for at least 6 months and the benefits for maximum treadmill workload and exercise endurance remained significant for 1 year. Some of the psychological benefits persisted for longer. For example, differences in self-efficacy for walking remained statistically significant for up to 18 months, while differences in rating of perceived breathlessness during exercise persisted for 24 months.

Outcomes for treadmill endurance, perceived breathlessness, and muscle fatigue are summarized in Fig. 4.7. Consistent with other rehabilitation studies, differences between rehabilitation and educational control groups on physiological measures of lung function were not statistically significant at any follow-up (Ries *et al.*, 1995).

Psychosocial Mediators of Outcome

Several chapters in this book concern important mediators of outcome in COPD, including dyspnea (see Chapter 5), compliance (Chapter 8), quality of life (Chapter 9), and other issues (Chapter 14). These and a variety of other psychosocial variables are important for understanding outcomes for patients with COPD. In the following sections we review several psychosocial variables that may be of importance for patients with COPD. We begin with variables that may be related to survival and

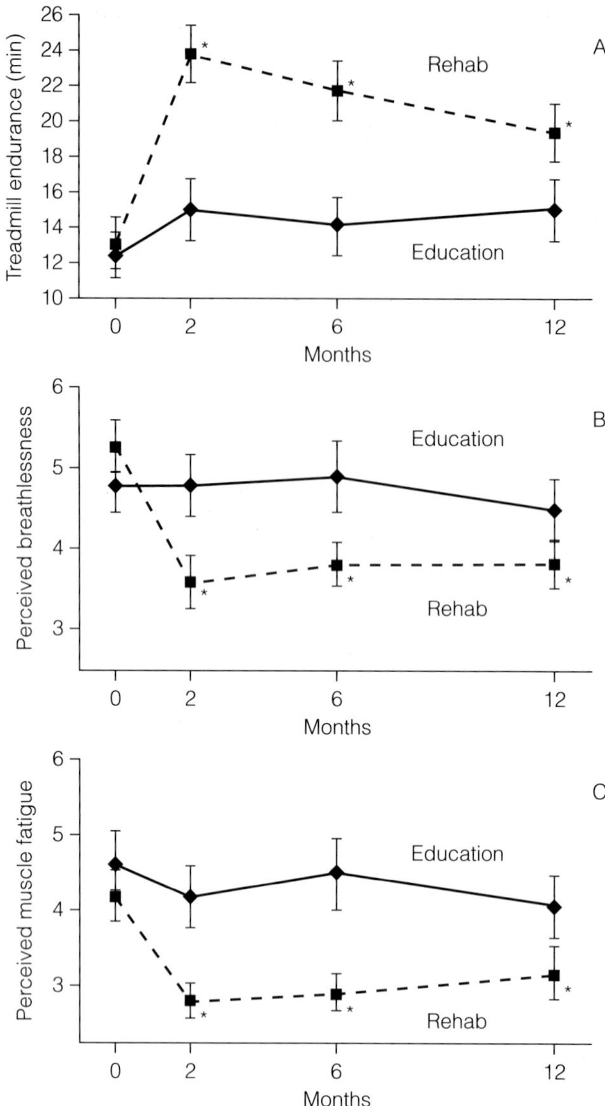

Figure 4.7

Results of treadmill endurance exercise tests for patients in the rehabilitation (Rehab) and education groups at baseline and for 12 months of follow-up. A, exercise endurance time; B, perceived breathlessness rating at the end of exercise; C, perceived muscle fatigue. Asterisks indicate $p < 0.05$ for within-group change from baseline; values and error bars represent the mean ± SE (From Ries *et al.*, 1995.)

proceed with discussion of variables that may mediate treatment outcomes.

Psychosocial Variables and Survival

We have found psychosocial variables to be related to survival for patients with COPD. These are quality of life, social support, and self-efficacy.

Quality of Life

Quality of life is now recognized as an important outcome in studies of medical care. The measurement of quality of life in lung disease is reviewed elsewhere in Chapter 9. In our studies, we have favored quality of life measures that can be used in cost-effectiveness analysis. Measures that incorporate morbidity and mortality in the same scale have the advantage of avoiding survivor and healthy subject biases inherent in other measures. In studies of patients with COPD, both disease-specific and general measures have been applied.

Disease-specific measures usually focus on shortness of breath (Eakin *et al.*, 1993, 1998; Eakin & Glasgow, 1996). Dyspnea is the subjective sensation of difficult or labored breathing. It is one of the most common symptoms of patients with COPD. Various authors have described a dyspnea–panic cycle in which the experience of breathlessness leads to anxiety, creates muscle tension, and results in increased dyspnea and panic (Kaplan *et al.*, 1985).

In addition to disease-specific measures that emphasize shortness of breath, general measures are used to provide a more comprehensive assessment of health status and well-being; one example is a general health status index known as the quality of well-being scale (QWB). The QWB is a utility weighted measure that classifies patients according to observed levels of functioning. These levels are represented by scales of mobility, physical activity, and social activity. In addition to classification according to observable function, individuals are also classified by their chief symptom or problem. On any particular day, nearly 80% of the general population is at an optimum level of function. However, fewer than half of the population experience no symptoms (Kaplan *et al.*, 1976). Symptoms or problems may be severe, such as serious chest pain, or minor, such as taking medications or a prescribed diet for health reasons. Preferences or values are used to map function states and symptoms onto a 'quality continuum ranging between 0.0 (for death) and 1.0 (for optimum function).' The quality-adjusted life year (QALY) is defined as the equivalent of a completely well year of life or a year of life free of any symptoms, problems, or health-related disabilities. The QWB scale has been validated for patients with COPD (Kaplan *et al.*, 1984) as well as for patients with other lung diseases (Orenstein *et al.*, 1989).

Quality of life is an important outcome for patients with COPD. However, it is also an important predictor of outcomes. One study predicted survival among 74 patients selected for lung transplantation (Squier *et al.*, 1995). While on a waiting list to receive lung transplant, patients completed the QWB along with a variety of measures of lung function. The Beck Depression Inventory was also administered. These 74 patients were followed prospectively. Forty-nine of the patients eventually received a lung transplantation. Of the original 74 patients, 24 died: 13 who had received lung transplant and 11 who were still on the waiting list. Survival analysis was used to determine predictors of survival.

These analyses demonstrated that the QWB was the best prospective predictor of survival. Interestingly, whether or not the patients received lung transplant did not significantly predict survival. Figure 4.8 summarizes these results. The figure shows that a higher proportion of patients who obtained QWB scores above the median survived compared with patients whose initial QWB scores were below the median (relative risk = 0.45, $p < 0.05$). These findings suggest that quality of life may be an important predictor of survival for patients with severe lung disease. It

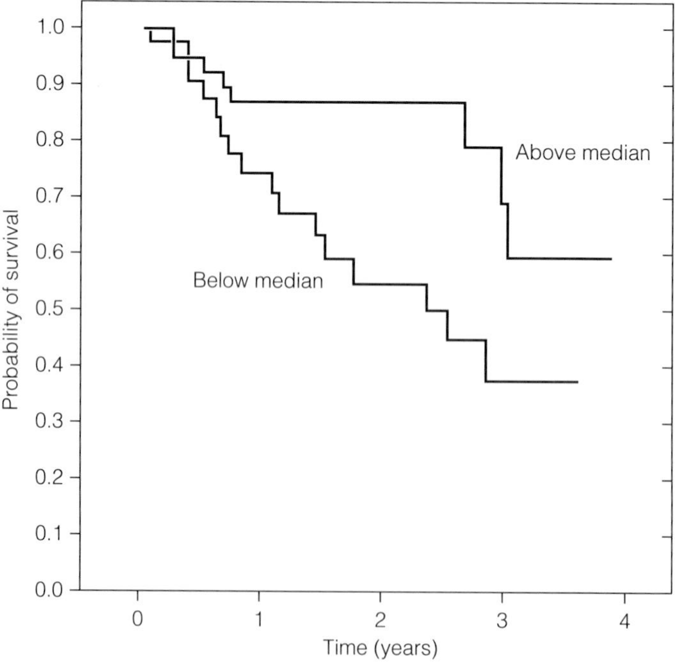

Figure 4.8

Kaplan–Meier proportional estimate survival curves: Above median quality of well-being (QWB) scores versus Below median QWB scores. (From Squier *et al.*, 1995.)

is important to emphasize that the patients in this analysis included those with other lung diseases such as cystic fibrosis and vascular lung disease in addition to those with COPD (Squire *et al.*, 1995).

Social Support

Several papers have argued that older adults with COPD often have difficulty with social relationships. For example, Leidy & Traver (1996) reported that family members of patients with COPD are often dissatisfied with their social relationships with the patient. In particular, they disliked disruptions of free-time activity. A variety of other studies have documented the importance of psychosocial adjustment for patients with COPD (Leidy & Traver, 1995; Lewis & Bell, 1995; Büchi *et al.*, 1997).

One factor that may be particularly important is social support. A growing literature suggests that supportive social relationships are associated with positive health outcomes (Pierce *et al.*, 1996). Most studies define social support as the number of persons in a social network. However, recent conceptualizations go beyond network size and consider quality of social relationships. Thus, in addition to quantity, quality is also important. In order to evaluate the role of social support in patients with COPD, we used measures developed by Sarason *et al.* (1983). These investigators developed a social support questionnaire that measures the number of persons in the social network (SSQ-N) and the self-perception of satisfaction with available support (SSQ-S). In one investigation, we considered the relationship between social support and survival for patients with COPD. The study found significant correlations between both the SSQ-N and SSQ-S with a variety of measures, including exercise tolerance, shortness of breath, and lung function. Among the patients with COPD followed over the course of 6 years, there were 68 survivors and 42 nonsurvivors. Survival analysis was conducted using the Cox proportional hazard model. The analysis demonstrated that SSQ-S (but not SSQ-N) was related to longer survival (Hazard ratio = 0.79, 95% CI = 0.63–0.99). In other words, those who were satisfied with their social support experienced a 21% increase in the chance of survival over 6 year (Grodner *et al.*, 1996).

Survival functions for males and females are shown separately in Figs 4.9 and 4.10. For males, there was a trend for improved survival for those who had high SSQ-S scores; however, the differences were nonsignificant. For females, there was a significant benefit of social support satisfaction: women with low social support satisfaction were significantly more likely to die within 6 years compared with women who had high satisfaction with their social relationships (Grodner *et al.*, 1996). Other studies have also suggested a relationship between social support and survival for women but not men. For instance, the Tecumseh Community Health Study demonstrated a relationship between social support and survival among women (House *et al.*, 1982). The Framingham Heart

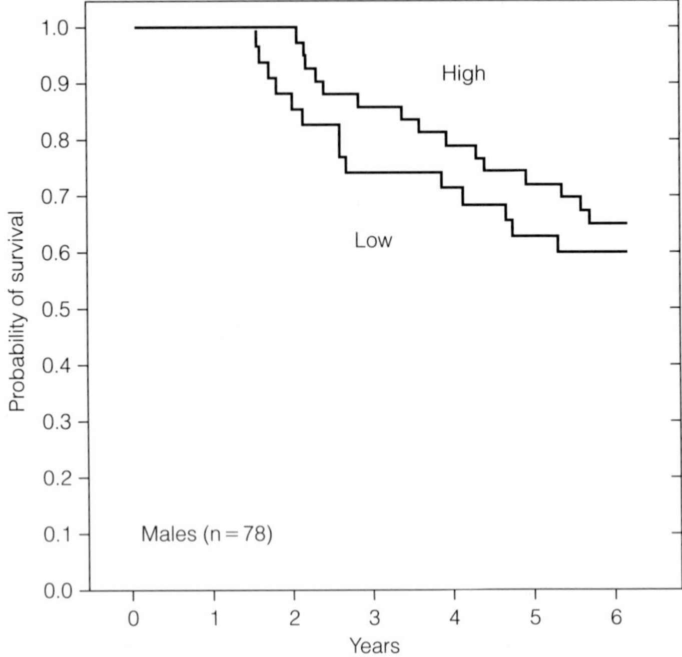

Figure 4.9

Survival of 78 males for high versus low social support satisfaction. (Reprinted from Grodner *et al.*, 1996.)

Study reported that women (but not men) with nonsupportive spouses were more likely to be victims of heart disease (Haynes & Feinleib, 1980).

Self-Efficacy

A third variable that may predict survival for patients with COPD is self-efficacy expectation. Self-efficacy expectancies are defined as expectations that a particular behavior can be executed or completed (Bandura, 1977). A substantial literature suggests that self-efficacy expectations play an important role in the execution and maintenance of complex behaviors (Schwarzer, 1992). We have performed several studies demonstrating that specific rather than generalized efficacy expectations mediate changes in patients with COPD (Kaplan *et al.*, 1994).

To measure self-efficacy, we adapted a self-efficacy scale that was originally developed to measure expectations for completing activities that imposed burden for patients who had experienced uncomplicated myocardial infarction (Ewart *et al.*, 1983). For studies of patients with COPD the self-efficacy questionnaire was modified to more accurately

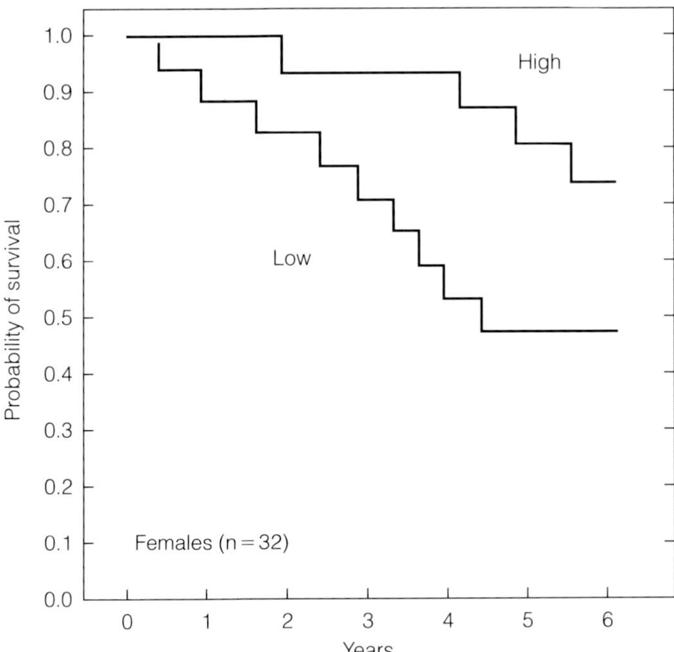

Figure 4.10

Survival of 32 females for high versus low social support satisfaction. (From Grodner *et al.*, 1996.)

represent disabilities associated with this condition. In a series of studies, we demonstrated the validity of the self-efficacy construct by showing systematic correlations with lung function and exercise variables. For example, simple self-efficacy ratings for exercise are systematically related to measures of pulmonary function (Fig. 4.11). The efficacy for walking measures were also associated with diffusion capacity (Fig. 4.12) and exercise tolerance. For example, in the study of exercise tolerance, patients by lowest, middle, or highest tertile of each efficacy category are related to $Vo_{2\,max}$ as assessed in treadmill tests by blind observers (Toshima *et al.*, 1992b).

Self-efficacy ratings are simple to obtain. There has been a predominant tradition in medical science to disregard patient self-reports. Often, self-reports are regarded as unreliable and of low validity. These amateur reports provided by patients are typically devalued in relation to objective tests. However, self-evaluated health status tends to be a good prospective predictor of survival (Mossey & Shapiro, 1982). In one study, we

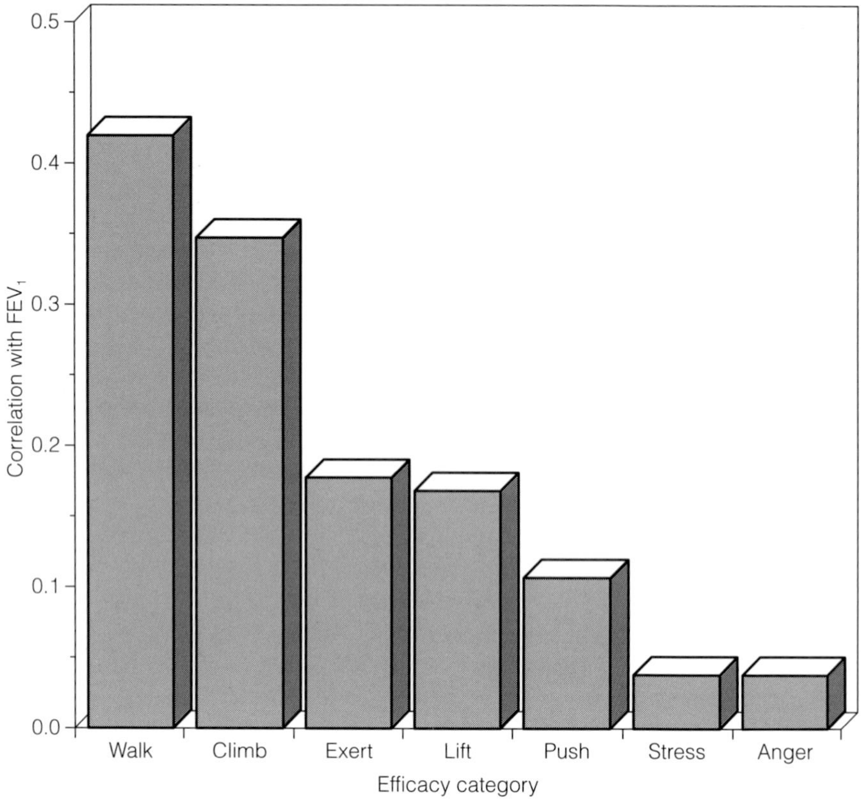

Figure 4.11

Correlations between categories of self-efficacy and FEV_1. Exercise efficacy expectations are more highly correlated with pulmonary function. (Adapted from Toshima *et al.*, 1992b.)

compared the predictive value of simple self-efficacy ratings for exercise against a series of physiological variables. In an earlier study, 28 physiological indicators of disease severity for COPD were factor analyzed. The analysis demonstrated that physiological measurements were highly redundant and are best summarized by four constructs: pulmonary function, diffusing capacity, maximum exercise tolerance, and arterial oxygen level (Ries *et al.*, 1991).

Using data from our prospective study, we developed a predictive model that included these four physiological parameters along with self-efficacy expectations. These variables were assessed at baseline and patients were followed prospectively for 5 years. Death certificates were obtained for all deceased patients. The analysis included 75 patients who survived for 5 years and 33 who died. In a univariate analysis,

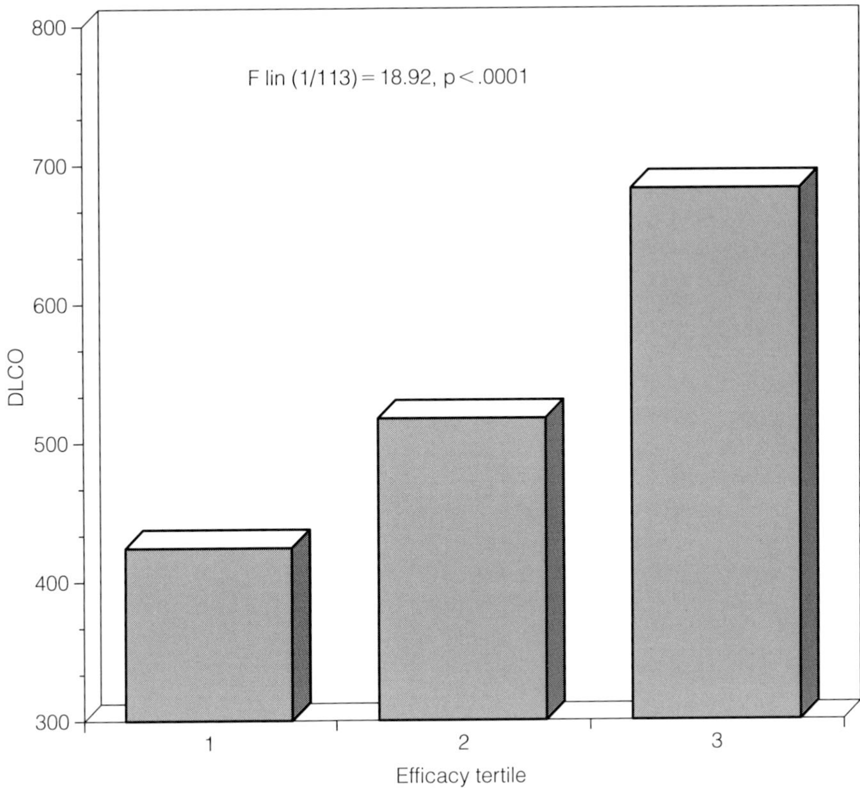

Figure 4.12

Relationship between diffusing capacity (DLCO) and tertile of self-efficacy. (Adapted from Toshima *et al.*, 1992b.)

self-efficacy for walking was a significant predictor of survival ($\chi^2 = 9.01$; d.f. = 1; $p < 0.01$) (Fig. 4.13). The analysis also showed that three other variables were also significant predictors of mortality (FEV_1, $Vo_{2\,max}$, and DLCO). Arterial blood oxygen was not a significant predictor of survival. Multivariate analysis was used to estimate the effects of physiological variables after self-efficacy had been removed. In this analysis, only pulmonary function (FEV_1) added significant information beyond self-efficacy.

These analyses are interesting because they suggest that a simple self-rating of efficacy expectation significantly predicts survival for patients with COPD. The finding compliments other observational studies that have shown that simple patient ratings provide a significant amount of information. It could be argued that the self-efficacy ratings are unimportant because they are only proxies for disease severity. On the other

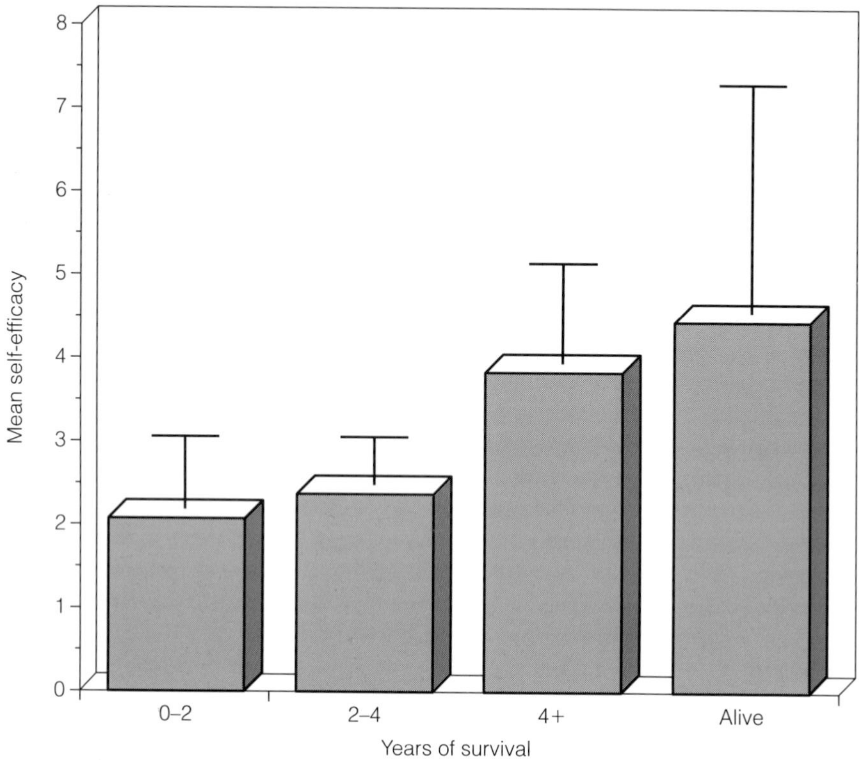

Figure 4.13

Mean self-efficacy for walking by years of survival. (From Kaplan *et al.*, 1994.)

hand, these simple ratings, which literally take a few seconds to assess, compete favorably with expensive laboratory tests when used as predictors of survival. Other studies have shown that simple self-reports provide significant information about survival. In one review, Idler & Kasl (1995) found that simple self-reports have predicted survival in 11 separate studies. These analyses typically use statistical control for other risk factors. Clearly, efficacy expectations are driven by severity of illness. Nevertheless, these findings support the validity of simple self-reports for predicting survival.

Mediating Variables

Several variables may help explain the relationship between behavioral intervention and health outcome; these include dyspnea, compliance and depression.

Dyspnea

Dyspnea, the clinical term for shortness of breath, is defined as the subjective sensation of difficult or labored breathing. Dyspnea is one of the most common and disabling symptoms of people with COPD (Eakin *et al.*, 1993). The sensation of labored breathing can be extremely distressing and may be perceived as life threatening in addition to limiting the function and quality of life of people with COPD. In addition to COPD, dyspnea is common in other medical conditions (e.g., cardiac disease, obesity, neuromuscular disorders affecting the respiratory system).

The sensation of dyspnea is often accompanied by fear and anxiety (Eakin *et al.*, 1993). Several authors have described a dyspnea–panic cycle in which the experience of breathlessness leads to anxiety, which creates muscle tension, resulting, in turn, in increased dyspnea and panic (Dudley *et al.*, 1980). The distress caused by dyspnea can become part of a vicious cycle, leading to fear of future shortness of breath. This may cause patients with COPD to slowly decrease their activity level. In turn, patients become deconditioned, leading to greatly limited independent functioning and quality of life (Ries, 1990).

One hypothesis is that treatment that focuses on dyspnea will result in improved functional outcomes. To address this hypothesis, we evaluated a treatment program centered on training patients to cope with this one symptom. Eighty-nine patients with COPD were randomly assigned to either 6 weeks of treatment or to a general health education program. The treatment was specifically designed to help patients cope with dyspnea. Patients assigned to the treatment protocol were given instruction in progressive muscle relaxation, breathing exercises, pacing, self-talk, and panic control.

To evaluate the effectiveness of the treatment, all patients were evaluated by a 6-min walk test, the QWB, and a series of psychological measures. In addition, they completed six different measures of dyspnea. The measures were administered before the treatment, after the treatment, and 6 months following the intervention.

Following the 6-week treatment, there were no differences between the treatment and control groups on any outcome measure. At the 6-month follow-up, there was a significant difference for only one variable: the dyspnea index (Mahler & Wells, 1988). The results of this study suggest that management of dyspnea alone is not enough to produce significant outcome changes for patients with COPD. Although the program may have some mild effect on the symptom of dyspnea, it did not have an effect on exercise tolerance, quality of life, or any measure of anxiety or depression. As a result of this experience, we now believe that programs must include other behavioral components. In particular, we believe that exercise training is probably one of the most important components of any program (Sassi-Dambron *et al.*, 1994).

Compliance

The rehabilitation programs prescribed for patients with COPD are often difficult to follow. Typically, patients are asked to participate in education, physical and respiratory therapy, and exercise training. Several of our studies have focused on the exercise training component. This is of particular interest because exercise causes discomfort and produces anxiety for many patients. In one study, patients assigned to a rehabilitation program participated in 12 exercise training sessions. During these sessions, the patients walked on a treadmill and performed upper body exercises. The speed of the treadmill was individually determined on the basis of a maximum exercise tolerance test. Patients were individually instructed in translating the treadmill walk into a free-walking regimen that included the number of minutes to be walked and the steps per minute. The patients were then asked to implement this prescription in their daily routines. Specifically, they were asked to walk twice daily at the prescribed pace and duration for the 2 months' duration of the program. In addition, they were asked to keep a daily log of the time and distance they had walked for at least 8 weeks.

Each week the logs were reviewed and the average minutes per day walked was calculated for each patient by dividing the total number of recorded minutes walked during the 8-week period by the total number of days that the patient could have walked. To determine whether compliance was related to outcome, an exercise endurance walk was performed prior to the program and after 12 weeks. During this test, the patients were urged to walk on the treadmill for as long as possible, up to a maximum of 20 min at the target work load, and an additional 10 min at a higher work load.

The results of the study showed there was a dose–response relationship between compliance with walking prescriptions and improvements in exercise endurance. Thus, compliance with the exercise program was a significant predictor of improved exercise endurance. A linear equation was fit to the data. This analysis suggested that each 0.35 min change in compliance resulted in a 1-min improvement in exercise endurance (Fig. 4.14). A variety of analyses were conducted to determine if other variables explained these improvements. The relationship was not diminished by statistical controls for initial levels of disease severity or for any other patient characteristic. Thus, it appears that volitional patient behavior is an important component of improvements in exercise endurance for patients undergoing pulmonary rehabilitation; i.e., patients' choices to comply with daily exercise prescriptions may have a significant effect upon health outcome (Eakin *et al.*, 1992).

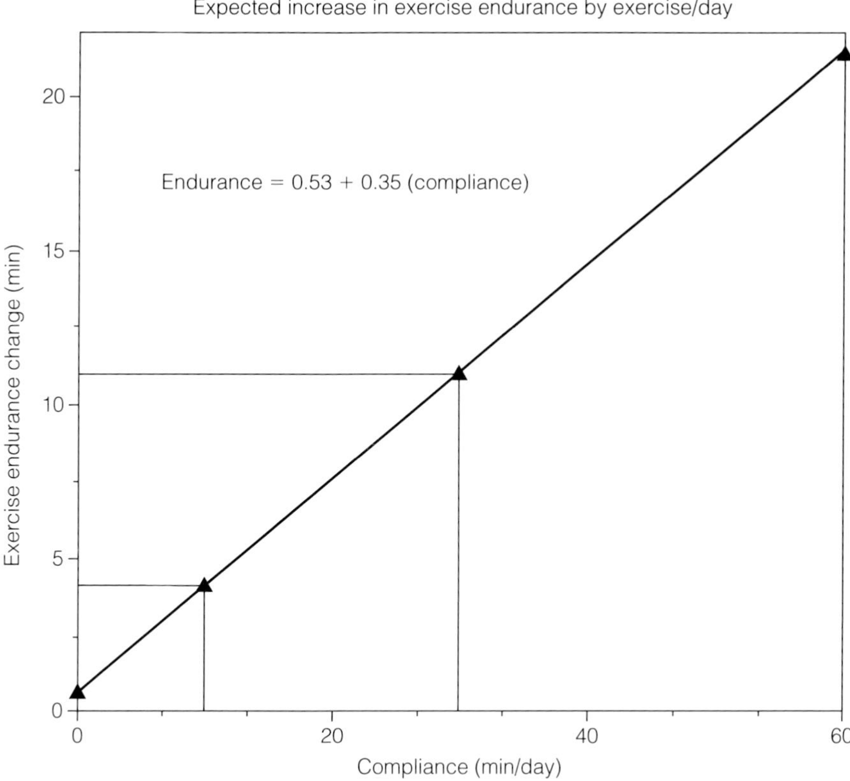

Figure 4.14

Regression of compliance on exercise. Each 0.35 unit change in compliance resulted in a 1-min change in exercise endurance. (From Eakin *et al.*, 1992.)

Depression

A variety of studies demonstrate that patients with chronic illness experience more psychological distress than nondisabled populations. This has clearly been shown in a variety of studies involving patients with COPD (Dudley *et al.*, 1980; Maillé *et al.*, 1994; Herbert & Gregor, 1997; Tu *et al.*, 1997). One explanation of the high levels of depression in patients with COPD is that disability prevents patients from obtaining the reinforcers of everyday life. Abramson *et al.* (1989) defined hopeless depression as an individual expectation that highly desired outcomes will not occur or highly aversive outcomes will. This definition emphasizes that depression will result when people have no control over important events. If this theory is correct, then behavioral interventions that give patients more control and improve their activities of daily living might result in reduced depression.

This hypothesis was evaluated in our experimental trial on rehabilitation. Depression was measured using the CES-D scale. This is a 20-item scale that assesses dimensions of depressed mood, feelings of guilt and worthlessness, appetite loss, sleep disturbance, and energy level (Weissman *et al.*, 1977).

Although patients randomly assigned to rehabilitation improved on functional outcomes, they did not demonstrate lower levels of depression. Comparisons between the education and rehabilitation groups were nonsignificant. Within each treatment group, however, other comparisons were made. The patients were subdivided into two groups based on their changes in depression. One group included those who had increased depression (50 patients) and the other group included those who had a decrease between the baseline and the post-treatment follow-up (52 patients). The data were reanalyzed as a function of treatment circumstances, with depression (increased versus decreased) serving as a categorical independent variable. In the rehabilitation group, the patients who had decreases in depression levels showed a significant increase in exercise endurance performance. For those in the education group, increasing or decreasing depression was unrelated to improved exercise endurance (Fig. 4.15).

Another series of analyses separated the patients who were depressed at baseline ($n = 25$) and those who were not depressed ($n = 74$). The frequency of depression at baseline was approximately equal in the rehabilitation and the education groups. Depression was defined as a CES-D score greater than or equal to 18. Eight patients had to be eliminated from the analysis because of missing data. The analyses demonstrated that, for some variables, there was a differential response to treatment as a function of baseline depression. This was most apparent for changes in exercise tolerance ($V{O_2}_{max}$). For changes in this variable, there were no differences between the education and rehabilitation programs for those who initially had low depression scores. However, for patients who were initially depressed and assigned to the rehabilitation program, there were significant improvements in exercise tolerance; i.e., the rehabilitation program was particularly useful for patients who were initially depressed (Fig. 4.16). This finding is particularly interesting since several authors have suggested that depressed patients be screened out of rehabilitation programs. These data suggest that depressed patients may, indeed, gain even more from the rehabilitation interventions.

Depression is likely to be a comorbidity for patients with any chronic illness. Although it is difficult to make comparisons across studies, it appears that about 40% of patients with COPD experience depression (Isoaho *et al.*, 1995). In our work, 29% of patients reported clinically significant levels of depression at their initial assessment, as determined by

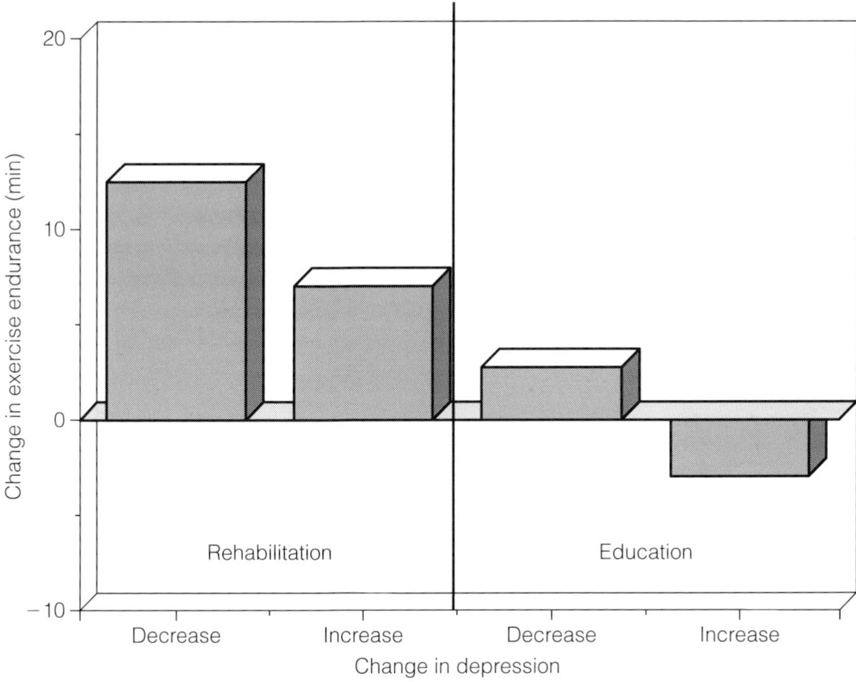

Figure 4.15

Changes in exercise endurance among rehabilitation and education patients who increased or decreased in depression. (From Toshima *et al.*, 1992a.)

CES-D scores greater than 18. The measurement of depression for patients with COPD is difficult because most assessments are based on the general population. For example, items on the CES-D and other depression measures assess decreased sleep, poor appetite, decreased energy, and so on. These are often symptomatic experiences of lung disease. It is not uncommon for patients with COPD to have trouble sleeping or decreased energy because of dyspnea. Further, many patients with COPD report decreased appetite because of the discomfort associated with a full stomach pressing on the diaphragm. Therefore, scores on depression measures may not accurately reflect the level of clinical depression in patients suffering from chronic diseases such as COPD. We do not yet understand whether responses to some items represent the lung disease or depression, so it is impossible to determine how many patients who report depression-like symptoms actually have a major affective disorder. Considerably more work on the importance of depression and the role of the behavioral intervention is needed (Toshima *et al.*, 1992a).

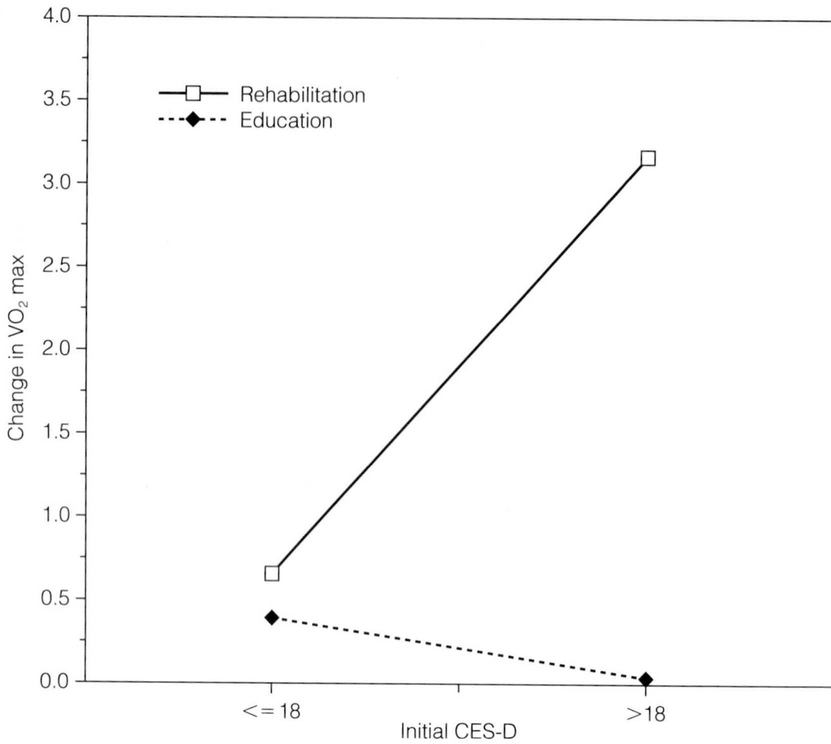

Figure 4.16

Changes in $VO_{2\,max}$ as a function of initial depression for rehabilitation and education patients. (From Toshima *et al.*, 1992a.)

Conclusion and Future Directions

Chronic obstructive pulmonary disease has received relatively little attention from behavioral scientists. Several important challenges await investigators interested in this field. First, behavioral risk factors for COPD have been well studied, but deserve ongoing attention. Changes in the prevalence of tobacco use might effect future epidemic patterns. Further, environmental exposures and unique interactions between genotypes and lifestyle might define future populations at risk.

A second important area of investigation involves behavioral interventions. Rehabilitation has now become common practice for patients with COPD. However, the components of rehabilitation need additional study. It is unclear whether benefits attributable to intervention result from exercise, compliance with medications, psychosocial support, relaxation training, or some combination of interventions. Further, additional study is required to maintain behavior change over the course of time.

Finally, outcome measurement deserves continuing attention. Benefits of both surgical and medical treatments are often represented as changes in quality of life. In addition, measures of shortness of breath and psychosocial mediators must be validated in continuing studies. A variety of behavioral and psychosocial variables may mediate outcome for patients with COPD, including depression, social support, and self-efficacy expectations. Ultimately, treatments might be tailored to patients with particular psychosocial needs.

References

Abramson, L.Y., Metalsky, G.I., & Alloy, L.B. (1989). Hopelessness depression: a theory-based subtype of depression. *Psychological Review*, 96, 358–372.

ACCP/AACVPR Pulmonary Rehabilitations (1997). Guidelines Panel. Pulmonary rehabilitation: Joint ACCP/AACVPR evidence-based guidelines. *Chest*, 112, 1363–1396.

Albert, R.K. (1997). Is pulmonary rehabilitation an effective treatment for chronic obstructive pulmonary disease? No. *American Journal of Respiratory and Critical Care Medicine*, 155, 784–785.

Ambrosino, N., Paggiaro, P.L., Macchi, M., *et al.* (1981). A study of short-term effect of rehabilitative therapy in chronic obstructive pulmonary disease. *Respiration*, 41, 40–44.

American Thoracic Society (1987). Standards for the diagnosis and care of patients with chronic obstructive pulmonary disease (COPD) and asthma. *American Review of Respiratory Disease*, 136, 225–244.

American Thoracic Society (1995). Standards for the diagnosis and care of patients with chronic obstructive pulmonary disease (COPD) and asthma. *American Review of Respiratory Disease*, 152, S78–S121.

Atkins, J.C., Kaplan, R.M., Timms, R.M., Reinsch, S., & Lofback, K. (1984). Behavioral exercise programs in the management of chronic obstructive pulmonary disease. *Journal of Consulting & Clinical Psychology*, 52, 591–603.

Austin, T. W. (1976). Cigarette smoking & chronic bronchitis. *British Medical Journal*, 2, 1261.

Bach, J.R. (1996). *Pulmonary rehabilitation. The obstructive & paralytic condition.* Philadelphia, PA: Hanley & Delfus.

Bandura, A. (1977). Self-efficacy: toward a unifying theory of behavioral change. *Psychological Review*, 84, 191–215.

Bell, C.W. & Jensen, R.H. (1977). Physical conditioning. In: R.H. Jensen & I. Kass (Eds), *Pulmonary rehabilitation home programs.* Omaha: University of Nebraska Medical Center.

Belman, M.J. & Wasserman, K. (1981). Exercise training and testing in patients with chronic obstructive pulmonary disease. *Basics of Respiratory Diseases*, 10, 1–6.

Büchi, S., Villiger, B., Sensky, T., Schwarz, F., Wolf, C., & Buddeberg, C. (1997). Psychosocial predictors of long-term success of in-patient pulmonary rehabilitation of patients with COPD. *European Respiratory Journal*, 10, 1272–1277.

Celli, B.R. (1997). Is pulmonary rehabilitation an effective treatment for chronic obstructive pulmonary disease? Yes. *American Journal of Respiratory and Critical Care Medicine*, 155, 781–783.

Cooper, J.D., Trulock, E.P., Triantafillou, A.N., *et al.* (1996). Bilateral pneumectomy (volume reduction) for chronic obstructive pulmonary disease. *Journal of Thoracic Cardiovascular Surgery* 109, 106–116.

Dudley, D.L., Glaser, E.M., Jorgenson, B.N., & Logan, D.L. (1980). Psychosocial concomitants to rehabilitation in chronic obstructive pulmonary disease: Part 1. Psychosocial and psychological considerations. *Chest*, 77, 413–420.

Eakin, E.G. & Glasgow, R.E. (1996). The physician's role in diabetes self-management: helping patients to help themselves. *The Endocrinologist*, 6, 1–10.

Eakin, E.G., Sassi-Dambron, D., Kaplan, R.M., & Ries, A.L. (1992). Clinical trial of rehabilitation in chronic obstructive pulmonary disease: compliance as a mediator of change in exercise endurance. *Journal of Cardiopulmonary Rehabilitation*, 12, 105–110.

Eakin, E.G., Kaplan, R.M., & Ries, A.L. (1993). Measurement of dyspnoea in chronic obstructive pulmonary disease. *Quality of Life Research*, 2, 181–191.

Eakin, E.G., Resnikoff, P.M., Prewitt, L.M., Ries, A.L., & Kaplan, R.M. (1998). Validation of a new dyspnea measure: the UCSD shortness of breath questionnaire. *Chest*, 113, 619–624.

Eiser, N., West, C., Evans, S., Jeffers, A., & Quirk, F. (1997). Effects of psychotherapy in moderately severe COPD: a pilot study. *European Respiratory Journal*, 10, 1581–1584.

Ewart, C.K., Taylor, C.B., Reese, L.B., & DeBusk, R.F. (1983). Effects of early postmyocardial exercise testing on self-perception and subsequent physical activity. *American Journal of Cardiology*, 51, 1076–1080.

Fishman, A.P. (Ed.) (1996). *Pulmonary rehabilitation*. New York: Marcel Dekker.

Grodner, S., Prewitt, L.M., Jaworski, B.A., Myers, R., Kaplan, R.M., & Ries, A.L. (1996). The impact of social support in pulmonary rehabilitation of patients with chronic obstructive pulmonary disease. *Annals of Behavioral Medicine*, 18, 139–145.

Guyatt, G.H., Berman, L.B., & Townsend, M. (1987). Long-term outcome after respiratory rehabilitation. *Canadian Medical Association Journal*, 137, 1089–1095.

Haynes, S.G. & Feinleib, M. (1980). Women, work and coronary heart disease: prospective findings from the Framingham Heart Study. *American Journal of Public Health*, 70, 133–141.

Herbert, R. & Gregor, F. (1997). Quality of life and coping strategies of clients with COPD. *Rehabilitation & Nursing*, 22, 182–187.

Higgins, M.W. (1989). Chronic airways disease in the United States. Trends and determinants. *Chest* 96(Suppl), 328S–334S.

Hodgkin, J., Connors, G.L., & Bell, C.W. (Eds) (1993). *Pulmonary rehabilitation: guidelines to success* 2nd edn (pp. 86–101). Philadelphia, PA: Lippincott.

House, J.S., Robbins, C., & Metzner, H.L. (1982). The association of social relationships and activities with mortality: prospective evidence from the Tecumseh Community Health Study. *American Journal of Epidemiology*, 116, 123–140.

Idler, E.L. & Kasl, S.V. (1995). Self-ratings of health: do they also predict change in functional ability? *Journals of Gerontology. Series B, Psychological Sciences & Social Sciences*, 50, S344–S353, 18.

Isoaho, R., Keistinen, T., Laippala, P., & Kivela, S.L. (1995). Chronic obstructive pulmonary disease and symptoms related to depression in elderly persons. *Psychological Reports*, 76, 287–297.

Kaplan, R.M., Bush, J.W., & Berry, C.C. (1976). Health status: types of validity and the index of well-being. *Health Services Research*, 11, 478–507.

Kaplan, R.M., Atkins, C.J., & Timms, R. (1984). Validity of a Quality of Well-being Scale as an outcome measure in chronic obstructive pulmonary disease. *Journal of Chronic Diseases*, 37, 85–95.

Kaplan, R.M., Ries, A., & Atkins, C.J. (1985). Area review: behavioral management of chronic obstructive pulmonary disease. *Annals of Behavioral Medicine*, 7, 5–10.

Kaplan, R.M., Ries, A.L., Prewitt, L.M., & Eakin, E. (1994). Self-efficacy expectations predict survival for patients with chronic obstructive pulmonary disease. *Health Psychology*, 13, 366–368.

Kaptein, A.A. (1997). Behavioral interventions in COPD: a pause for breath. *European Respiratory Review*, 7, 88–91.

Leidy, N.K. & Traver, G.A. (1995). Psychophysiologic factors contributing to functional performance in people with COPD: are there gender differences? *Research in Nursing & Health*, 19, 535–546.

Leidy, N.K. & Traver, G.A. (1996). Adjustment and social behavior in older adults with chronic obstructive pulmonary disease: the family perspective. *Journal of Advanced Nursing*, 23, 252–259.

Lewis, D. & Bell, S.K. (1995). Pulmonary rehabilitation, psychosocial adjustment, and use of healthcare services. *Rehabilitation Nursing*, 20, 102–107.

Lisansky, D.P. & Clough, D.H. (1996). A cognitive-behavioral self-help educational program for patients with COPD. A pilot study. *Psychotherapy & Psychosomatics*, 65, 97–101.

Mahler, D.A. & Wells, C.K. (1988). Evaluation of clinical methods for rating dyspnea. *Chest*, 93, 580–586.

Maillé, A.R., Kaptein, A.A., Koning, C.J., & Zwinderman, A.H. (1994). Developing a quality-of-life questionnaire for patients with respiratory illness. *Monaldi Archives for Chest Diseases*, 49, 76–78.

Maillé, A.R., Kaptein, A.A., de Haes, J.C., & Everaerd, W.T.A.M. (1996). Assessing quality of life in chronic non-specific lung disease – a review of empirical studies published between 1980 and 1994. *Quality of Life Research*, 5, 287–301.

McGavin, C.R., Gupta, S.P., Lloyd, E.L., & McHardy, G.J. (1997). Physical rehabilitation for the chronic bronchitic: results of a controlled trial of exercise in the home. *Thorax*, 32, 307–311.

McKenna, R.J.J., Brenner, M., Fischel, R.J., *et al.* (1997). Patient selection criteria for lung volume reduction surgery. *Journal of Thoracic Cardiovascular Surgery*, 114, 957–964.

Mertens, D.J., Shepard, R.J., & Kavenagh, T. (1978). Long-term exercise therapy for chronic obstructive pulmonary disease. *Respiration*, 35, 96–107.

Mossey, J.M. & Shapiro, E. (1982). Self-rated health: a predictor of mortality among the elderly. *American Journal of Public Health*, 72, 800–808.

Murray, C.J. & Lopez, A.D. (1996). Evidence-based health policy – lessons from the Global Burden of Disease Study. *Science*, 274, 740–743.

National Center for Health Statistics (1995). *Advance report of final mortality statistics.* Hyattsville, MD: Centers for Disease Control and Prevention.

National Heart, Lung, and Blood Institute (1996). *Morbidity and mortality chartbook on cardiovascular, lung and blood diseases.* Bethesda, MD: National Institutes of Health.

Orenstein, J.M., Nixon, P.A., Ross, E.A., & Kaplan, R.M. (1989). The quality of well-being in cystic fibrosis. *Chest*, 95, 344–347.

Pierce, G., Lakey, B., Sarason, I.G. & Sarason, B.R. (Eds) (1996). *Sourcebook of social support and personality.* New York: Plenum.

Ries, A.L. (1990). Scientific basis of pulmonary rehabilitation: position paper of the American Association of Cardiovascular and Pulmonary Rehabilitation. *Journal of Cardiopulmonary Rehabilitation*, 10, 418–441.

Ries, A.L., Kaplan, R.M., & Blumberg, E. (1991). Use of factor analysis to consolidate multiple outcome measures in chronic obstructive pulmonary disease. *Journal of Clinical Epidemiology*, 44, 497–503.

Ries, A.L., Kaplan, R.M., Limberg, T.M., & Prewitt, L.M. (1995). Effects of pulmonary rehabilitation on physiologic and psychosocial outcomes in patients with chronic obstructive pulmonary disease. *Annals of Internal Medicine*, 122, 823–832.

Sarason, I.G. & Sarason, B.R. (1982). Concomitants of social support: attitudes, personality characteristics, and life experiences. *Journal of Personality*, 50, 331–344.

Sassi-Dambron, D.E., Eakin, L., Ries, A.L., & Kaplan, R.M. (1994). The effect of compliance on exercise training in pulmonary rehabilitation. *Rehabilitation Nursing Research*, 3, 3–10.

Schwarzer, R. (Ed.) (1992). *Self-efficacy: thought control of action.* Washington, DC: Hemisphere.

Squier, H.C., Ries, A.L., Kaplan, R.M., *et al.* (1995). Quality of Well-being predicts survival in lung transplantation candidates. *American Journal of Respiratory and Critical Care*, 152, 2032–2036.

Toevs, C.D., Kaplan, R.M., & Atkins, C.J. (1984). The costs and effects of behavioral programs in chronic obstructive pulmonary disease. *Medical Care*, 22, 1088–1100.

Toshima, M.T., Blumberg, E., Ries, A.L., & Kaplan, R.M. (1992a). Does rehabilitation reduce depression in patients with chronic obstructive pulmonary disease? *Journal of Cardiopulmonary Rehabilitation*, 12, 261–269.

Toshima, M.T., Kaplan, R.M., & Ries, A.L. (1992b). Self-efficacy expectancies in chronic obstructive pulmonary disease rehabilitation. In: R. Schwarzer (Ed.), *Self-efficacy: thought control of action* (pp. 325–354). Washington, DC: Hemisphere.

Tu, S.P., McDonell, M.B., Spertus, J.A., Steele, B.G., & Fihn, S.D. (1997). A new self-administered questionnaire to monitor health-related quality of life in patients with COPD. Ambulatory Care Quality Improvement Project (ACQUIP) Investigators. *Chest*, 112, 614–622.

van den Broek, A. (1995). *Patient education and chronic obstructive pulmonary disease – Health psychology Series No. 1* (p. 13). Den Haag: Cip-Data Koninklijke Bibliotheek.

Vital and Health Statistics, Series 10, #193, 1986.

Weissman, M.M., Sholomskas, D., Pottenger, M., Prusoff, B.A., & Locke, B.Z. (1977). Assessing depressive symptoms in five psychiatric populations: A validation study. *American Journal of Epidemiology*, 106, 203–214.

World Health Organization (1999). *World Health Report, 1999. Making a difference.* Geneva: World Health Organization.

Yang, G., Fan, L., Tan, J., *et al.* (1999). Smoking in China. Findings of the 1996 National Prevalence Survey. *Journal of the American Medical Association*, 282, 1247–1253.

5
Symptom perception in asthma

Simon Rietveld and Walter Everaerd

Editors' note—*In most cases, patients detect the onset of asthma or chronic obstructive pulmonary disorder (COPD) exacerbations and react by initiating the appropriate treatment, which is the sequence of events that constitutes treatment in most patients. However, what seems a simple discrimination task – detecting the onset of an exacerbation – is not always simple. As Simon Rietveld and Walter Everaerd point out, the act of detecting the onset of a respiratory exacerbation can be complex, both across patients and individual episodes. Symptom discrimination is based on patient interpretation of environmental, physiological, cognitive, and behavioral variables that interact to generate a context that signals a change in breathing. Simon and Walter are ideal investigators to explain the complexities of symptom discrimination, as they have revived interest in the topic of symptom discrimination in the past decade; by doing so, they have made enormous contributions to our understanding of the phenomenon.*

Periodically over the years, symptom discrimination of exacerbations in respiratory disorders, particularly asthma, has prompted considerable interest and research. Perhaps the strangest approach taken toward solving the problem of symptom discrimination came with bilateral carotid body resection in patients with asthma and COPD. The approach as a treatment for asthma was simultaneously reported by Nakayama (1961) and Overholt (1961). Nakayama (1961) described 3914 cases where unilateral removal of the carotid body produced a 'cure' for asthma in 81% of the patients; Overholt (1961) reported similar findings.

Winter (1972) has been the strongest champion of surgical removal of the carotid body in the United States. He presented data on 57 patients following unilateral carotid body resections according to the criteria of Nakayama (1961) and Overholt (1961). Six months following the operation, Winter (1972) reported failure in 47% of the patients, equivocal results in 33%, and success in 20%. Winter continued by claiming that bilateral resection performed on 18 failures, at intervals ranging from 1 to 26 months, yielded success in 78% and equivocal results in the remaining 22% of patients. Less than a decade ago, Winter (1991) remained a fervent advocate of carotid body resection in asthma and COPD.

The irony is that this radical approach not only failed to solve the problem of symptom discrimination in patients with asthma or COPD but generated a number of unfortunate consequences to patients. Simply put, carotid body resection killed the physiological message that a patient was beginning to experience a change in his or her breathing. The result, as most notably described by Kirkuchi et al. (1994), was reduced chemosensitivity to hypoxia and blunted perception of dyspnea. This basic deficit resulted in other serious consequences, including the predisposition to fatal asthma attacks (Kikuchi et al., 1994), vulnerability to hypoxic death in sleep (Sullivan, 1980), severe obstructive sleep apnea (Parisi et al., 1987), poor gas exchange even with use of the medication almitrine bismesylate (de Backer et al., 1983), and episodes of cyanosis in a 12-year-old boy who, while disoriented, experienced no subjective feelings of discomfort or dyspnea (Chang et al., 1978). Attempts to improve symptom discrimination, while avoiding negative consequences, is the purpose of the exciting research described in this chapter by Rietveld and Everaerd.

Introduction

The limitation of human symptom perceptual accuracy becomes apparent when patients with asthma fail to perceive airways obstruction. They therefore do not use bronchodilator medication and may suffocate as a consequence. Despite the increasing progress in pharmacology, the occurrence of near-fatal asthma attacks is rising globally, with poor symptom perception being a key issue (Barnes, 1994). A life-threatening attack of airways obstruction can develop within 1 hour. Rapid awareness of symptoms and taking the required medications can be decisive (Jones, 1992; Garden & Ayres, 1993).

Apart from a blunted perception of physical information that indicates airways obstruction, a common phenomenon is overperception of physical information, characterized by excessive breathlessness without sufficient cause (Rietveld & Brosschot, 1999). Inaccurate symptom perception is generally associated with poor asthma management and a negative prognosis with respect to hospitalization (Kotses *et al.*, 1980; Creer, 1983, 1987; Creer & Gustafson, 1989). Moreover, sudden asthma attacks are likely to decrease the sense of control over symptoms, enhancing distress and helplessness (Pennebaker *et al.*, 1977; Ahles *et al.*, 1983; Bandura, 1990). Specific problems characteristic of overperception of symptoms include excessive use of medicines, unwarranted illness behavior and negative emotions (Dirks & Schraa, 1983; Creer, 1987).

In clinical reality, patients with asthma may consider themselves symptom-free in the middle of an asthma attack, or suffer from severe breathlessness either with mild airways obstruction or with no obstruction at all (Boulet *et al.*, 1991; Rietveld *et al.*, 1999a). Patients with asthma may feel particular sensations during airways obstruction without knowing what is wrong. In fact, they may attribute their condition to having flu or fatigue (Rietveld & Prins, 1998a). Certain patients may be aware of marked airflow obstruction, but are not bothered by it, do not feel breathless, and do not take medication (McFadden *et al.*, 1973; Rubinfeld & Pain, 1976; Wolkove, 1992; Rietveld, 1998). Breathlessness in asthma is an ambiguous symptom, but it can often be extremely noxious in its manifestation. Breathlessness is not specific for airways obstruction but common in normal individuals after physical exercise and in patients with agoraphobia, panic disorder, or hyperventilation syndrome (Carr *et al.*, 1992; Saisch *et al.*, 1996). Breathlessness in asthma, as a function of airways obstruction, is not well understood (Pratter & Bartter, 1991; Muers, 1993).

This chapter provides an overview of the relevant literature about symptom perception in asthma and attempts to explain perceptual phenomena in terms of biased processing of information. First, we give common definitions and the various methods of studying symptom perception in respiratory disease. Next, we summarize physiological influences in symptom perception, from the afferent information associated with airways obstruction to the secondary physiological factors contributing to breathlessness. Despite the afferent information underlying a breathlessness response, the intensity of breathlessness is determined by psychological factors. We focus on three different influences:

- a competition of cues that determines the unconscious processing of information
- the response tendencies that patients acquire in the course of their living with asthma
- negative emotions.

In addition, we discuss methodological problems in symptom perception research. Finally, we discuss how symptom perception can be improved in patients with asthma, and summarize our views on future research.

Definitions and Research Methods

Symptom perception encompasses a broad field of processing of information, ranging from unconscious receptor stimulation to high-order evaluation of symptom consequences and coping strategies (Petrie & Weinman, 1997). A symptom is defined as the conscious awareness of physical information that follows unconscious processing of information. Symptom perception in this chapter is restricted to the factors that influence the perception process underlying the conscious awareness of symptoms.

Asthma is characterized by recurrent attacks of airways obstruction, which is measured through lung-function testing. There are various neural pathways that provide afferent information, resulting in breathlessness, tendency to cough, fatigue, or negative emotions. The major symptom, however, is breathlessness or dyspnea. Many scientists prefer the term 'dyspnea,' which refers to respiratory or ventilatory dysfunction rather than to a symptom. The term 'breathlessness' properly covers the subjective sensations associated with airways obstruction.

Symptom perception in respiratory disease has been investigated in three ways:

1 through signal detection experiments
2 via the parallel assessment of breathlessness and lung function
3 via a comparison between recorded lung function and lung function as estimated by the subject.

In signal detection experiments the capacity to detect increases in the flow-resistive component to breathing is measured under controlled circumstances. The subjects breathe through a mouthpiece (with a noseclip on), coupled with a tube device, while a series of external resistive loads to breathing are applied. The subjects are instructed to respond to detection by pressing a button or to estimate stimulus intensity by means of self-reports. The perceptual accuracy is expressed in a 'receiver operating characteristic' curve that reflects the subject's responses as a function of the stimuli presented. Response options are correct responses (hits) and false positive responses (Green & Swets, 1966; Harver *et al.*, 1993; Rietveld *et al.*, 1996b). The respiratory adjustment up to metabolic needs is dissimilar during real airways obstruction and external airflow interruption. During airways obstruction, ventilation, inspiratory airflow, and respiratory rate increase, and arterial carbon dioxide is reduced. Contrarily, during external airflow obstruction, the respiratory rate and inspiratory flow are reduced, but ventilation and carbon dioxide remain unaltered (Kelsen *et al.*, 1981). However, the increased respiratory labor during external obstruction is conjunct with the major model on the origin of breathlessness, legitimizing this method.

The second method for studying symptom perception focuses on the relationship between breathlessness and lung function during spontaneous or induced airways obstruction. When several of these measurements have been taken during fluctuations in airways obstruction, a significant negative correlation between breathlessness and lung function would generally indicate accurate symptom perception. Some research has been conducted under natural circumstances, but the problem is that actual exacerbation of asthma can be relatively rare (Ergood *et al.*, 1985; Fritz *et al.*, 1990).

Rietveld and Everaerd (2000) compared the relationship between breathlessness and airways obstruction in the homes of asthma patients by means of 24-hour recording of breathsounds with telemetry equipment (indicative of airways obstruction). Results indicated that breathlessness related to acute airways obstruction, but poorly with chronic obstruction. However, chronic airways obstruction related significantly to negative mood, whereas acute obstruction did not.

Hence, most research has been conducted with induced airways obstruction in the hospital during an airways challenge test. These tests are primarily conducted for the assessment of airways hypersensitivity, the major characteristic of asthma. Airways obstruction is induced by means of inhalation of a series of doubling concentrations of histamine or methacholine. The concentration required to induce a reduction in lung function of >20% is an indication of the sensitivity of the airways and may instigate changes in prescribed medication. During this test, breathlessness is repeatedly measured from baseline to posttest, usually 10 min after bronchodilator medication, used to relieve the induced airways obstruction (Marks *et al.*, 1996; Spinhoven *et al.*, 1997).

The third method for studying symptom perception is the comparison between estimated lung function and the actually recorded lung function, usually the peak expiratory flow (Reader *et al.*, 1990). One can conclude that there is a capacity for accurate symptom perception when patients can accurately estimate their own lung function. As we shall see in the final section of this chapter, this method has particularly been applied to train patients with asthma to cope better with their symptoms.

Despite the different methods for studying symptom perception, accurate symptom perception implies that patients should always and only feel breathlessness during airways obstruction. Moreover, the degree of breathlessness should positively relate to the degree of airways obstruction as indicated by lung-function tests, with the highest breathlessness reported during extreme airways obstruction.

Perceptual Mechanisms

For decades, breathlessness has been attributed to increased arterial carbon dioxide that results from insufficient ventilation (Remmers *et al.*, 1968). However, in a series of classic psychophysical experiments, Campbell *et al.* (1989) demonstrated that breathlessness is also caused by afferent information from the respiratory muscles. They blocked the afferent neuromuscular pathway with curare and found that the paralysis this caused significantly lengthened the time that the subjects could hold their breath without breathlessness (Campbell *et al.*, 1969). Their model postulates that the intensity of breathlessness increases not only as the tension in the inspiratory muscles increases but also as their length becomes smaller and inspiratory flow increases (Gandevia *et al.*, 1981).

Despite the explanatory power of the model, some researchers maintained that respiratory muscle contraction is not necessary to evoke breathlessness (Banzett *et al.*, 1989). Paralysed quadriplegics, fully dependent upon mechanical ventilation, reported breathlessness when the level of carbon dioxide in the administered gas mixture was increased. Subsequent replication studies provided mixed results, favoring or refuting the predictions of the two models (Adams *et al.*, 1985). Breathlessness does not relate to oxygen uptake, but may arise during actual hypoxemia. An additional influence in the origin of breathlessness would be efferent information from the breathing center in the brain stem (MacBugler *et al.*, 1993). Barnes (1994) hypothesized that absence of breathlessness during excessive airways obstruction might be a result of an insensitivity to hypoxemia.

To summarize, the adequacy of respiration is maintained and guarded by at least three neural systems, although these often seem to copy only modestly to the sensory cortex for conscious awareness. In other words, the physical information underlying breathlessness often seems neither clear nor specific. Breathlessness is a subjective experience and the unconscious processing of information underlying this experience is influenced by biomedical and psychological factors.

Contributing Physiological Factors

Several physiological factors are likely to influence breathlessness and are not always reflected in lung-function parameters.

1. Central versus peripheral airways obstruction is likely to influence the afferent information underlying breathlessness. McFadden (1984) suggested that central obstruction accounts for more symptoms than peripheral airways obstruction. Late or gradually developing asthmatic reactions are also less accurately perceived and reflected in breathlessness than are acute reactions (Turcotte *et al.*, 1990). It seems a general phenomenon that phasic physiological changes are less well perceived than are tonic changes (Pennebaker, 1982). In asthma, acute airways obstruction through smooth muscle contraction would be more accurately perceived than gradually developing obstruction with a relatively important contribution of edema and excessive mucosal secretion (McFadden, 1984).

2. Existing, modest airways obstruction may interfere with the perception of additional, artificially induced airways obstruction (Burdon *et al.*, 1982). More severe pathophysiology may interfere with symptom perception, although this has not been investigated with breathlessness. Excessive mucosal secretion in the airways of patients with cystic fibrosis results in a heightened threshold for cough when exposed to cough-provoking agents (Chang *et al.*, 1997).

3. Particular breathing maneuvers may disproportionately increase breathlessness, irrespective of airways obstruction (Killian *et al.*, 1984). During emotional stress or perceived airways obstruction, breathing may turn into a pattern of increased inspiratory frequency and expiratory prolongation. The result is a dynamic hyperinflation of the lungs, which is associated with thoracic pressure and breathlessness (Lougheed *et al.*, 1993).

4. Different agents to induce airways obstruction may differentially stimulate receptors and influence breathlessness (Marks *et al.*, 1996). Turcotte *et al.* (1990) found no difference in breathlessness after exposure to allergens, histamine, or physical exercise. Rietveld *et al.* (2001) observed higher breathlessness during airways obstruction induced with histamine than with physical exercise. Different neural pathways, as well

as additional symptoms such as excessive saliva due to histamine inhalation, could have been involved. Moreover, the authors emphasized the influence of negative emotions during the more stressful histamine test. Other support for the influence of different pathways comes from studies where airways obstruction and breathlessness were treated with different medication. Corticosteroids have been reported to improve symptom perception, whereas cromoglycate had no effect, although both act against airways inflammation (Higgs & Laszlo, 1996).

5. Secondary symptoms such as nasal congestion, excessive secretion of mucus or saliva, or persistent cough may influence respiratory distress and enhance breathlessness (Freestone & Eccles, 1997; Rietveld & Rijssenbeek-Nouwens, 1998).

6. Rapid breathing during emotional stress may turn into hyperventilation, with the eventual state of hypocapnia causing a wide range of symptoms, including breathlessness (Saisch *et al.*, 1996).

7. The influence of beta-endorphin levels, one of the opioid peptides that modulates high cortical functioning, may influence symptom perception in asthma. This hypothesis has hardly been investigated, however (Isenberg *et al.*, 1997).

8. Some researchers have emphasized the influence of a biological or circadian rhythm on the accuracy of symptom perception, although conclusions are diffuse (Bagg & Hughes, 1980; Peiffer *et al.*, 1989). The correlation between breathlessness and lung function seems to be lower in the afternoon than in the early morning (Peiffer *et al.*, 1989). Children's complaints of breathlessness at night are generally higher than during the day, irrespective of lung function (Weiss, 1966).

The above factors may suggest that patients with more severe asthma are more vulnerable to inaccurate symptom perception than patients with mild asthma. Signal detection experiments have indeed suggested that patients with more severe obstructive problems (chronic obstructive pulmonary disease, COPD) perform less well than patients with asthma or normal controls (Gottfried *et al.*, 1981; Noseda *et al.*, 1992). The differences between asthmatics and normal controls seem to be small but consistent, with asthmatics being less accurate (Burki *et al.*, 1978; Côté *et al.*, 1987; Harver *et al.*, 1993; Rietveld *et al.*, 1996b). However, in contrast with this assumption of influential pathophysiology, recent studies have shown that children with mild asthma were as inaccurate in symptom perception as adults with severe asthma (Ergood *et al.*, 1985; Sly *et al.*, 1985; Fritz *et al.*, 1990; Rietveld *et al.*, 1996b).

Moreover, the accuracy of symptom perception seems to be independent of reduction in lung function, airways hyperresponsiveness or prescribed medication (Janson-Bjerklie *et al.*, 1987). In addition, the airways of fatal asthma cases seem to be relatively clean, without obvious pathology (Barnes, 1994). This suggests that severe airways pathophysiology is not a substantial factor in blunted perception of airways obstruction.

Perceptual differences within individuals may further dismiss the notion of lung pathology as an important factor in inaccurate symptom perception (Hudgel *et al.*, 1982; Wilson & Jones, 1990). It can be concluded that physiological factors and secondary symptoms are determinants of symptom perception in asthma, although they are insufficient to explain the extreme manifestations of inaccurate symptom perception.

The Psychological Perspective

The integration of receptor stimulation with preset knowledge in the memory is subject to learned responses on various unconscious cognitive levels. The vast majority of visceral afferent information remains beyond conscious awareness but may be capable of instigating physiological adaptation or mood change (Hoelzl *et al.*, 1996). Perceptual strategies or mechanisms could likewise be mobilized to direct the subsequent flow of physical information and determine processing of information toward conscious perception of a symptom. Experience with symptoms and knowledge of asthma is stored in cognitive recall schemata to influence consecutive symptom perception, as well as thinking about symptoms in full awareness (Lacroix *et al.*, 1991; Petrie & Weinman, 1997). Symptom perception can be viewed as an unconscious psychological construction of scratches of information from different internal and external domains (Pennebaker & Skelton, 1981; Rietveld & Brosschot, 1999). Hence, it is the individual whose knowledge and experience modulates information by giving meaning to specific physical information. The cognitive influence may disproportionately increase when symptoms are neither clear nor specific but are associated with a harmful situation (Pennebaker, 1982).

During exacerbations of asthma, stimulation of receptors in airways or the chest wall, as well as chemoreceptors, provide afferent information indicating airways obstruction. If the initial encoding of this sensory information in terms of a match with mental representations in the memory falls short, additional information is sampled to constitute a 'clear' representation of the physical state. The following paragraphs describe how many factors may unconsciously influence symptom perception and favor either blunted or overperception of physical information. Conscious, selective monitoring for relevant information may contribute to the role of unconscious mechanisms, but this topic remains beyond the scope of this chapter (Cioffi, 1991).

The conscious awareness of symptoms and breathlessness are considered to be analogous, hence the term 'breathlessness perception' (Jones, 1992; Barnes, 1994). From a psychological viewpoint, Heim *et al.* (1972) emphasized that breathlessness comprises the awareness of airways obstruction and the reaction to this awareness. The reaction to particular physical information is a learned response. As elaborated later in this chapter, sensory information that is associated with (but not causally related to) airways obstruction is often integrated into the symptom–perception process and may enhance breathlessness. Hence, there can be two parallel systems: a circuit from actual airways obstruction to breathlessness, and a circuit from perceived physical information to breathlessness. These different pathways are better known as 'bottom-up' and 'top-down' directed processing of sensory information. By relying on learned cues that are merely secondary to asthma, blunted perception could occur when these learned cues are occasionally absent during actual airways obstruction.

The distinction between different perceptual systems was clearly suggested by two signal detection experiments. Both used the same apparatus to block airflow externally in adolescents with asthma. The accuracy of detection correlated significantly with the intensity of airflow obstruction, whereas breathlessness related only modestly to intensity (Rietveld *et al.*, 1996b). Obviously, different levels of perceptual consciousness may differentially influence the outcome of the symptom perception process (Hoelzl *et al.*, 1996).

Simon *et al.* (1990) interpreted their experimental results in terms of the possibility that different respiratory conditions are associated with different 'types' of breathlessness. These differences could primarily be accounted for by psychological influences. The following subsections describe the three major psychological factors that influence symptom perception.

Internal versus External Cues

The concept of a 'competition between internal and external cues' (or asthmatic versus nonasthmatic cues in the current context) has been proposed to explain differences in symptom perception (Pennebaker & Lightner, 1980). Because the human capacity to process sensory information is limited, the probability of detecting internal cues depends on the ratio between available internal and external information. Pennebaker (1982) extrapolated their experimental results to lifestyle and use of medicines. However, in general, the experimental support for the concept of a competition of cues is limited. Presumably, the meaning of sensory information as perceived by a subject, i.e., in terms of learned possible harm, will stimulate cognitive elaboration in favor of internal cues, thus reducing the role of the concept (Fillingim *et al.*, 1988; Williams & Lees-Haley, 1993). The accuracy of signal detection in an experiment with external airflow obstruction was actually improved during external distraction. The presentation of film clips reduced the number of false responses among asthmatics, but not their correct responses (Rietveld *et al.*, 1997b). This shows that, in patients with a chronic disease, the learned meaning of particular information may be dominant, thus emphasizing the impact of acquired response tendencies in symptom perception.

Acquired Response Tendencies

The lay assumption might be that the accuracy of symptom perception increases with the acquisition of knowledge of, and experience with, a disease (Bishop, 1987; Pennebaker, 1982). Consequently, patients with chronic diseases and a long history of symptoms would be more accurate in symptom perception than novices. In clinical reality, the opposite may often be true when the symptom perception in chronic disease becomes less accurate over time. The increase of selective perceptual mechanisms and other acquired response tendencies, structured in illness schemata, would be the major reason for this decline. Although acquired response tendencies may be adaptive in many patients, a minority would respond toward blunted or overperception of physical information. Clinical observations by Yellowlees and Ruffin (1989) have confirmed the existence of two contradictory coping strategies in adults with a near-fatal asthma experience: either they were highly anxious and excessive users of medicines or they ignored symptoms and neglected their asthma. Acquired symptom perception tendencies would be mediators between previous experience with symptoms and current coping with symptoms.

At least six acquired response tendencies can be distinguished.

1. Selective processing and cognitive elaboration of information that possibly refers to asthma enhances the likelihood that symptoms of asthma are perceived (Pennebaker & Skelton, 1981; Rietveld & Prins, 1998a).

2. The asthma-congruent interpretation of nonasthma-related information may certainly enhance breathlessness (Dirks & Schraa, 1983; Rietveld & Prins, 1998b). This implies that indirect, situational information or associated physical information is interpreted in terms of asthma and contributes to breathlessness. Children with asthma in a physical exercise setting reported unrealistically high breathlessness after receiving false feedback of negative lung-function information or respiratory 'wheezing' sounds, suggestive of airways obstruction (Rietveld *et al.*, 1996a, 1997).

3. The repression of sensory information associated with symptoms of asthma has been proposed to explain blunted symptom perception (Steiner *et al.*, 1987). Confirming this proposition remains a problem. The difference between repression and inaccurate symptom perception on the one hand, and conscious neglect of symptoms on the other, remains possibly beyond testing.

4. Some patients with asthma seem to be aware of airways obstruction but are not bothered by it. Previous experiences and perceived control over symptoms could be decisive influences in the neglect of asthma symptoms and coincide with the absence of negative emotions (Wilson & Jones, 1991; Rietveld, 1997).

5. Both blunted and overperception of physical information may be the result of a false interpretation of physical information. As Cioffi (1991) pointed out, noxious sensations cannot be ignored for long, and attempts to distract from them either ultimately or intermittently fail. Considering

that sensory input is elaborated beyond cortical control, 'repression' or neglect of serious symptoms of asthma could possibly be incurred through false interpretation of signals. What happens is that signals of airways obstruction are interpreted in terms of general sensations, such as fatigue, hyperventilation, irritability, or flu (Dirks & Schraa, 1983; Rietveld & Prins, 1998b). With respect to overperception, the opposite effect would be involved. Signals underlying general sensations, associated with airways obstruction, are interpreted as signals of airways obstruction. In other words, general sensations are mistaken for breathlessness or vice versa (Rietveld & Prins, 1998a; Rietveld *et al.*, 1999a).

6. Habituation to physical information may occasionally explain blunted perception of airways obstruction. In a study with normal adults, breathlessness in some subjects decreased after prolonged exposure to external airflow obstruction, supporting the possible involvement of habituation (Rietveld, 1997). In clinical practice, habituation and behavioral adaptation are difficult to distinguish. Patients who diminish the metabolic demand of oxygen by keeping calm may feel less breathless than those pacing up and down in distress (Bonnel *et al.*, 1987).

Overall, the effect of perceptual mechanisms on overperception would be most apparent in an ambiguous situation with asthmatics being uncertain about the condition of their airways. The influence of indirect or situational information in symptom perception could be restricted to information that matches established stimulus–response relationships or existing expectations (Rietveld & Prins, 1998a). The influence of perceptual mechanisms in blunted perception is less clear, but situational factors could be decisive. It is the context that may trigger selective perceptual mechanisms and give direction to processing of information.

In an attempt to demonstrate that context or situational effects on symptom perception can be automatic and unconscious, cough responses were manipulated in asthma patients (Rietveld, Van Beest & Everaerd, 2000). One patient group was recruited for asthma research, presented to them as the determination of cough thresholds. A second group of patients was recruited without reference to asthma and the experiment was presented as signal detection, that is the estimation of flavors. Actually, participants from both groups underwent the same procedure: inhalation of doubling concentrations of citric acid to evoke cough. The results showed that participants in the asthma condition coughed significantly more often, and reported more 'tendency to cough' than participants in the signal detection condition. Clearly, the experimental context dominated the intensity of objective and subjective cough responses. Thus, a particular situation or setting that patients have learned to associate with symptoms may unconsciously dominate symptom perception.

Moreover, asthmatics who have learned to rely on indirect information or secondary symptoms would be vulnerable to blunted perception when such cues are absent.

In summary, symptoms may often be the interpretation of aspecific sensations in a particular context. Perceptual mechanisms may have an immense impact in symptom perception. In clinical reality, this influence is usually associated with negative emotions. Consequently, emotions may interact with perceptual mechanisms in complex patterns (Easterling & Leventhal, 1989; Rietveld & Prins, 1998b).

Negative Emotions

Negative emotions influence the process of symptom perception but are also a distinct concomitant of breathlessness. Although the subjective sensations during asthma exacerbations are assessed in the single sensation of breathlessness, factor analysis showed that breathlessness may comprise up to five distinct factors, with a dominance of worry and negative emotions (Brooks *et al.*, 1989). Clinical observations may confirm that negative emotions can completely dominate the subjective expression of asthma (Dirks *et al.*, 1982; Wilson & Jones, 1991; Lehrer *et al.*, 1993). Approximately two-thirds of children undergo panic when noticing the first signs of airways obstruction (Janson *et al.*, 1994). Naturally this affects a subjective state such as breathlessness.

The multifactorial structure of breathlessness subscribes to the suggestion that different factors in breathlessness are associated with different respiratory conditions (Simon *et al.*, 1990). In other words, the presence of factors such as emotions alone may account for a discordance between breathlessness and airways obstruction. When, for instance, anxiety increases, the relationship between breathlessness and lung function changes and so does the accuracy of symptom perception.

Subjects in the carbon dioxide study by Banzett *et al.* (1990) admitted that the 'air hunger' during induced hypercapnia was 'colored' by test anxiety and discomfort. They felt various sensations such as warmth, pounding heart, irritability, and headache. Although they claimed that these sensations did not actually contribute to breathlessness, it is doubtful that subjects can reliably differentiate the concomitants of how they feel. For example, adolescents with asthma in an exercise setting could not distinguish induced itching and breathlessness, and somehow 'added' these sensations when reporting excessive breathlessness (Rietveld *et al.*, 1999a). Either way, emotional influences are likely to dominate the symptom perceptual process in many patients with asthma. Six overlapping influences of emotions can be distinguished.

1. Emotions interfere with perception. The accuracy of symptom perception correlates negatively with emotional state (Hudgel *et al.*, 1982; Spinhoven *et al.*, 1997). However, although anxiety interferes unconsciously with perception, worry and modest anxiety may instigate conscious monitoring. Although the latter may often result in overperception of symptoms, quite often patients may accurately evaluate the state of their airways (Rietveld, 1998).

2. Emotional distress and breathlessness overlap broadly. Negative emotions directly enhance the magnitude of breathlessness. The negation would be that the absence of negative emotions may result in low levels or even absence of breathlessness, irrespective of airways obstruction. This could thereby explain blunted symptom perception (Rietveld & Prins, 1998b). An indication of this effect was observed in an experiment where normal control subjects reported very modest breathlessness during an extreme external airflow obstruction, analogous to a reduction of 64% in lung function (Rietveld, 1997). The subjects could take off the face mask when feeling distressed, probably decreasing anxiety and improving control over symptoms.

3. Some researchers have suggested that a subgroup of patients with asthma may repress symptoms of asthma (see earlier subsection Acquired Response Tendencies). An explanation would be that negative emotions associated with asthma are inhibited in order to prevent the occurrence of emotion-induced asthma attacks (Hollaender & Florin, 1983; Yellowlees & Kalucy, 1990). Although the existence of emotion-induced airways obstruction is a topic of dispute, patients themselves (65%) believe in the effect of emotion on their symptoms of asthma (Busse *et al.*, 1995; Rietveld *et al.*, 1999b). The secondary effect of repressed or inhibited emotions would be that symptoms of asthma attract less attention, thereby increasing the likelihood of blunted perception (Rietveld & Brosschot, 1999).

4. Asthmatics in a negative emotional state are inclined to evaluate the severity of asthma symptoms negatively (Costa & McCrae, 1987). Watson and Pennebaker (1989) argued that patients with high levels of negative affectivity would be vulnerable to excessive self-reporting of their physical symptoms.

5. Dirks and colleagues (Dirks *et al.*, 1982; Dirks & Schraa, 1983) assumed that negative emotions can be falsely interpreted as symptoms of asthma: example emotions would be worry, irritability, and anxiety.

6. Emotions that are associated with asthma may trigger selective symptom–perception processes, and facilitate breathlessness even when there is no airways obstruction. Rietveld and Prins (1998b) hypothesized that the occurrence of negative emotions, associated with asthma, may facilitate biased symptom perception. They compared breathlessness in children with asthma in four experimental conditions and observed the highest breathlessness in children in whom negative emotions were induced first, and general symptoms after physical exercise second. The effect was attributed to negative emotions enhancing the probability that exercise-related general symptoms, such as fatigue, sighing, and heart pounding, were interpreted in terms of asthma, thus enhancing breathlessness.

It can be concluded that emotional influences can determine symptom perception from various directions and often in subtle ways. Because of many overlapping and interacting factors, it usually remains very difficult to attribute manifestations of symptom perception to emotional influences. In a recent study on the effect of stress on asthma symptoms, adolescents, both with and without asthma, reported high levels of stress and negative emotions. However, only adolescents with asthma experienced breathlessness, which could not be accounted for by changes in lung function or blood gas values (Rietveld *et al.*, 1999b). In fact, all subjects with asthma at least doubled self-reported breathlessness, and the mean values increased from 0.3 to 4.9 points on a 10-point scale. Three girls actually believed that they were having an asthma attack and could hardly believe that there was objectively nothing wrong with their airways. In the light of scores on state and trait anxiety, this study highlighted that emotional dominance in asthma is to be expected in each patient and not particularly in those with emotional problems, neuroticism, or somatoform disorder.

Methodological Factors

Although methodological factors have nothing to do with actual symptom perception, their influence may affect empirical conclusions about symptom perception.

Green & Swets (1966) stressed that at least 100 or more stimulus–response pairs are required for the proper assessment of a subject's perceptual capacity. This criterion is impossible to accomplish with the method of relating lung function to breathlessness. Generally, only a few observations are made and the conclusion about the accuracy of symptom perception is based on the difference between pretest and posttest measures. Moreover, the assessment of airways obstruction by means of forced lung-function parameters should often be questioned. These measures involve the motivation of subjects, and thereby violate methodological criteria. Although lung-function testing is a generally accepted method, some patients may develop airways obstruction after forced breathing maneuvers during testing (Moran, 1991).

The assessment of breathlessness has also been the subject of serious critiques, centering around multifactorial sensations measured with the single measure of breathlessness, and a modest test–retest reliability of scales (Morton *et al.*, 1983; Killian, 1988; Skevington *et al.*, 1997). The problems associated with the assessment of airways obstruction and breathlessness are joined in symptom perception research, probably affecting the credibility of conclusions. On the other hand, the external validity of signal detection experiments for actual asthma may be questioned (Yamamoto *et al.*, 1978; Kelsen *et al.*, 1981). Signal detection experiments may have little validity with respect to actual asthma attacks. Labored breathing through a mouthpiece may be exhausting or unpleasant but may often be distinct from the suffering during an actual asthma attack.

The third method of studying symptom perception, the estimation of lung function, hardly resembles the natural perception of airways obstruction. Estimating physical performance is different from reporting breathlessness, as has been shown by Silverman *et al.* (1987). These researchers successfully trained asthmatic patients to estimate their lung function better, but they were not able to get them to report breathlessness accurately during fluctuations in lung function (Silverman *et al.*, 1987). The main problem with symptom perception of asthma under natural circumstances may be the unexpected occurrence of symptoms when there is no research assistant prompting introspection for lung-function estimation.

As a general disadvantage, convergent measures in symptom perception research are rarely available. Some good exceptions may be lung sound analysis and blood gas analysis for lung-function testing and a battery of questionnaires for the assessment of breathlessness (Rietveld & Dooijes, 1996; Skevington *et al.*, 1997).

In summary, symptom perception research leaves much to be desired. New methods should be found to heighten the validity of measuring variables. In this respect, the in-vivo assessment of symptoms and physical signs is promising because many methodological problems are avoided. However, obstacles are a lack of asthma exacerbations, excessive consumption of time and effort, and patient compliance.

Improving Symptom Perception

The influence of psychological factors in inaccurate symptom perception may suggest that patients can learn to improve their perception of airways obstruction. Remarkably, there have been only modest attempts to improve actual symptom perception (Silverman *et al.*, 1987). A first method seems to be information about symptom perception, possibly with some insight into the perceptual characteristics of a given patient. Unfortunately, it seems to be the case that indicating to patients the perceptual errors they are likely to make does not actually prevent these errors from being made during subsequent occasions. Gonder-Frederick & Cox (1991) reported the case of a woman with diabetes who consistently interpreted headache as an indication of excessive blood glucose, and continued to do so after she had been informed of her false interpretation. It should be noted that research in asthma is not available.

Harver (1994) successfully trained subjects to detect the presence of resistive loads during breathing through external apparatus by giving them feedback about load presentation. The effect of this training was similar in patients with asthma and normal controls. Stout *et al.* (1993) achieved comparable results with a sample of normal controls. It seems clear that patients with asthma can be taught to estimate aspects of their own respiration under laboratory conditions; however, this does not automatically mean that they also learn to better perceive actual airways obstruction. It seems important to test the degree to which laboratory tests can predict the accuracy of symptom perception under natural circumstances.

The use of peak flow meters in the assessment of lung function by patients themselves is widely accepted in Western society. These handy devices can be used on a regular basis and provide insight in fluctuations in airways obstruction. Moreover, peak flow meters are used when patients feel unhealthy and the peak expiratory flow rate should be the basis for bronchodilator medication or emergency room (ER) visit. In other words, although patients may be capable of properly perceiving airways obstruction, the results of objective assessment should be preferred. There are two problems. First, patients may grow careless in the proper handling of the device, particularly children. Secondly, patients have a tendency to stop using the peak flow meter after a period without symptoms. The question as to whether the use of peak flow meters eventually improves symptom perception has been confirmed by some studies, but rebutted by Silverman *et al.* (1987).

Training patients with asthma to improve their symptom perception may have a general effect that they become more involved with their disease and hence become vulnerable for an overperception of symptoms. False positive responses from an evolutionary perspective are probably less adverse than are false negative responses ('blunted' perception), although the implication may be that patients become overly anxious and preoccupied with their symptoms. Ignoring the problem of inaccurate symptom perception, however, increases the risks for ER visits and fatal asthma. More research is obviously required to guide the way for patients and healthcare providers.

Conclusions and Recommendations

Physiological factors and secondary symptoms are determinants of the perception of airways obstruction in asthma, although they cannot sufficiently explain the various manifestations of inaccurate symptom perception. The respiratory adjustments to compensate for metabolic demands during airways obstruction are insufficiently copied to the sensory cortex. Consequently, the physical information underlying breathlessness is often neither clear nor specific. However, human beings are equipped to cognitively and emotionally elaborate on sensory information associated with a harmful situation such as asthma. Psychological factors may influence symptom perception by means of (a) a competition of cues, influencing the unconscious flow of sensory information; (b) response tendencies based on the learned meaning of information as patients have stored it in the memory; and (c) negative emotions. Patients are bound to make mistakes when integrating indirect, external information or physical signs secondary to airways obstruction in their symptom perception. The output of the symptom perception process is a response which can be inaccurate in opposite directions: i.e., blunted perception or overperception of physical information. In other words, although extensive elaboration of information may be adaptive in many patients with asthma, a minority is bound to make perceptual mistakes. It is almost certain that all patients with asthma are vulnerable to a biased perception of asthma-related information.

Several recommendations for asthma management can be drawn. The clinical application of assessing the accuracy of symptom perception in individual asthmatics should be recommended. Testing the perceptual accuracy may be particularly relevant for asthmatics who commonly complain of symptoms secondary to asthma, i.e., dizziness, fatigue, or irritability. When impaired symptom perception can be expected, continuous medication should be preferred over 'if needed' bronchodilator medication. Regular assessment of peak expiratory flow with a mini peak flow meter should be a basis for 'if needed' medication. Peak flow assessment can be particularly warranted when asthmatics feel themselves weak or sick, or complain of having a cold or the flu. There is evidence that asthmatics are most vulnerable to impaired symptom perception when they are emotionally aroused. Consequently, the assessment of negative emotions in asthmatics can be essential and instigates specific intervention.

Some methodological points of attention in future research would be

1 Subjects should be naive with respect to the aims of a study and should not be aware of the importance of their motivation to perform.
2 Actual asthma attacks can not be replaced by analogous methods. Even the induction of actual airways obstruction precludes that natural, everyday responses can be measured.
3 Emotions should be measured in symptom perception research; these comprise self-reported emotions and physiological measures of emotional arousal.
4 Convergent measures for both subjective and objective variables of asthma should be included.
5 Respiratory variables should be assessed, particularly the respiratory frequency and breathing pattern.

Acknowledgment

The authors thank Cedric Sands and James Boutos for commenting on drafts of the manuscript.

References

Adams, L., Lane, R., Shea, S.A., Cockcroft, A. & Guz, A. (1985). Breathlessness during different forms of ventilatory stimulation: a study of mechanisms in normal subjects and respiratory patients. *Clinical Science*, 69, 663–672.

Ahles, T., Blanchard, E. & Leventhal, H. (1983). Cognitive control of pain: attention to the sensory aspects of the cold pressor stimulus. *Cognitive Therapy and Research*, *7*, 159–177.

Bagg, L.R. & Hughes, D.T.D. (1980). Diurnal variation in peak expiratory flow rate in asthmatics. *European Journal of Respiratory Disease*, 61, 298–302.

Bandura, A. (1990). Perceived self-efficacy in the exercise of control over AIDS infection. In: K.L. Kaemingle & L. Sechrist (Eds), *The primary prevention of AIDS: psychological approaches* (pp. 128–141). Newbury Park: Sage.

Banzett, R.B., Lansing, R.W., Reid, M.B., Adams, L. & Brown, R. (1989). 'Air hunger' arising from increased PCO_2 in mechanically ventilated quadriplegics. *Respiration Physiology*, 76, 53–68.

Banzett, R.B., Lansing, R.W., Brown, R., *et al.* (1990). 'Air hunger' from increased PCO_2 persists after complete neuromuscular block in humans. *Respiration Physiology*, 81, 1–18.

Barnes, P.J. (1994). Blunted perception and death from asthma (editorial comments). *New England Journal of Medicine*, 330, 1383–1384.

Bishop, G. (1987). Lay conceptions of physical symptoms. *Journal of Applied Social Psychology*, 17, 127–146.

Bonnel, A.M., Mathiot, M.J., Jungas, B. & Grimaud, C. (1987). Breathing discomfort in asthma: role of adaptation level. *Bulletin Europeèn de Physiopathology Respiratoire*, 23, 23–29.

Boulet, L.P., Deschesnes, F., Turcotte, H. & Gignac, F. (1991). Near fatal asthma, clinical and physiologic features, perception of broncho-constriction and psychologic profile. *Journal of Allergy and Clinical Immunology*, 88, 838–846.

Brooks, C.M., Richards, E.J., Bailey, W.C., Martin, B., Windsor, R.A. & Soong, S.J. (1989). Subjective symptomatology of asthma in an outpatient population. *Psychosomatic Medicine*, 51, 102–108.

Burdon, J.G.W., Juniper, E.F., Killian, K.J., Hargreave, F.E. & Campbell, E.J.M. (1982). The perception of breathlessness in asthma. *American Review of Respiratory Disease*, 126, 825–828.

Burki, N.K., Mitchel, K., Chaudhary, B.A., Zechman, F.W. & Campbell, E.J.M. (1978). The ability of asthmatics to detect added resistive loads. *American Review of Respiratory Disease*, 117, 71–00.

Busse, W.W., Kiecolt-Glaser, J.K., Coe, C., Martin, R.J., Weiss, S.T. & Parker, S.R. (1995). NHLBI workshop summary: stress and asthma. *American Journal of Respiratory and Critical Care Medicine*, 151, *249–252.*

Campbell, E.J.M., Godfrey, T.J.H., Clark, T.J.H., Freedman, S. & Norman, J. (1969). The effect of muscular paralysis induced by tubocurarine on the duration and sensation of breath-holding during hypercapnia. *Clinical Science*, 36, 323–328.

Carr, R.E., Lehrer, P.M. & Hochron, S.M. (1992). Panic symptoms in asthma and panic disorder: a preliminary test of the dyspnea-fear theory. *Behaviour, Research and Therapy*, 30, 251–261.

Chang, A.B., Phelan, P.D., Sawyer, S.M., ElBrocco, S. & Robertson, F. (1997). Cough sensitivity in children with asthma, recurrent cough, and cystic fibrosis. *Archives of Disease in Childhood*, 77, 331–334.

Chang, K.C., Morrill, C.G. & Chai, H. (1978). Impaired response to hypoxia after bilateral carotid body resection for treatment of bronchial asthma. *Chest*, 73, 667–669.

Cioffi, D. (1991). Beyond attentional strategies: a cognitive perceptual model of somatic interpretation. *Psychological Bulletin*, 109, 25–41.

Clark, T.J.H., Godfrey, S. & Lee, T.H. (Ed.) (1992). *Asthma*. London: Chapman and Hall.

Costa, P.T. Jr. & McCrae, R.R. (1987). Neuroticism, somatic complaints and disease; is the bark worse than the bite? *Journal of Personality*, 55, 299–316.

Côté, J., LeBlanc, P. & Boulet, L.P. (1987). Perception of bronchospasm in normal and asthmatic subjects. *American Review of Respiratory Disease*, 135, 231–000.

Creer, T.L. (1983). Response: self-management psychology and the treatment of childhood asthma. *Journal of Allergy and Clinical Immunology*, 72, 607–610.

Creer, T.L. (1987). Self-management in the treatment of childhood asthma. *Journal of Allergy and Clinical Immunology*, 80, 500–506.

Creer, T.L. & Gustafson, K.E. (1989). Psychological problems associated with drug therapy in childhood asthma. *Journal of Pediatrics*, 115, 850–855.

De Backer, W., Bogaert, E., Van Maele, R. & Vermeire, P. (1983). Effect of almitrine bismesylate on arterial blood gases and ventilatory drive in patients with severe chronic airflow obstruction and bilateral carotid body resection. *European Journal of Respiratory Disease*, 126, 239–242.

Dirks, J.F. & Schraa, J.C. (1983). Patient mislabelling of symptoms and rehospitalization in asthma. *Journal of Asthma*, 20, 43–44.

Dirks, J.F., Schraa, J.C. & Robinson, S.K. (1982). Patients mislabelling of symptoms: implications for patient–physician communication and medical outcome. *International Journal of Psychiatry in Medicine*, 12, 15–27.

Easterling, D.V. & Leventhal, H. (1989). Contribution of concrete cognition to emotion: neutral symptoms as elicitors of worry about cancer. *Journal of Applied Psychology*, 74, 787–796.

Ergood, J.S., Epstein, L.H., Ackerman, M. & Fireman, P. (1985). Perception of expiratory flow by asthmatics and non-asthmatics during rest and exercise. *Health Psychology*, 4, 545–554.

Fillingim, R.B., Roth, D.L. & Haley, W.E. (1988). The effects of distraction on the perception of exercise-induced symptoms. *Journal of Psychosomatic Research*, 33, 241–248.

Freestone, C. & Eccles, R. (1997). Assessment of the antitussive efficacy of codeine in cough associated with common cold. *Journal of Pharmacy and Pharmacology*, 49, 1045–1049.

Fritz, G.K., Klein, R.B. & Overholser, J.C. (1990). Accuracy of symptom perception in childhood asthma. *Developmental Behavior in Pediatrics*, 11, 69–72.

Gandevia, S.C., Killian, K.J. & Campbell, E.J.M. (1981). The effect of respiratory muscle fatigue on respiratory sensations. *Clinical Science*, 60, 463–466.

Garden, G.M. & Ayres, J.G. (1993). Psychiatric and social aspects of brittle asthma. *Thorax*, 48, 501–505.

Gonder-Frederick, L.A. & Cox, D.J. (1991). Symptom perception, symptom beliefs, and blood glucose discrimination in the self-treatment of insulin-dependent diabetes. In: J.A. Skelton and R.T. Croyle (Eds), *Mental representation in health and illness* (pp. 220–246). New York: Springer.

Gottfried, S.B., Altose, M.D., Kelsen, S.G. & Cherniack, N.S. (1981). Perception of changes in airflow resistance in obstructive pulmonary disorders. *American Review of Respiratory Disease*, 124, 566.

Green, D.M. & Swets, J.A. (1966). *Signal detection theory and psychophysics*. New York: Wiley.

Harver, A. (1994). Effects of feedback on the ability of asthmatic subjects to detect increases in the flow-resistive component to breathing. *Health Psychology*, 13, 52–62.

Harver, A., Humphries, C.T. & Baker, D. (1993). Perception of added resistive loads in children with asthma. *American Journal of Respiratory & Critical Care Medicine*, 155, A260.

Heim, E., Blaser, A. & Waidelich, E. (1972). Dyspnea: psychophysiologic relationships. *Psychosomatic Medicine*, 34, 405–423.

Higgs, C.M.B. & Laszlo, G. (1996). Influence of treatment with beclomethasone, cromoglycate, and theophylline. *Clinical Science*, 90, 227–234.

Hoelzl, R., Erasmus, L.P. & Moeltner, A. (1996). Detection, discrimination and sensation of visceral stimuli. *Biological Psychology*, 42, 199–214.

Hollaender, J. & Florin, I. (1983). Expressed emotion and airway conductance in children with bronchial asthma. *Journal of Psychosomatic Research*, 27, 307–311.

Hudgel, H.D., Cooperson, D.M. & Kinsman, R.A. (1982). Recognition of added resistive loads in asthma; the importance of behavioral styles. *American Review of Respiratory Disease*, 126, 121–125.

Isenberg, S., Lehrer, P. & Hochron, S. (1997). Defensiveness and perception of external inspiratory resistive loads in asthma. *Journal of Behavioral Medicine*, 20, 461–472.

Janson, C., Bjornsson, E., Hetta, J. & Boman, G. (1994). Anxiety and depression in relation to respiratory symptoms and asthma. *American Journal of Respiratory & Critical Care Medicine*, 149, 930–934.

Janson-Bjerklie, S., Ruma, S.S., Stulbarg, M., Kohlman, K. & Carrieri, V.K. (1987). Predictors of breathlessness intensity in asthma. *Nursing Research*, 36, 179–183.

Jones, P.W. (1992). Breathlessness perception in airways obstruction. *European Respiratory Journal*, 5, 1035–1036.

Kelsen, S.G., Prestel, T.F., Cherniack, N.S., Chester, E.H. & Chandler Dale, E. (1981). Comparison of the respiratory responses to external resistive loading and broncho constriction. *Journal of Clinical Investigation*, 67, 1761–1768.

Kikuchi, Y., Okabe, S., Tamura, G., *et al.*. (1994). Chemosensitivity and perception of dyspnea in patients with a history of near-fatal asthma. *New England Journal of Medicine,* 330, 1329–1234.

Killian, K.J. (1988). Assessment of dyspnoea. *European Respiratory Journal*, 1, 195–197.

Killian, K.J., Gandevia, S.C., Summers, E. & Campbell, E.J.M. (1984). Effect of increased lung volume on perception of breathlessness, effort and tension. *Journal of Applied Physiology*, 57, 686–691.

Kotses, H., Lewis, P. & Creer, T.L. (1980). Environmental control of asthma self-management. *Journal of Asthma*, 27, 375–384.

Lacroix, J.M., Martin, B., Avendano, M. & Goldstein, R. (1991). Symptom schemata in chronic respiratory patients. *Health Psychology*, 10, 268–273.

Lehrer, P.M., Isenberg, S. & Hochron, S.M. (1993). Asthma and emotion: a review. *Journal of Asthma*, 30, 5–21.

Lougheed, M.D., Lam, M., Forkert, L., Webb, C.A. & O'Donnall, D.E. (1993). Breathlessness during acute bronchoconstriction in asthma; pathophysiologic mechanisms. *American Review of Respiratory Disease*, 148, 1452–1459.

MacBugler, M., Roberts, P.D. & Spirer, J.P.(1993). The effect of arterial oxygen desaturation on six minute walk distance perceived effort and perceived breathlessness in patients with airflow limitation. *Thorax*, 48, 33–38.

McFadden, E.R. (1984). Pathogenesis of asthma. *Journal of Allergy and Clinical Immunology*, 73, 413–424.

McFadden, E.R., Kiser, R. & de Groot, W.J. (1973). Acute bronchial asthma; relations between clinical and physiological manifestations. *New England Journal of Medicine*, 288, 221–225.

Marks, G.B., Yates, D.H., Sist, M., Ceyhan, B., De Campos, M., Scott, D.M. & Barnes, P.J. (1996). Respiratory sensation during bronchial testing with methacholine, sodium metabisulphite, and adenosine monophosphate. *Thorax*, 51, 793–799.

Moran, M.G. (1991). Psychological factors affecting pulmonary and rheumatologic disease. *Psychosomatics*, 32,14–23.

Morton, P.B., O'Neill, P.A., Stark, R.D. & Stretton, T.B.(1983). A demonstration of methods for studying breathlessness. *Journal of Physiology*, 342, 8–9.

Muers, M. (1993). Understanding breathlessness. *The Lancet*, 342, 1190–1191.

Nakayama, K. (1961). Surgical removal of the carotid body for bronchial asthma. *Diseases of the Chest,* 40, 593–604.

Noseda, A., Schmerber, J., Prigogine, T. & Yernault, J.C. (1992). Perceived effect on shortness of breath of an acute inhalation of saline or terbutaline: variability and sensitivity of visual analogue scale in patients with asthma and COPD. *European Respiratory Journal*, 5, 1043–1053.

Overholt, R.H. (1961). Glucomectomy for asthma. *Diseases of the Chest,* 40, 605–610.

Parisi, R.A., Croce, S.A., Edelman, N.H. & Santiago, T.V. (1987). Obstructive sleep apnea following bilateral carotid body resection. *Chest,* 91, 922–924.

Peiffer, C., Marsac, J. & Lockhart, A. (1989). Chrono-biological study of the relationship between dyspnoea and airway obstruction in symptomatic asthmatic subjects. *Clinical Science*, 77, 237–244.

Pennebaker, J.W. (1982). *The psychology of physical symptoms.* New York: Springer.

Pennebaker, J.W. & Lightner, J.M. (1980). Competition of internal and external information in an exercise setting. *Journal of Personality and Social Psychology*, 39, 165–174.

Pennebaker, J.W. & Skelton, J.A. (1981). Selective monitoring of physical sensations. *Journal of Personality and Social Psychology*, 41, 213–223.

Pennebaker, J.W., Burnam, M.A., Schaeffer, M.A. & Harper, D.C. (1977). Lack of control as a determinant of perceived physical symptoms. *Journal of Personality and Social Psychology*, 35, 167–174.

Petrie, K.J. & Weinman, J.A. (Eds) (1997). *Perceptions of health and illness.* Amsterdam: Harwood Academic Publishers.

Pratter, M.R. & Bartter, T. (1991). Dyspnea: time to find the facts. *Chest*, 100, 1187.

Reader, K.P., Dolce, J.J., Duke, L., Kazynski, J.M. & Bailey, W.C. (1990). Peakflow meters: are they monitoring tools or training devices? *Journal of Asthma*, 27, 219–227.

Remmers, J.E., Brooks, J.G. & Tenny, S.M. (1968). Effect of controlled ventilation on the tolerable limit of hypercapnia. *Respiration Physiology*, 4, 78–90.

Rietveld, S. (1997). Habituation to prolonged airflow obstruction. *Journal of Asthma*, 34, 133–140.

Rietveld, S. (1998). Symptom perception in asthma, a multidisciplinary review. *Journal of Asthma*, 35, 137–146.

Rietveld, S. & Brosschot, J.F. (1999). Current perspectives on symptom perception in asthma: a biomedical and psychological review. *International Journal of Behavioral Medicine*, 6, 120–134.

Rietveld, S. & Dooijes, E.H. (1996). Characteristics and diagnostic significance of wheezes during exercise-induced airway obstruction in children with asthma. *Chest*, 110, 624–631.

Rietveld, S. & Everaerd, W. (2000). Perceptions of asthma by adolescents at home. *Chest*, 117, 434–439.

Rietveld, S., Everaerd, W. & VanBeest, I. (1999a). Can biased symptom perception explain false-alarm choking sensations? *Psychological Medicine*, 29, 121–126.

Rietveld, S. & Prins, P.J.M. (1998a). Children's perceptions of physical symptoms; the example of asthma. *Advances in Clinical Child Psychology*, 20, 153–183.

Rietveld, S. & Prins, P.J.M. (1998b). The relationship between negative emotions and acute objective and subjective symptoms of childhood asthma. *Psychological Medicine*, 28, 407–415.

Rietveld, S. & Rijssenbeek-Nouwens, L.H.M. (1998). Diagnostic significance of cough in childhood asthma; results of continuous monitoring in the homes of children. *Chest*, 113, 50–54.

Rietveld, S., Kolk, A.M.M. & Prins, P.J.M. (1996a). The influence of lung function information on self-reports of dyspnoea by children with asthma. *Journal of Pediatric Psychology*, 21, 367–377.

Rietveld, S., Prins, P.J.M. & Colland, V.T. (2001). Accuracy of symptom perception in asthma and illness severity. *Children's Health Care*, 30, 27–41.

Rietveld, S., Prins, P.J.M. & Kolk, A.M.M. (1996b). The capacity of children with and without asthma to detect external resistive loads on breathing. *Journal of Asthma*, 33, 221–230.

Rietveld, S., Kolk, A.M.M., Colland, V.T. & Prins, P.J.M. (1997a). The influence of respiratory sounds on breathlessness in children with asthma: a symptom-perception approach. *Health Psychology*, 16, 546–553.

Rietveld, S., Kolk, A.M.M., Prins, P.J.M. & VanBeest, I. (1997b). The influence of external stimulation on airflow detection by children with and without asthma. *Psychology and Health*, 12, 553–563.

Rietveld, S., Everaerd, W. & VanBeest, I. (in press). Can biased symptom perception explain false-alarm choking sensations? *Psychological Medicine*.

Rietveld, S., VanBeest, I. & Everaerd, W. (1999b). Stress-induced breathlessness in asthma. *Psychological Medicine*, 29, 1359–1366.

Rubinfeld, A.R. & Pain, M.C.F. (1976). Perception of asthma. *The Lancet*, 2, 882–884.

Rubinfeld, A.R. & Pain, M.C.F. (1977). Conscious perception of bronchospasm as a protective phenomenon in asthma. *Chest*, 72, 154–000.

Saisch, S.G.N., Wessely, S. & Gardner, W.N. (1996). Patients with acute hyperventilation presenting to an inner city emergency department. *Chest*, 110, 952–957.

Silverman, B.A., Mayer, D., Sabinsky, R., *et al.* (1987). Training perception of airflow obstruction in asthmatics. *Annals of Allergy*, 59, 350–354.

Simon, P.M., Schwartzstein, R.M., Weiss, J.W., Fencl, V., Teghtsoonian, M. & Weinberger, S.E. (1990). Distinguishable types of dyspnea in patients with shortness of breath. *American Review of Respiratory Disease*, 142, 1009–1014.

Skevington, S.M., Pilaar, M., Routh, D. & MacLeod, R.D. (1997). On the language of breathlessness. *Psychology and Health*, 12, 677–689.

Sly, P.D., Landau L.L. & Weymouth, R. (1985). Home-recording of peak expiratory flow rates and perception of asthma. *American Journal of Diseases of Children*, 18, 479–482.

Spinhoven, P., Van Peski-Oosterbaan, A.S., VanderDoes, A.J.W., Willems, L.N.A. & Sterk, P.J. (1997). Association of anxiety with perception of histamine-induced bronchoconstriction in patients with asthma. *Thorax*, 52, 149–152.

Steiner, H., Higgs, C.M.B., Fritz, G.K., Lazlo, G. & Harvey, J.E. (1987). Defense style and the perception of asthma. *Psychosomatic Medicine*, 49, 35–44.

Stout, C., Kotses, H. & Creer, T.L. (1993). Improving recognition of respiratory sensations in healthy adults. *Biofeedback and Selfregulation*, 18, 79–92.

Sullivan, C.E. (1980). Bilateral carotid body resection in asthma: vulnerability to hypoxic death in sleep. *Chest, 78,* 354.

Turcotte, H., Corbeil, F. & Boulet, L. (1990). Perceptions of breathlessness during bronchoconstriction induced by antigen, exercise and histamine challenges. *Thorax*, 45, 914–918.

Watson, D. & Pennebaker, J.W. (1989). Health complaints, stress, and distress: exploring the central role of negative affectivity. *Psychological Review*, 96, 234–254.

Weiss, J.H. (1966). Moodstates associated with asthma in children. *Journal of Psychosomatic Research*, 10, 267–273.

Williams, C.W. & Lees-Haley, P.R. (1993) Perceived toxic exposure: a review of four cognitive influences on the perception of illness. *Journal of Social Behavior and Personality*, 8, 297–308.

Wilson, R.C. & Jones, P.W. (1990). Influence of prior ventilatory experience on the estimation of breathlessness during exercise. *Clinical Science*, 78, 149–153.

Wilson, R.C. & Jones, P.W. (1991). Differentiation between the intensity of breathlessness and the distress it evokes in normal subjects during exercise. *Clinical Science*, 80, 65–70.

Winter, B. (1972). Bilateral carotid body resection for asthma and emphysema. *International Surgery, 57,* 455, 458–466.

Winter, B. (1991). Carotid body resection in chronic obstructive pulmonary disease. *Chest,* 100, 883.

Wolkove, N., Dajozman, E., Coalacone, A., *et al.* (1992). Relationship between spontaneous dyspnoea and liability of airways obstruction in asthma. *Clinical Science*, 82, 717–724.

Yamamoto, H., Inaba, S., Nishimura, M., Kishi, F. & Kawakami, Y. (1978). Relationship between the ability to detect added resistance at rest and breathlessness during broncho-constriction in asthmatics. *Respiration*, 52, 42–48.

Yellowlees, P.M. & Kalucy, R.S. (1990). Psychobiological aspects of asthma and the consequent research implications. *Chest*, 97, 628–634.

Yellowlees, P.M. & Ruffin, R.E. (1989). Psychological defenses and coping styles in patients following a life-threatening attack of asthma. *Chest*, 95, 1298–1303.

6

Self-management and respiratory disorders: Guiding patients from health counseling and self-management perspectives

Ilse Mesters, Thomas L. Creer and Frans Gerards

Editors' note—*Self-management of respiratory disorders has emerged in the past two decades as an approach for not only prompting patients to assume greater responsibility for their disorder but also for assisting them to become allies with their health care providers in controlling their disease. Ilse Mesters, Frans Gerards, and Thomas Creer describe this exciting research. In doing so, they point out that self-management programs must be tailored for individual patients. While some patients require intensive training in self-management, others possess knowledge of their disorder that can serve as the basis for assisting them to be more effective in applying the skills they know.*

Bailey et al. (1999) recently found that when state-of-the-art care, based on asthma guidelines, is provided by a specialist physician knowledgeable about self-management techniques, extra patient education components may be unnecessary. This finding supports the suggestions of Ilse, Frans, and Tom in the chapter that follows; however, as they emphasize, the acquisition of knowledge does not automatically translate into improved performance. When people know how to manage their asthma or COPD (chronic obstructive pulmonary disease), the task shifts toward attaining a more difficult outcome: insuring patients acquire self-efficacy and outcome expectations that their performance can make a significant contribution to the management of their condition.

The importance of self-efficacy and outcome expectations in motivating performance cannot be overestimated; this is a theme that runs through the writings of Albert Bandura (e.g., Bandura, 1997). Perhaps the best illustration of this point, however, is found in a recent study by Cabana et al. (1999). Literally thousands of clinical guidelines have been issued in an attempt to improve the clinical management of various diseases, including asthma (e.g., National Institutes of Health, 1995). The guidelines are systematically developed statements designed to assist practitioners and patients to make decisions about appropriate health care for specific disorders and circumstances. Despite the wide promulgation, these guidelines have had limited effect in changing patient behavior (Cabana et al., 1999). These investigators set about to determine why clinical guidelines were not being followed; in particular, they were interested to reviewing barriers that interfered with physician adherence to practice guidelines.

A review of 76 articles revealed 120 surveys that described 293 potential barriers to physician compliance to clinical guidelines. A number of common barriers were found in this review. Several of the major barriers might have been expected – lack of awareness and familiarity with the guidelines, and agreement with their systematically developed statements. If a physician doesn't know about a set of guidelines or doesn't perceive that they fit a practice, it would not be anticipated that he or she would use the guidelines. However, the next two major barriers were somewhat unexpected: the lack of self-efficacy – the belief that one can actually perform a behavior – and the lack of outcome expectancy – the expectation that a given behavior will result in a particular consequence. The fact that these were major barriers to physicians adopting clinical guidelines illustrates again the schism between teaching someone what to do and actually having them perform what they are taught, a theme that weaves its way throughout the chapter.

Introduction

People with a chronic disorder, such as asthma or chronic obstructive pulmonary disease (COPD), need to change or adjust their behavior and/or environment to reduce or prevent discomfort and disability from their illness. Health care professionals – physicians, nurses, behavioral scientists, physiotherapists, and dietitians – play an important role in guiding patients. It is increasingly necessary that these professionals work in an interdisciplinary fashion to treat the patient. Varni (1983, p. 5) emphasizes that 'the interdisciplinary approach is synergistic, integrating the knowledge and skills from the various disciplines into a coordinated plan for patient care.' Such an approach assumes that all professionals have a working knowledge of the skills and expertise of other team members; it also suggests that all team members will, at one time or another, counsel the patient. Therefore, in this chapter, all professionals who work on interdisciplinary teams are referred to as health counselors.

Learning to deal with a respiratory disorder involves the development of a host of new behaviors, such as taking prescribed medications; other behaviors, already in the repertoire of patients must be increased. This would include, for example, asthma and COPD patients improving their physical condition by exercising on a regular basis. At other times, patients with a respiratory disorder must quit performing certain behaviors, such as smoking or knowingly exposing themselves to stimuli that exacerbate their disorder. Which behaviors are most relevant for patients to perform or not to perform can be discovered during conversations and interactions between health counselors and individual patients.

There is reasonable consensus about the relevant behaviors patients must perform to control symptoms and to ameliorate the impact of asthma (Krutzch *et al.*, 1987; Wilson-Pessano & Mellins, 1987). These behaviors can be summarized as falling into three categories (Clark & Starr-Schneidkraut, 1994): (a) prevention of asthma episodes/attacks; (b) episode/attack management; and (c) the development and performance of appropriate social skills. Prevention entails such behaviors as identifying and controlling triggers, recognizing early signs of asthma episodes/

attacks, acting on early signs to halt attacks, and taking prescribed medications properly and on schedule. Attack/episode management includes such skills as using peak flow meters to predict or verify attacks, taking as-needed medications as prescribed, resting and remaining calm, adjusting treatment in a stepwise manner, and following other strategies outlined in cooperation with health care providers. Social skills refer to interpersonal strategies, such as communication and information-seeking skills, that patients need to perform in order to control their disorder and to avoid disruption of their daily lives.

Asthma and COPD patients must perform many different behaviors to control their disorder. Adherence to the advice of health counselors varies widely among asthma patients. For example, the adherence of adult asthma patients to prescribed medications was estimated at between 50 to 60% (Horn *et al.*, 1989). The rates of adherence to medication regimens by children with asthma was shown to range from 2 to 100%; overall, however, the compliance rate was less than 50% (Creer, 1993). The rate of adherence for other behaviors, such as adherence to exercise prescriptions like breathing maneuvers, physical exercise, and outdoor physical activity, is similarly low (Van den Heuvel, 1994).

Nonadherence to the advice of health counselors can sometimes be considered as a conscious decision of a patient; when this is the case, the decision should be respected. However, the role of health counselors, no matter what their discipline, is to make every effort to help patients attain the goal of experiencing the best possible health and quality of life. For most patients, nonadherence is rarely a conscious decision; rather, it is a result of misconceptions and/or lack of knowledge or skills about what activity to do and how to do it, when to do the activity, how long to perform the activity, and why the activity is necessary (Mesters *et al.*, 1991).

The task of health counselors is to teach the patients whatever is necessary in order for them to adhere to medical and health care instructions and, as a consequence, attain the improved health and an enhanced quality of life. This chapter presents two behavioral models – the Health Counseling Model and the Self-Management Model – that can effectively guide health counselors in this respect. The Health Counseling Model describes steps that can be taken by health counselors to build on preexisting strengths of patients to help them manage a chronic disorder, such as COPD or asthma. Specifically, counselors must learn to recognize and utilize the knowledge and skills, already in the patients' behavioral repertoire, to generate cooperative strategies that patients can use to manage a chronic disorder effectively. The health counselor can achieve this with a minimal amount of instruction or intervention. The Self-Management Model outlines and teaches patients skills they can perform to help manage their asthma. In many cases, the model assumes that the patients lack the basic skills required for collaborative management of the disorder; under these conditions, exposure to a formal educational and intervention program is needed. In reality, the two models should be regarded as complementary to one another. Both models offer suggestions useful for targeted and systematic counseling for any given asthma or COPD patient. The aim of such counseling is to tailor individualized programs to teach each patient to perform, master, and maintain whatever behavioral skills are required to control either disorder.

Health Counseling Model

Earlier, we pointed out that all professionals who work with patients, no matter what their background or training, are health counselors. We also emphasized that the interdisciplinary model (Varni, 1983) posits that each professional should have a working knowledge of the skills and expertise of other members of the treatment team. Such a background is necessary for two reasons. First, it provides a common basis for counseling patients across disciplines. A behavioral scientist who understands why a particular medical treatment has been prescribed for a given asthma patient knows what to accentuate in her contacts with that patient. The patient might clarify, for example, why controller medications are taken to prevent attacks and as-needed medications are taken to abort exacerbations. The behavioral scientist might also provide instruction in assisting the patient to establish cues for taking drugs and to monitor his behavior. Secondly, current treatments of asthma and COPD are so sophisticated that it is no longer possible for members of one discipline to practice their skills without knowledge of a patient's treatment goals and the specific strategies devised to achieve the goals. For example, a behavioral scientist would not wish to design and implement a program to improve medication adherence unless she knew the specifics of the treatment regimen, including type, schedule, and dosage level of the drugs prescribed for the patient. Previous research suggests that without this information, a behavioral scientist might improve adherence to a regimen but unwittingly generate serious harm in a patient (Creer & Levstek, 1996).

The interdisciplinary approach to treatment insures that all members of the treatment team are on the same page, so to speak, with respect to the treatment of individual patients. It is the only approach to take to assure that systematic health counseling and the positive outcomes it produces occur.

Figure 6.1 depicts processes of the Health Counseling and Self-Management models. As shown, there is considerable overlap with respect to patient goals and the processes followed to achieve the goals. This could be expected, considering that the purpose of both models is to insure patients learn and perform the skills they need to help manage their condition.

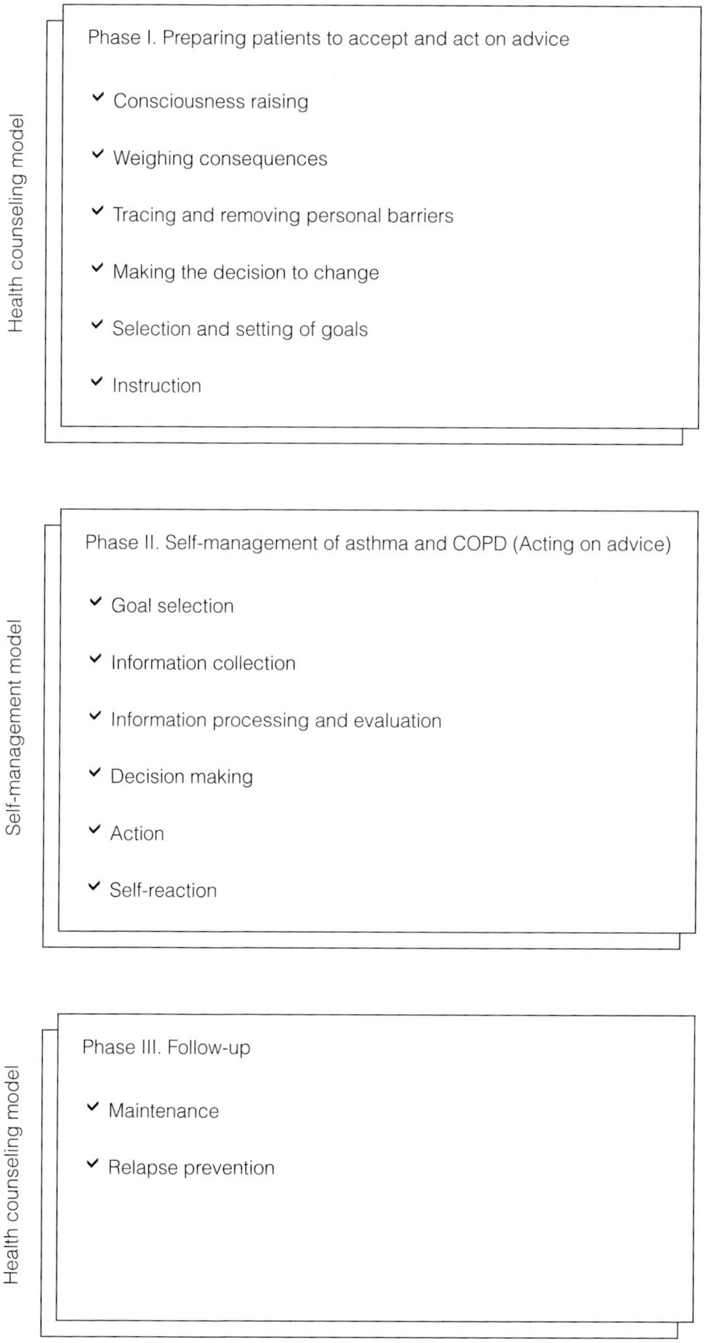

Health counseling model

Phase I. Preparing patients to accept and act on advice

- Consciousness raising
- Weighing consequences
- Tracing and removing personal barriers
- Making the decision to change
- Selection and setting of goals
- Instruction

Self-management model

Phase II. Self-management of asthma and COPD (Acting on advice)

- Goal selection
- Information collection
- Information processing and evaluation
- Decision making
- Action
- Self-reaction

Health counseling model

Phase III. Follow-up

- Maintenance
- Relapse prevention

Figure 6.1

The integration of processes of Health Counseling and Self-Management Models.

Characteristics of the two models permit elements of each to be used to complement one another. For example, components of the Self-Management Model can be added to the Health Counseling Model or, by the same token, preparatory steps of health counseling can be used prior to the introduction of self-management training. How each model is used – or how they are combined – depends upon a number of variables, including the unique characteristics and abilities of the individual patient.

With patients who appear less motivated to follow the suggested regimen or whose problems with managing asthma or COPD are unclear, for example, the Health Counseling Model would probably be the best model to use. The Health Counseling Model would also be the approach to use with patients who have already developed, in part through advice offered by health counselors, effective self-management skills and tactics to control their respiratory disorder. These are patients who, regardless of their illness, have consciously complied with their health counselors' advice and demonstrated they can manage their disorder in a successful manner. Formal self-management training with respect to asthma or other respiratory conditions might help them perform in a more systematic manner; indeed, these patients often volunteer for such programs because they want both to learn more about their disorder and to improve their management of the condition. However, in many cases, such patients and their health care providers may conclude that the time and costs of self-management training are not worth the limited benefits they anticipate will follow formal self-management training. We would agree with this conclusion because it is based upon empirical evidence, gathered by members of the treatment team, that the patient can generally manage his condition. In these cases, however, the Health Counseling Model would remain useful in reinforcing and maintaining the patient's performance.

Processes of Health Counseling

The processes of the Health Counseling Model are shown in Fig. 6.1. Significant processes in the model include (a) preparing the patient to accept and act on advice; (b) establishing goals; (c) patient action; and (d) providing follow-up to insure that the patient continues to follow and use advice provided by health counselors.

Preparing Patient to Accept and Act on Advice (Phase I)

Before patients are advised what to do, there are preparatory steps that should be considered by a health counselor. These include the following:

Consciousness Raising. Guidance by the health counselor in this phase is aimed at working with patients to optimize the chances of their accepting the need to modify their behavior, to produce change, and to maintain such behavioral adjustments. Success in consciousness raising implies that health counselors have the ability to communicate about the disorder at the reading and comprehension level of the patient. Health counselors must be constantly aware of the fact that they probably differ from a particular patient in many ways, including background, level of language, and perceptual perspective on the disease. As Anderson (1985, p. 32) cautioned, 'While many health-care practitioners see the treatment regimen as a solution, patients may see it as another part of the problem of having a chronic disease.' Attribution theory recognizes that health counselors and patients may have different beliefs about the cause of the illness, its severity, or the side effects of medication; these beliefs dictate how the patients will be treated (Weiner, 1986). For instance, during focus groups with parents of young children with asthma, it was revealed that parents believed that drug side effects were indicative of some kind of irreparable damage to the body; thus, parents thought that asthma medications should be avoided as much as possible (Mesters *et al.*, 1991). These beliefs were expressed, although most side effects of asthma medication can be considered as an inconvenience but are not damaging to patients. When this difference was explained to parents, their beliefs about the medication changed in a positive direction; these positive beliefs, in turn, improved medication adherence (Mesters *et al.*, 1994). Another common example of differing viewpoints between health counselors and patients is that a physician might consider a certain asthma patient as nonadherent because he took less medication as prescribed, while the same asthma patient might perceive himself as doing well because he is experiencing no symptoms or no increase of symptoms. Consciousness-raising activities are aimed at helping the asthma patient gain insight into how behaviors are related to the occurrence, the continuation, and the relief of asthma symptoms. Patient teaching is essential for consciousness raising, and for optimizing patients' knowledge about their condition.

Weighing Consequences: the Pros and Cons. In the second step of the preparation phase of the Health Counseling Model, the advantages (pros) and disadvantages (cons) of performing suggested behaviors should be discussed before goal selection occurs (Ajzen & Fishbein, 1980; Janz & Becker, 1984; Vries de & Mudde, 1998). Although health counselors tend to motivate people to change by using negative appeals such as fears they will die from a disorder, the literature shows that positive appeals, such as improved health and quality of life, are more likely to result in adherence. In general, it is suggested that negative appeals may provoke a social desirability bias; individuals may feel the need to say they understood the message and are changing their ways, but feel no motivation to actually change their behavior. Positive appeals make people feel better about themselves and can be persuasive in generating behavioral change (Monahan, 1995). For example, if COPD patients can be motivated to change their behavior, such as by quitting smoking and exercising more, specific goals for their treatment can be established. However, before goals can be set, it is necessary to discover what personal rewards help the patient both reach these goals and meet his personal expectations.

Tracing and Removing Personal Barriers. The next step in the preparation phase is concerned with tracing and removing barriers that might block a patient's decision to perform a behavior or set of behaviors. Barriers can be of diverse origins. A number of common barriers will be identified. Emotions, such as anxiety, guilt, shame, or pain, can block a decision to perform a behavior. For example, if an asthma or COPD patient has to exercise but fears getting out of breath, he will think twice before getting involved in such an activity. Some patients might believe they lack the willpower to adhere to a recommended medication schedule. An instance might be, 'I know I am sloppy, so I know that I will never take my medicines daily.' Other patients might underestimate their self-efficacy and say, 'I can take my medicine at home, but I am not sure whether I will manage when I am at school among friends.' Because patients have to perform behaviors, independent of health counselors, at home and in other areas of their environment, it is not enough for them to learn and practice skills; they also have to gain the confidence to apply these skills on a day-to-day basis (Bandura, 1986). To gain the confidence to apply skills, a graduated approach is required; we only acquire efficacy beliefs through successful performance, usually over a period of time. Sometimes, inadequate skills might block performance of a behavior: e.g., an asthma patient might incorrectly inhale medication while having an attack. Some beliefs or misconceptions might hinder the performance of self-management behaviors by a person, say, 'I should take those medicines, but I don't want to get dependent on them.' The social environment might hinder a patient in a couple of ways, including: 'My colleagues will laugh at me when I tell them not to smoke when I am there,' or 'I'll have nobody I can talk to when I don't feel like doing exercises.' Craving, especially, might be relevant for those patients who must quit smoking, 'I want to stop smoking, but when I don't have an alternative to relieve tension, I just have to smoke.' Finally, practical opportunities are sometimes missing through lack of money, time, or nearby gyms, or because of a busy lifestyle. If no barriers exist or existing barriers can be removed, the preparation phase can continue by setting specific goals and providing patient instruction. Thus, when patients have made a positive decision, the actual performance of the behavior can be discussed in more detail.

Making the Decision to Change. After patients have received advice from health counselors, they must decide if they are willing to act on the advice. This involves decision making. According to Janis and Mann (1978), a decision may be based on five decision-making steps. The steps emerged from research on people who displayed vigilance in reaching a difficult personal decision that they subsequently carried out successfully, such as giving up smoking, losing weight, or undergoing a prescribed medical treatment. As can be noted, the first steps show some overlap with the previous steps described in the Health Counseling Model. The decision-making steps are (1) appraising the challenge; (2) surveying alternatives; (3) weighing alternatives; (4) deliberating about commitment; and (5) adhering despite negative feedback. In step 1, a person is exposed to information about a threat or opportunity that effectively challenges a current course of action. This information can be an event that disturbs the person's equanimity because a particular threat can no longer be ignored, such as a significant drop in peak flow. Once the decision maker makes a positive response to the challenging information, such as 'I have to take action,' he proceeds to search for alternatives. Step 2 is largely devoted to discovering and selecting viable alternatives. Self-care algorithms might help patients in getting a quick overview of possible alternatives. In the case of experiencing a drop in peak flow, a patient might decide to get away from the trigger if possible, take medications, or decide that the problem requires medical attention. In step 3, the decision maker proceeds on to a thorough evaluation by focusing on the pros and cons of each of the options: the goal is to select the best-available course of action by weighing the advantages and disadvantages of each alternative. After the decision maker decides which is the best option, he begins to deliberate (step 4) about implementation and conveying his intentions to others. In the last stage (step 5), the decision maker implements his choice.

Selecting and Setting of Goals. As the Health Counseling model continues, it shows some overlap with the Self-Management Model (phase II, Fig. 6.1) in that both models explicitly stress the importance of goal selection. If a patient is made aware that a certain behavior, such as smoking, is responsible or related to the prevention, occurrence, and exacerbation or duration of airway symptoms, and the patient is motivated to change, the next step is to jointly select specific goals the health counselor and patient want to achieve by quitting smoking. It is essential that patients recognize that their active participation is required in selecting and setting goals. A study in the Netherlands showed that this process was often unclear to patients (Mesters *et al.*, 1991), who often believed that 'treating' asthma symptoms was something only doctors could do. Based on this finding, derived from focus group interviews with parents of children with asthma (0–4 years), new educational materials of the Netherlands Asthma Foundation explicitly state what information is required by patients if they are (a) to learn what to do and (b) to perform behaviors necessary to managing their asthma. After a goal has been jointly selected by health counselors and patients, the performance of whatever behaviors are required to attain the goal becomes the responsibility of the patient.

A goal can be defined as the end state which both patient and health counselor want to achieve; it concerns a valued and future destination (Lee *et al.*, 1989). Goals can vary by (a) degree of actual and/or perceived difficulty; (b) degree of specificity; and (c) degree of complexity (Strecher *et al.*, 1995). A prerequisite is that the respiratory patient should be interested in achieving a certain goal, such as to quit smoking or to take medications as prescribed. Mutual participation of the health counselor and the patient in setting goals provides information on whether or not a patient is interested in a certain outcome. Once a person is interested in achieving a goal, there is the assumption that setting goals to achieve a specific end state leads to higher performance than would occur, either with no set goals or with ambiguous goals. Another assumption is that the higher and more difficult the goals established for the patient, the less likely the patient is to attain them. The commitment of the patient toward attaining the goals may also be weaker; motivation to change is the prerequisite for the achievement of goals. To conclude, selected goals should be proximal, attainable, and specific (e.g., walk eight blocks three times a week for the next 2 months) in order to enable patients to implement and maintain the regimen (Burke & Dunbar-Jacob, 1995).

Instruction. Before patients can act on the advice they are provided by health counselors, they must learn about their respiratory condition. In most cases, patients' knowledge about asthma or COPD needs to be changed, particularly their misconceptions about the disorders. With respect to asthma, topics for education include basic knowledge about the disorder and how it can be prevented and/or managed. However, improving knowledge about asthma will not automatically result in behavioral change and improved control over the disorder; any acquired knowledge must be translated into performance (Bandura, 1986). Many attitudes patients have toward asthma also require change. Finally, patients invariably need training in order to perform selected behaviors, such as monitoring airway obstruction with a peak flow meter or taking medication via an inhaler. In monitoring peak flow or using an inhaler correctly, verbal instruction should be augmented with demonstration either by the health counselor or by utilizing other instructional media. Furthermore, providing opportunities for practice and demonstration during repeat visits must be considered as an educational strategy that will enable the asthma patient to implement a prescribed regimen.

When teaching patients during any interaction, it should be remembered that, as occurs with us all, the ability of patients to process information is limited. This implies that verbal instruction should be delivered in small amounts, should be specific to an activity, and should be distributed over time. In general, it is helpful to dispense printed instructions to reinforce verbal instructions. Joos & Hickham (1990), as suggested by social–psychological perspectives on patient–provider interactions, summarized primary behaviors for enhancing communication. For a detailed description of this approach, the reader is referred to the article by Joos & Hickham (1990) and to the publication by Burke & Dunbar-Jacob (1995).

In attempting to convey information, health counselors should be aware that research has shown that primacy information – information presented to patients first – and recency information – information presented last – is remembered best (Ley, 1982). A physician who wants a patient to remember when to take the medication will not present this information in the middle of the consultation. One approach, as suggested by Spector (1985), is that the physician presents the major topics she wants the patient to remember at the beginning of the meeting. Then, continued Spector, the physician should ask the patient to repeat what she has been told just before the meeting is concluded. This approach not only takes advantage of primacy and recency effects, but it repeats and reiterates the learning of key topics presented during the session.

In summary, patients must first acquire knowledge about asthma or COPD and how the conditions can be managed. Health counselors can, through formal educational programs and informal consultation, teach patients about their specific disorder and how it can be controlled. In addition, health counselors must assess whether patients can actually act on the advice they have been given to help control their condition. Only when patients have shown some mastery of actions they have been advised to perform, can goal selection occur.

Acting on Advice (Phase II)

Patients who have demonstrated they can manage their disorder because of instruction concerning their chronic disorder and their self-management, use skills similar to those taught in a self-management program (see Fig. 6.1 phase II). They have learned, by interacting with their health counselors and by their own performance, how to use peak flow meters, to inhale medications correctly, and to take other steps to manage their asthma or COPD. When this is the case, the role of the health counselor is to reinforce the patient's performance and, whenever possible, help the patient to refine and maintain his or her skills. If the patient needs additional instruction, he might be referred to a self-management program or, if the problem centers around the inappropriate performance of specific skills, given extra training. Additional instruction can be provided during a patient's regularly scheduled appointment with a health counselor.

The mechanism that guides patients in performing the actions they take is identical to that followed by patients in self-management: self-generated self-statements that guide the patient through the steps he needs to take to prevent or manage respiratory distress. We each use different forms of self-statements to guide ourselves through our daily lives (Creer, 1997). We might use self-talk to take us through the steps required to inhale medications correctly; self-generated stimulus change to prompt us to change our environment, such as by escaping from cigarette smoke; or self-generated response change, such as halting exercise if it is making us tight, to help control our behavior.

In most cases, the verbal self-statements we use are automatic; from the time the alarm goes off in the morning until we fall asleep, we talk to ourselves. Patients who are skilled at managing their respiratory disorders may report that they automatically perform the steps they need to control respiratory distress. However, this state only comes with considerable training, successful performance, and the development of self-efficacy. Even then, there are likely to be situations where the patient experiences distress that is beyond his boundaries of expertise. It is then that advice from health counselors is needed to assist and guide the patient.

Follow-up (Phase III)

We constantly evaluate our performance, no matter what we are doing. If what we did works the way we expected, great; we are probably going to do the same thing under the same circumstances in the future. If what we did failed to produce the results we expected, then we will probably want to try another strategy. The whole process of evaluating our performance is referred to as self-reaction. If self-reaction leads the patient to conclude that he needs help from the health counselor, then an appointment with the latter should be made. Results from patients' self-reaction will be discussed during the regular follow-up visits. In the Health Counseling Model, follow-up is especially important when dealing with behaviors that have to be performed over long periods of time.

Two steps are distinguished in the follow-up phase: (i) maintenance of behavior; and (ii) prevention of relapse. Guidance with respect to maintenance of behavior focuses on the following. First, the outcomes of the behavior can be evaluated jointly by health counselors and the patient. The question is whether patient's expectations were met. If so, this will be an important reinforcer to maintain the behavior in the future. Secondly, patient successes should be verbally reinforced by health counselors (e.g., a health counselor can praise the patient for his attempts and progress in meeting goals when reviewing the patient's self-monitoring records). From a meta-analysis conducted by Mullen *et al.* (1992), it appeared that reinforcement was seldom or only partially applied in patient education interventions; consequently, the skills taught in the intervention were not strengthened or maintained. Reinforcement should be designed and added in the counseling process to reward the behavior after it has occurred. Rewards can be diverse, such as receiving social support when interacting with fellow patients or health counselors. Thirdly, for patients who find it difficult to maintain their performance of appropriate behaviors, family and friends can be mobilized to support the patient if that is considered helpful. Information can also be given to patients about available community services, such as respiratory disorder support groups, where additional help can be obtained.

Lapses in behavior should be treated as opportunities to analyze and subsequently control the factors that caused the lapse (Marlatt & Gordon, 1985). For asthma patients, it is known that they tend to cut down on their medication intake when they feel well. Several research projects acknowledged this phenomenon and investigated the possibilities of self-treatment by asthma patients (van der Palen *et al.*, 1998). Furthermore, for respiratory patients who try to reduce behaviors such as smoking or remain at a certain weight, extra attention to lapses is required. If patients' expectations are unmet, this should be discussed by patients and health counselors; if not the patient's motivation to continue the behavior will dramatically decrease. Several tactics can be used. First, it may be that the advice needs to be adjusted: for example, the patient's regimen might be simplified so as to be easier to follow. Secondly, it may be essential to detect, via conversations with the patient, if there are high-risk situations in which performance of the behavior was difficult: patients must learn an appropriate response to cope with such situations. Thirdly, it may be that the patient did not succeed in integrating the 'new' behavior into his daily routine or that behaviors failed to be maintained because the patient's daily routine had changed. Better or refined tailoring of the desired behavior to more closely fit the patient's lifestyle may be required; this might include recommended diet changes with more sensitivity to cultural and/or personal food preferences, or the development of a medication schedule to accommodate a work/school schedule. Fourthly, it may be that patients are not performing the behavior in an adequate way. A study in the Netherlands showed that of the 316 patients attending a pulmonary outpatient department, only 11.1% completed the assessment of their inhalation technique without making any mistakes (van Beerendonk *et al.*, 1998). This finding is comparable to percentages found in studies conducted in other countries (Larsen *et al.*, 1994; Thompson *et al.*, 1994). Regular checks of the inhalation technique lower the risk of incorrect inhalation technique habits being established. Studies show that patient education, either by verbal instructions or instructional media such as videotapes, can improve the inhalation technique of asthma patients (van der Palen *et al.*, 1997). For patients who still have difficulties performing the correct inhalation technique, an inhalation chamber or a nebulizer is recommended to facilitate their performance (van Beerendonk *et al.*, 1998).

Strengths and Limitations of the Health Counseling Model

Strengths of the Model

The Health Counseling Model is a practical model with proven value in that there are many patients, including those with asthma or COPD, who learn how to control their condition through the interactions they have with health counselors. The patients already have the behavioral repertoire needed to manage a chronic condition. These patients often use what is tantamount to an idiosyncratic set of self-management techniques that they may be unable to fully describe, but which nevertheless help them to manage their asthma or COPD. In these cases, either health counselors or patients may examine the costs/benefits of additional self-management training and conclude that the costs outweigh the gains. The model is also applicable where there are limited resources for providing self-management training or in settings where interdisciplinarian treatment teams effectively work with patients. It is impossible to overemphasize the significance of an interdisciplinary treatment team: Not only does it consist of health counselors who, working in a cooperative fashion, help manage the patient's respiratory condition but also it integrates the patients as active members of the team. Under these ideal circumstances, patients are able to bridge the time between appointments by successfully managing their asthma or COPD.

The Health Counseling Model is also a rational model in that diverse aspects of the counseling process are clearly distinguished. Every aspect of the counseling process receives attention. Furthermore, in this model, the type of advice provided is fine tuned to fit the phases of behavior change. A further strength of the model is that presentation and adherence to advice is presented as a continuous decision-making process in which the management of a respiratory disorder is achieved and maintained.

Although the advantages of active participation are often stressed in the literature, it appears difficult for health counselors to put this aspect into practice. Hopefully, the Health Counseling Model will give these care providers more insight into how to activate patients during their consultation. Working according the Health Counseling Model makes a strong appeal for the active participation of the patient in order to achieve adequate self-management. The patient is considered responsible for the final choices that are made; the health counselor, on the other hand, remains responsible for the professional guidance and support of the self-management process. Furthermore, the model forces health counselors and patients to anticipate diverse problems or difficulties that can occur in the execution and consolidation of an advised behavior. The idea behind the model is to search for solutions to these problems before they occur.

The final aim of this model is to help optimize adherence on the part of patients. We do not deny patients their right to consciously nonadhere to advice; however, by applying the model, it is possible to detect why patients display a lack of interest or motivation in complying to advice provided by health counselors, which can prevent feelings of frustration among patients and health counselors at an early stage.

Limitations of the Model

There are several limitations to the Health Counseling Model:

1. The success of the model is dependent upon members of the treatment team working in an interdisciplinary fashion to counsel the patient. When this occurs, the team combines the knowledge and skills of each member in a coordinated fashion for the benefit of the patient. Achieving this aim, however, is easier said than done. For example, much of the success of the team is a function of the knowledge and skills of the physician who serves on the team. Yet, as suggested by Creer *et al.* (1999), evidence indicates that many physicians do not follow established guidelines for treatment of asthma. In fact, many primary care physicians do not know of the existence of these guidelines. Knowledge and expertise is an essential ingredient in establishing control over the patients asthma; if the ingredients are not present, how can appropriate advice be provided patients? The situation with COPD is equally disturbing: there remains a controversy as to whether pulmonary rehabilitation, including the advice given to patients in helping to manage their disorder, is effective in the treatment of the COPD (Albert, 1997). Unless a coordinated team strategy is taken with asthma and COPD patients, any advice offered by members of a treatment team is apt to be fragmented and of little value to patients in assisting them to systematically manage their disorder.
2. As with any chronic disorder, much of the success of a treatment regimen is a function of the motivation and actions of the patients themselves. The processes of the Health Counseling Model are designed to insure patients play an active role in their own treatment. How successful they will be, in turn, depends not only on how well team members work together but also on the constant advice and reinforcement they provide to patients. We have acknowledged that many patients do very well at managing either asthma or COPD; this is a basic tenet of the Health Counseling Model. What we need to know is how patients have translated the advice they received over the years from health counselors to help control their disorders. This data would greatly enhance the role played by health counselors in the future management of both disorders.
3. The Health Counseling Model originated as an approach to extinguish behaviors that have a strong habitual character; e.g., smoking, overeating, and excessive alcohol intake. Today, the model is applied to other problems, including urinary incontinence (Alewijnse, 1999). What we need to know is how effective the model will be in helping to manage COPD and asthma.
4. Although the model describes processes by which patients can be motivated to perform adequate self-management, the diverse techniques

involved in communication with patients are not systematically addressed by this model. For this kind of information, readers are referred other sources (Lloyd & Bor, 1996; Buckman *et al.*, 1998; Northhouse & Northouse, 1998; Silverman *et al.*, 1998). As noted, we have yet to determine how effective these techniques will be with respiratory disorders.

5. There is the need for information on how to maintain patient performance and to prevent relapse. This is a nascent area of research in the management of chronic disease. Yet, the ultimate success of either the Health Counseling Model or the Self-Management Model depends upon the long-term maintenance of patient skills taught in both approaches. Thus far, little attention has been paid to long-term maintenance of patient skills in asthma (Creer *et al.*, 1998); this omission must be corrected if either of the two models is to be successful. The situation regarding rehabilitation of COPD is even bleaker: any benefits attained in such programs, including those provided by patients themselves, dissolve over time, with measurable loss after the first year (Tiep, 1997). Reversing this trend will require, in the words of Tiep (1997, p. 1652), 'creative attention.' We think that both the Health Counseling Model and the Self-Management Model provide imaginative solutions for maintaining patient performance and avoiding relapse.

Self-Management Model

A plethora of self-management models have been proposed for the management of chronic illnesses such as asthma, cystic fibrosis, and COPD (e.g., Creer, 2000). These models are often highly theoretical (e.g., Glanz *et al.*, 1997), however, and omit discussions of the practical problems faced in developing and initiating a self-management program for a chronic disorder. Furthermore, what is meant by the term 'self-management' is often a source of confusion. Some writers reserve the term self-regulation for implying that patients follow self-set goals and self-management for a patient who follows goals set by others; however, this flies in the face of reality for two reasons. First, as emphasized in recent asthma guidelines (e.g., National Institutes of Health, 1997), it is recommended that health counselors and patients jointly set treatment goals. In these cases, the patient is guided neither by the goals he sets nor by the goals set by others; rather, the patient attempts to attain goals that he has helped set. Secondly, there is little evidence that behavioral scientists have distinguished between the terms self-regulation and self-management. Rather, the tendency in writing about chronic diseases has been to treat such terms as self-management, self-regulation, self-care, self-control, self-change, and self-directed behavior change as synonyms (Creer, 2000).

Another problem with the term self-management has been the unwillingness of many health counselors to recognize that it means what it says: i.e., the patient manages his disorder by accepting personal agency and taking whatever actions are necessary to guide his own behavior in appropriate ways. An approach taken by some medical personnel has been to say that patients are performing 'guided self-care' or that they are 'co-managing' their asthma (Creer, 1998). This tactic is not only fallacious, but it generates unrealistic and dangerous expectations on the part of both patients and some health counselors. An analogy of what happens in the self-management of asthma is to compare such processes to what happens in driving an automobile. Driving instructors teach people the mechanics of driving a car, as well as the do's and don'ts of driving. After so much training and an assessment of a person's competence to drive an automobile, the person is given a license and turned loose on the highway. How well that person then drives becomes a matter of the choices, decisions, and skills of that individual. Fortunately, most people do try to operate their vehicle correctly and to drive safely. However, as we know too well, others often create a menace for themselves and for others on the road. They may speed, drive in a reckless manner, or drive when physically impaired. The point is this: ultimately, it is the individual's choice how he drives. There is no driving instructor sitting next to the individual to take over control of the automobile if necessary. It is this way in asthma, cystic fibrosis, or COPD self-management: the patient alone takes over the management of his disorder. He will occasionally need help, but, as Anderson (1995) noted in discussing diabetes, patients are asked to be responsible for up to 95% of the care for their disorder. More will be noted later about the demands made of patients with asthma and COPD.

Figure 6.2 presents several definitions of self-management. All are useful; they should be considered given the purposes of individual health counselors in working with a patient. For this chapter, however, a definition adapted from Creer (2000) will be used:

> *Self-management is a procedure where asthma patients change some aspect of their own behavior. It involves processes including: (a) goal selection; (b) information collection; (c) information processing and evaluation; (d) decision making; (e) action; and (f) self-reaction. Successful mastery, performance, and maintenance of self-management skills results in the following outcomes: (a) reduction in mortality and morbidity due to asthma or COPD; (b) improvement in the quality of life in patients and family members; and (c) the development of self-efficacy beliefs on the part of patients that they can make a contribution to the management of their asthma or COPD, in part through their becoming partners with their physicians and other health counselors in controlling the disorder (e.g., Rutten-Van Mölken et al., 1992; Wigal et al., 1993; Clark, 1994; Mesters et al., 1994, 1995; Clark & Nothwehr, 1997).*

Karoly (1993): Self-management refers to those processes, internal or transactional, that enable individuals to guide goal-directed activities over time and across settings. Self-management entails modulation of thought, affect, behavior, or attention through use of specific mechanisms and skills.

Creer & Holroyd (1997): Self-management is defined as the individual's performance or assumption of preventive therapeutic health activities, often in collaboration with health care professionals.

Tobin *et al.*, (1986): Self-management is the concept that individuals can monitor a health behavior goal by keeping records of their own target behavior and factors associated with the behavior, and provide self-rewards or reinforcements that will help to increase the likelihood of achieving the goal.

Modeste (1996): Self-management entails (a) dealing with the consequences of disease and illness, not just physiological; (b) being concerned with problem solving, decision making, and patient confidence, rather than prescription and adherence; and (c) placing patients and health professionals in partnership relationships.

Sulzer-Azaroff & Mayer (1992): Procedure in which individuals change some aspect of their own behavior. One or more major components are generally involved: (a) self-selection of goals; (b) monitoring one's own behavior; (c) selection of procedures; and (d) implementation of procedures.

Figure 6.2

Definitions of self-management.

Processes of Self-Management

The Expert Panel 2 Report (National Institutes of Health, 1997) underscored the point that education for all asthma patients should begin at the time of diagnosis and be integrated into every step of their care. The aim of patient instruction is to teach patients self-management skills they can perform to help control their asthma or COPD. Once patients have acquired knowledge about asthma or COPD and its control, joint goal selection and the tailoring of a program for a given patient can take place. Many of the techniques described earlier in the Health Counseling Model can be used to instruct patients in asthma or COPD self-management.

Processes of self-management have been detailed in several sources (e.g., Thoresen & Mahoney, 1974; Thoresen & Kirmil-Gray, 1983; Bandura, 1986; Holroyd & Creer, 1986; Zimmerman, 1986; Ford, 1987; Karoly, 1993; Clark & Zimmerman, 1990; Creer & Holroyd, 1997; Creer, 2000). While different terminology has often been used, there is considerable commonality among different descriptions of self-management. As Creer & Holroyd (1997) pointed out, apparent differences occur because of the way specific processes are categorized, not from actual differences in conceptualization. Processes identified as significant in the self-management of asthma include (a) goal selection; (b) information collection; (c) information processing and evaluation; (d) decision making; (e) action; and (e) self-reaction (see Fig. 6.1, phase II).

Goal Selection

Many of the processes described in the Health Counseling Model are applicable to goal selection in self-management. It is often necessary, for example, for health counselors to move through the preparatory steps outlined earlier. In addition, successful goal selection should involve negotiation between patients and health counselors. The latter must be willing to engage in give-and-take in discussing treatment goals with patients; if they are all agreeable, then any set goals will incorporate the wishes of both patients and health care counselors, which increases the likelihood that the goals will be reached. If health counselors are unwilling to negotiate goals with patients, then any goals are unlikely to be reached. The patient may feel that as his wishes and desires were ignored, the goals are not worth attaining, or that they are the goals of the health counselor and not the patient.

There are three positive aspects to goal selection in self-management (Ford, 1987; Karoly, 1993; Creer & Holroyd, 1997):

- it establishes preferences among patients and health counselors about desirable goals and outcomes;
- it increases the commitment of patients to perform goal-relevant self-management skills; and
- it establishes expectancies on the part of patients that trigger their effort and performance.

In the case of chronic illness, including asthma and COPD, goal selection can have a final positive consequence: it establishes goals for managing the disorder that can be reached only through the collaborative efforts of patients and health counselors (Creer, 2000). Ideally, patients begin to believe that by developing self-management competencies, they can become allies with their health counselors in managing a chronic illness (Creer & Holroyd, 1997).

Perhaps the most ignored or overlooked aspect of self-management is that goal selection is the only activity where there is true collaboration between patients and health counselors (Creer, 2000). From the time agreement is reached, it becomes the responsibility of individual patients to perform whatever self-management skills are required to attain the goals. Thereafter, as we described with our driving instructor's analogy, physicians and other health counselors are restricted to tracking the behavior of patients. Health counselors can offer advice and suggestions, but they cannot perform the self-management skills needed to control asthma or COPD. After the health counselors and patients have discussed, negotiated, and determined jointly set goals, they should be described, as precisely as possible, in a patient treatment or action plan.

Written action plans are invaluable to asthma patients because they provide a blueprint for them to follow in treating their disorder (Lieu *et al.*, 1997; National Institutes of Health, 1997).

Information Collection

The foundation of information collection is self-monitoring, or the self-observation and self-recording of data; it may be considered as a behavioral supportive action in the Health Counseling Model (Gerards, 1993). Programs on asthma self-management often include strategies designed to optimize self-monitoring, such as symptom self-management plans or peak expiration flow graphs (Turner *et al.*, 1998). Self-monitoring is essential for successful self-management; it is a necessary, although not sufficient activity, that must be performed by patients if goals are to be reached (Creer & Bender, 1993; Lorig, 1996; Creer, 2000). Lorig (1996) pointed out that self-monitoring can provide an insight into the problem that is being monitored, such as keeping track of when asthma attacks occur, and/or feedback to patients on their progress with respect to established goals, such as by keeping track of lung function or exercise-induced symptoms. This also implies that the health counselor reviews the data recorded with the patient during consultation to identify patterns threatening adherence and to solve problems (see 'Follow-up' of the Health Counseling Model). In general, feedback is essential for skill mastery.

Creer & Bender (1993) offered three suggestions on self-monitoring that might be considered by health counselors with regards to the self-management of asthma.

1 Patients should only monitor phenomena that have been operationally defined as target behaviors related to the goals or objectives they are pursuing. Anyone, including asthma or COPD patients, would be overwhelmed if asked to monitor too many classes of phenomena, including their own behavior.
2 Whenever possible, an objective standard – such as a peak flow meter to measure airway obstruction or the number of cigarettes smoked per day – should be used to assess targeted behaviors. Objective data is useful in supporting subjective assessment of progress.
3 It is important that patients observe and record information only during specified periods of time, as agreed on with their health counselors. Continuous monitoring should be avoided to prevent the possibility that patients center their lives around their disorder.

Information Processing and Evaluation

Patients have to be counseled on how to process and evaluate the information they have gathered about themselves and their asthma. Five steps may be distinguished in this respect (Creer & Bender, 1993; Creer & Holroyd, 1997).

1. Individuals must be able to detect relevant changes in the information they observe, record, and process about themselves. This may not be difficult when objective measures are used, such as a peak flow meter. However, in most instances, patients do not have a peak flow meter with them when they begin to have an attack. They must, therefore, compare the changes in breathing of the experience against some sort of personal breathing level to which they have become adapted. Their adaptation level, or benchmark of breathing, is private information available only to the patient; some patients are good at detecting changes from this level, but others are not (Kendrick *et al.*, 1993; Fritz *et al.*, 1994; Rietveld, 1998). With the patients not good at detecting changes, training in symptom detection or discrimination is warranted (Creer, 1983).

2. Standards should be established to help patients evaluate data they gather and process about themselves. For example, asthma patients are asked to compare the peak flow values they gather daily against their personal best peak flow value (e.g., National Institutes of Health, 1995, 1997), which is the highest peak flow value blown by the patient over a period of time, usually 2 weeks or more.

3. Patients must learn to interpret, evaluate, and make judgments about the data they collect and process about themselves. For example, having standards with peak flow meters not only permits patients to readily compare their readings against their personal best, but can be used as a method of predicting whether or not they are likely to experience asthma within a prescribed period of time (e.g., Taplin & Creer, 1978). Or, using the scheme of green, yellow, or red levels incorporated into their asthma action plan, patients may judge whether their peak flow values are in the safe, warning, or alarm stages.

4. Individuals must learn to analyze any changes they observe in terms of the ABC's of the change: A = antecedent factors that led to the change, such as asthma triggers; B = behaviors they might perform to control the episode, such as specific self-management skills; and C = consequences of their actions, such as the halting of the attack and its outcomes. The ABC analysis provides essential information for decision making with respect to the most appropriate action to take. For example, a patient may have targeted exposure to cat allergens as leading to asthma symptoms. In doing so, she has identified the trigger of the attack. Escaping from the trigger or taking a reliever medication are behaviors that provide short-term solutions to the problem. However, upon considering the consequences of having a pet to which she is allergic, the patient may decide that the best long-term solution is to find a new home for the cat. Such a solution would probably reduce the number of attacks suffered by the patient in the future.

5. Contextual factors must be considered when processing and

interpreting information about asthma. A good example is provided by the asthma patient who is attempting to quit smoking. He may find it to be easy not to smoke when he is at home; perhaps he can occupy himself with a hobby that is incompatible with smoking. Being around others, such as occurs at work, however, creates another context: here the patient may find it difficult to refuse a cigarette when one is offered to him.

Decision Making

The earlier discussion of decision making is relevant to the Self-Management Model. Patients must make decisions as to what actions to take in the management of asthma or COPD. No matter what the decision-making strategy taken by patients – the suggestions by Janis & Mann (1978) are but one proven approach – decision making is a critical function in self-management. It could be tragic if a patient made a poor decision based upon valid and reliable information he gathered regarding his asthma. Despite the importance of the process, however, there is a paucity of information regarding decision making and asthma or COPD. Creer (2000) declared this was ironical for two reasons. First, patients are being asked not only to make more accurate judgments about their condition but also to make more complex decisions. The demands made on asthma patients have increased sharply with the advent of new and better treatment strategies. Secondly, evidence continues to mount that patient decision making is at the center of successful self-management. Creer (1990) reported this in a study that compared a set of data, including physicians regarded as a gold standard group by their peers, to a set of data collected from patients regarded as a gold standard group by their ability to manage asthma (Creer *et al.*, 1988).

The results were striking similarities in the way both gold standard groups described how they managed asthma. Both groups utilized effective judgment rules or heuristics in that they:

- considered each attack as a separate event;
- generated a number of testable treatment alternatives;
- used their personal data base in selecting the most efficacious treatment strategy;
- adjusted treatment in a stepwise manner to fit changes in the severity of attacks;
- avoided preconceived notions about attack management;
- thought in terms of probabilities regarding the effect of their actions; and
- avoided an overreliance on memory regarding asthma and how it should be treated.

The tactics used by both groups are identical to those heuristics recommended by Arkes (1981) as important in decision making. In addition, both gold standard groups used advanced cognitive strategies, coupled with considerable flexibility in processing and evaluating information, to generate potential treatment approaches and in making decisions regarding these hypotheses.

Action

Action entails the performance of self-management skills to control asthma or COPD. How successful individual patients will be is, to a major extent, a function of the self-instruction they provide to themselves to initiate, direct, and maintain a behavior needed to achieve the goal they are pursuing (Creer & Bender, 1993). As described earlier, self-instruction involves self-generated self-statements, self-generated stimulus change, and self-generated response change. Contextual factors interact with the performance of the patients because they enable or limit the performance of behavior (Ajzen & Fishbein, 1980).

Self-instruction is important in two other ways if patients are to control their asthma. First, patients must perform, in a stepwise manner, whatever steps are required to control their asthma. These are the steps that they and their health counselors have agreed on beforehand and described in a patient's asthma action plan. Secondly, self-instruction can prompt other strategies for managing or coping with a disorder. Common steps taken in asthma include using an inhaler correctly, attempting to remain calm, thinking about what steps to do, seeking help if necessary, etc. In short, the patient would probably perform whatever skills were taught to him in the education stage of a self-management program. Karoly (1993) suggested other coping strategies that might be considered, including attentional resource allocation, effort mobilization, planning and problem-solving, verbal self-cueing, facilitative cognitive sets or expectations, stimulus control, and mental thought or cognitive control. Other strategies that could be taken are relaxation, self-desensitization, skill rehearsal, modeling, linking or unlinking behavioral chains, and self-reinforcement (Creer, 2000).

Self-Reaction

Self-reaction refers to the attention individuals direct toward evaluating their performance (Bandura, 1986). When reviewing records of their activities, patients might identify patterns threatening adherence or other problems that need to be solved. On the basis of this personal appraisal, patients can establish realistic expectations about their performance. They might find out that they were unable to manage aspects of their asthma or behavior that require control. Self-reaction might prompt them to seek extra training, such as obtaining more relaxation training, receiving better instruction in taking medications properly, or seeking medical care in case of serious problems they are unable to manage by themselves. Patients will also acquire realistic expectations regarding the limitations of asthma self-management. For example, despite taking preventive steps to control an asthma trigger, such as pollen, they might still experience some degree of discomfort from asthma symptoms. However, it is impossible that anyone, including asthma and COPD patients, can control everything in their lives by performing self-management behaviors.

A major component of self-reaction is self-efficacy (e.g., Bandura, 1977, 1986, 1997). The acquisition and knowledge of self-management skills, as occurs in self-management programs, are not enough to guarantee that the skills will be performed in an appropriate manner; patients must also believe they can do these skills in order to reach whatever goals they have jointly set with health counselors. Self-efficacy arises, in part, because of performance achievements; it guides and regulates future action (Creer & Holroyd, 1997). Self-efficacy is not only a basic ingredient in the performance of self-management skills, but is crucial to the maintenance of these skills over time. It is necessary if patients are to control their asthma across settings and over time, because self-efficacy is basically the fuel that drives the performance of self-management skills.

Strengths and Limitations of the Self-Management Model

Strengths of the Model

There are a number of strengths of self-management, particularly when applied to a chronic disorder such as asthma or COPD.

1. It places the major responsibility of managing asthma upon the patient. As it is the patient who has the greatest knowledge about his disorder – often only the patient has such knowledge – of when an attack occurred and how it was controlled, it is only logical that there be a shift away from an overreliance upon the medical and health care system back toward the patient. This may sound revolutionary, but it is not: in many ways, it reflects a return to the health care practiced by patients for centuries – including each one of us, as we all have dual citizenship in the kingdoms of the well and the sick (Sontag, 1976). What is revolutionary is that the model assumes that there will be interactions between health counselors and patients to the effect that the most recent knowledge on the management of asthma can be tailored to specific characteristics of the patient and his respiratory disorder.

2. Self-management fits within the paradigm of managed health care currently used throughout much of the world. As we have reiterated throughout the chapter, the ideal strategy is that patients are treated by an interdisciplinary team of experts, who not only apply their particular expertise, but who understand and respect each others skills (Varni, 1983). The result should, theoretically, be the development and implementation of the best possible treatment package for a given patient. Under the best of

circumstances, the patient will be taught skills that will effectively permit him to assume major responsibility for his asthma. In essence, patients become active participants in the interdisciplinary team that attempts to control the disorder. Under the worst of circumstances, particularly where the system is so stretched that patients spend little time with their primary care provider – in the United States, for example, it is estimated that physicians spend approximately 7 min with a patient during a typical visit (Moeller, 1998) – patients must assume greater responsibility for their own health care. They simply have no other recourse available to them.

3. Self-management is effective. Early self-management programs targeted pediatric asthma. The programs generated compelling evidence of their efficacy. For example, Wigal *et al.* (1990) reported that, to various degrees, the programs showed that when the children and their parents performed self-management skills, they prevented or reduced the rate of attacks, reduced financial costs incurred because of asthma, reduced the impact of the disorder upon the lives of children and their families – such as by reducing school absenteeism and hospital visits – and became allies with their physicians in the management of asthma. In working with adults, Kotses *et al.* (1995) demonstrated that short-term benefits of a self-management program included fewer asthma symptoms and physician visits, and an improvement in asthma management skills and cognitive abilities. On a long-term basis, the performance of self-management skills was related to lower asthma attack frequency, reduced medication use, improvement in cognitive measures, and increased use of self-management skills.

4. Asthma self-management programs for asthma are cost-effective (Rutten-Van Mölken *et al.*, 1992; Liljas & Lahdensuo, 1997). Data from the study by Kotses *et al.* (1995) were analyzed by Taitel *et al.* (1995). Comparison of the costs to the benefits of the program was a 1 : 2.28 cost : benefit; this indicated that the program more than paid for itself.

5. While a variety of approaches are available for teaching self-management, the processes that should be performed to self-manage asthma have repeatedly been proven (e.g., Kotses & Harver, 1998): they are the processes described earlier. Given the information that is available (e.g., Wigal *et al.*, 1990; Bailey *et al.*, 1998; Kotses, 1998) about asthma self-management, there is no need to reinvent the wheel and start from scratch in developing and applying such a program for a given group of asthma patients. The processes we've described work.

6. Data have been reported that attest to the maintenance of asthma self-management training over long periods of time. Creer *et al.* (1988) reported that all of the patients who needed to perform asthma self-management skills continued to do so 5 years after participating in a pediatric asthma self-management program. The data from the study have since been buttressed not only by surveying a larger sample of the participants but also by discussions with the physicians who referred the children and

their families to the program. Caplin (1998) recently contacted a high percentage of patients – a majority of them involved in the study by Kotses *et al.* (1995) – up to a decade after their participation in asthma self-management. Several findings were prominent in the follow-up data:

a. A majority of the patients continued to perform the skills they had been taught during self-management training. Most performed self-management skills each and every day; the remainder said they used self-management skills only when they noticed a change in their breathing that portended the possibility of an asthma attack. Skills commonly performed included self-monitoring, particularly self-observation; decision-making; action; and self-reaction. Of particular interest was the reported value of decision-making strategies to the patients.

b. Variables repeatedly cited by participants as contributing to their performance of asthma self-management skills included self-efficacy; cognitive beliefs, such as outcome expectations; and emotional well-being. Self-efficacy, or the patient's beliefs that they can do what they have to manage their asthma, was the variable most often identified by patients. The variables were described as being more significant in promoting and maintaining their performance than either physician instructions or illness characteristics.

c. Patients who frequently experienced relapse used conscious decision making in making the choice to stop performing self-management skills (although they all continued to use self-observation in tracking their asthma). They used the information they had accumulated about their disorder to assess their treatment and self-management needs. This finding suggests that patients followed a process-oriented approach to decision making rather than a simple skill-oriented approach. The data supports findings by Creer (1990), who reported that patients who had mastered the performance of asthma self-management skills were often surprisingly sophisticated in making decisions about their disorder and how it should be treated.

d. Lapses in the performance of asthma self-management tended to occur as a natural process in the long-term maintenance of these skills, regardless of relapse status. In other words, when asymptomatic, patients often do not perform asthma self-management; when they felt they were becoming symptomatic, however, they resume the performance of self-management skills as needed.

e. Caplin (1998) was able to compare patients taught self-management skills over a short period of time (three sessions) with those taught the skills over eight sessions: patients taught over eight sessions showed greater maintenance of self-management skills. They credited their success not only to the fact that the instructors were able to assess their acquisition and performance of self-management skills over a longer period of time but also to the constant support and reinforcement they received during this critical phase of self-management skills mastery. A common finding was that participants asked to be remembered to the instructors who had taught them self-management skills. The bond with the instructors had apparently served to maintain the performance of self-management skills by participants.

f. Relapse of asthma self-management is difficult to define, measure, and understand. The study by Caplin (1998) was only the first attempt to link cognitive, affective, and behavioral processes to the maintenance of patient's decision making regarding asthma and its management.

Limitations of the Model

Among the limitations to using self-management, many of which are also applicable to the Health Counseling Model, are the following conditions.

Organismic Boundary Conditions. Ford (1987) pointed out that we each consist of a matrix of anatomical, physical, and functional characteristics and capabilities that provide us with some options, but prohibit others. In most cases, asthma patients possess the necessary options to learn about changes in their breathing and how they should react to these changes. It is difficult, however, for a patient with asthma to sense the onset of an attack if he lacks the lung receptors required to detect such breathing changes (Harver & Mahler, 1998). Limitations with COPD are more serious in that the disorder is both chronic and progressive (Tiep, 1997).

Ford (1987) noted that we often use cognitive potential as a criterion of organismic boundary conditions in others. With asthma, for example, we might decide that patients lack the potential required to learn how to manage their asthma. However, argued Ford, the limits may lie less in the individual than within the context we select for instruction. The best strategy, he cautioned, is to assume that there are few organismic boundaries to learning and to design methods and environments to develop the capabilities of different individuals. This would include helping as many patients as possible to reach the goals of successfully performing asthma or COPD self-management. It would also permit us to overcome racial and cultural factors that must be often be addressed in asthma self-management (Creer, 2000).

Environmental Boundary Conditions. Developmental and performance capabilities are facilitated and constrained by the kinds and organization of the environmental conditions within which each of us develops and lives (Ford, 1987). This is not only a significant factor in how patients acquire self-management skills but also in how they perform these skills across time and over settings. What is referred to as context represents the interaction of environmental boundary conditions and the personal variables of a given patient; in many ways, it is the determining factor in the performance of self-management skills, including those needed to control asthma and COPD (Creer & Christian, 1976).

Selective Action. Conditions around and within each of us are constantly shifting and changing; consequently, we are always attempting to adapt to new conditions (Ford, 1987). Some of the conditions are irrelevant to what we are attempting to do at a particular moment in time; they merely belong to the stream of internal and external events that comprise our lives. Other conditions, however, are relevant to our efforts. We organize our lives in relation to selected and current aspects of our internal and external environment. Patients with asthma must be able to organize their behavioral repertoire and skills in relation to stimuli, both external and internal, that impinge upon them at any given moment, as well as to any changes these stimuli produce. Patients don't react, they transact (Ford & Urban, 1998). An important role of health counselors is to teach patients the aspects of their external and internal environment that they should attend to and act upon.

Individual Differences. Individual differences are important in all aspects of our life. They become of critical value, however, in the treatment of asthma and COPD. Attention to individual differences, in the form of tailoring self-management programs for specific patients, is a variable that should be considered by all health counselors in helping a patient tailor and execute a self-management program. COPD also affects patients in different ways. Some patients may be more than willing to assume greater personal responsibility for their own condition; others may not. Without considering individual differences, a viable program for a given patient is unlikely.

Performance Variability. No one behaves exactly the same way twice, even under the same circumstances. As Ford (1987) noted, all of the performance possibilities of which a person is capable is in that individual's behavioral repertoire. No patient can be expected to use self-management skills to manage each attack that he experiences. However, as health counselors, we can discuss performance variability so that it can be an asset to a patient in treating separate attacks that, like behavior itself, differ in various ways from episode to episode.

Interdependent Hierarchical Organization. Ford (1987) describes a person as a unit or system defined by an organization of structural and functional components. In order for a person to function effectively, these components must be constrained and coordinated to support and facilitate the maintenance and functioning of the larger unit: the person. Social learning theory posits the role of such an organization scheme – reciprocal determinism – in the self-management of behavior (e.g., Bandura, 1977, 1997). Applying this schemata to asthma, Creer et al. (1988) described the action and interaction of four components in asthma management: environmental, physiological, cognitive, and behavioral. In asthma, an environmental trigger impinges upon the physiology of a patient and precipitates an attack. Recognition, a cognitive event, of the impending episode can lead the patient to escape from the trigger or to initiate treatment, both behavioral events. Successful management of the episode requires the reciprocal interaction of these components until the attack is aborted. A similar situation exists with COPD. Patients must not only recognize exacerbations of their condition but also be aware of such changes and initiate behaviors to reverse the worsening of their health.

Expectancies of Patients and Health Counselors. If self-management is ever to be widely accepted and implemented in asthma or COPD, there must be a synthesis of the expectancies both of patients and health counselors (Creer, 2000). This has not occurred. As we described earlier, however, the performance of self-management skills is analogous to what occurs when someone begins to drive. Once a person has received driving instruction and been proclaimed to be an adequate driver, the choices on how to operate a motor vehicle are made by the driver alone. A major paradigmatic shift away from health counselors treating patients like parents treat their children, toward health counselors accepting patients as partners in an interdisciplinary manner, must occur. Until the shift occurs, the expectancies of patients and health counselors will serve as a major impediment and restriction on asthma or COPD self-management.

Task Demands. We noted that, in many cases, patients are being asked to do too many things to help control their asthma. The number and variety of tasks, if performed, would consume much of the waking time of the patients. With all the demands made upon them, it is easy to see how asthma or COPD could be at the center of their existence. The reason for the increase in task demands has been the inappropriate application of treatment guidelines for the disorder (e.g., National Institutes of Health, 1995, 1997). The fault is not with the guidelines per se: they offer proven and prudent methods for the management of asthma. However, instead of tailoring treatment regimens for individual patients, there has been a tendency to simultaneously hit patients with too much of the guidelines.

Let us put the problem into perspective: Sontag & Richardson (1997) reported that many physicians refuse to consign some HIV patients to regimens that require their taking medications, sometimes with food and sometimes without food, at specific intervals six or more times a day. As many patients did not comply with the regimen, they were taken off the drugs. Why? Because missing doses, it was feared, could lead to making HIV more resistant to future treatments. However, the treatment regimens of many patients with asthma is much more demanding than it is for HIV patients (Creer *et al.*, 1999). Take the following example which, unfortunately, is not atypical. A child with asthma was asked to take:

(a) an inhaled steroid twice a day;
(b) a long-lasting β-agonist drug twice daily;
(c) an anti-leukotriene medication twice a day;
(d) a long-lasting anti-allergy drug twice daily;
(e) a short-term β-agonist inhaled drug to be taken as needed; and
(f) a nasal corticosteroid to be taken daily.

In addition, the child was asked to take an aerosol twice a day, to take an antacid tablet with meals and before bedtime, and to use his inhaler before exercising. With such demands, the self-management of asthma and related conditions becomes a full-time job. If adhered to, the patient's asthma would be at the center of the lives of the child and his family. Eventually, the regimen is likely to fail and the patient will be labeled as noncompliant.

Unpredictability of Behavior. Behavior is highly complex. Even under the best of circumstances, our actions may or may not produce the results we wish. Patients and health counselors can agree on a program to optimize control over asthma or COPD. Patients, in turn, may faithfully adhere to every aspect of the action plan. Still, they are apt to experience exacerbations of asthma, in part because of the capricious course the disorder can take. This suggests that, in discussing asthma with patients, health counselors emphasize two points. First, they should point out the probabilistic nature of behavior, and stress that attacks are likely to occur despite the best efforts of patients. It is impossible to control all internal and external stimuli that impinge upon an individual, including those involved with asthma. Secondly, there is always uncertainty underlying the treatment received by patients with chronic disorders, including asthma and COPD (Creer, 2000). As there is no cure for either condition, physicians and other health counselors are uncertain as to what will work to control asthma in a given patient. All that can be done is to select what appears to be the best treatment option for a patient. If it works, great; if it doesn't, health counselors and patients must consider other treatment options. A trial-and-error approach, requiring the patience and persistence of all parties, is the only option available in the treatment of asthma and COPD.

Discussion

Two models for teaching patients to manage a chronic disorder – the Health Counseling Model and the Self-Management Model – were discussed. Neither model is a separate entity nor mutually exclusive; as emphasized, the two models serve to compliment one another. The first model, the Health Counseling Model, was designed to take advantage of skills that patients have in their behavioral repertoire when they are diagnosed with a chronic disorder. These abilities become the foundation upon which to refine the abilities the patient already possesses or to add further skills as needed. Capitalizing upon the existing competencies of patients means providing systematic and targeted education specifically tailored to help manage asthma or COPD. The literature shows that patient education, using a systematic and planned approach, is effective (e.g., Kok, 1992; Kok *et al.*, 1997). To maximize this effectiveness, patient education should be initiated as soon as possible after the diagnosis of asthma or COPD. By doing so, the health counselors, as part of an interdisciplinarian treatment team, can integrate their educational and counseling efforts into the action plan developed for a given patient. The regular interactions that occur between health counselors and patients become learning opportunities to help systematically teach patients to manage asthma or COPD. In addition, these learning opportunities allow health counselors to monitor and reinforce patients for acquiring the skills required for them to help manage their condition.

The Self-Management Model is an approach whereby patients provide much of the treatment required to control asthma or COPD. By assuming a major role in helping to manage their own condition, patients become part of the interdisciplinarian team that treats their asthma or COPD. This status can be achieved through building upon the existing strengths of patients, through effective use of the interactions among health counselors and patients – the Health Counseling Model – or by teaching patients the specific skills required to help manage their disorder – the Self-Management Model. Regardless of which approach is taken – we encourage the use of elements of both models to help tailor the best approach for a given patient – the outcome should be both better control of asthma or COPD and improved health for the patients.

The models provide three additional functions. First, they serve as guidelines to help health counselors direct patients and, in turn, to assist patients to manage their asthma or COPD. The models permit health counselors and patients to tailor and track the different skills and competencies required for a given patient to achieve optimal self-management over his condition. Secondly, the models fulfill a heuristic function in that they permit instruction and education of patients in an economical and efficient manner. With the ever-widening acceptance of managed health care throughout the world, this is increasingly important. Finally, the models serve as an integrative framework that not only synthesizes our existing knowledge of how patients can help manage their chronic disorder, particularly asthma and COPD, but also stimulates questions that can only be answered through additional research. Overbye (1999, p. 180) recently observed that:

> *History teaches that most ideas are flops, in science and otherwise. But, every once in while a hunch that began as pure thought, a wild gem of poetry about the way nature should be, blossoms into a theory that turns out to fit the world so miraculously that its authors cannot help feeling that they have tapped into the secret order of reality.*

Our hope is that future research shows the two models of self-management fit the world of health care in a way that provides better health and quality of life to anyone with a chronic respiratory condition, including those with asthma and COPD.

References

Ajzen, I. & Fishbein, M. (1980). *Understanding attitudes and predicting social behavior.* Englewood Cliffs, NJ: Prentice Hall.

Albert, R.K. (1997). Is pulmonary rehabilitation an effective treatment for chronic obstructive pulmonary disease? *American Journal of Respiratory and Critical Care Medicine*, 155, 784–785.

Alewijnse, D. (1999). Sex-specific health education on the promotion of adherence with pelvic floor muscle exercise therapy for women with urinary incontinence. Paper presented at the Second International Interdisciplinary Conference on Women and Health, 12–14 July, Edinburgh, UK.

Anderson, R.M. (1985). Is the problem of noncompliance all in our heads? *Diabetes Educator*, 11, 31–34.

Anderson, R.M. (1995). Patient empowerment and the traditional medical model. *Diabetes Care*, 18, 412–415.

Arkes, H.R. (1981). Impediments to accurate clinical judgments and possible ways to minimize their impact. *Journal of Consulting and Clinical Psychology*, 49, 323–330.

Bailey, W.C., Davies, S.L. & Kohler, C.L. (1998). Adult asthma self-management programs. In: H. Kotses & A. Harver (Eds), *Self-management of asthma* (pp. 293–308). New York: Marcel Dekker.

Bailey, W.C., Kohler, C.L., Richards, J.M., Jr., *et al.* (1999). Asthma self-management. Do patient education programs always have an impact? *Archives of Internal Medicine*, 159, 2422–2428.

Bandura, A. (1977). Self-efficacy: toward a unifying theory of behavioral change. *Psychological Review*, 84, 191–215.

Bandura, A. (1986). *Social foundations of thought and action, a social cognitive theory.* Englewood Cliffs, NJ: Prentice Hall.

Bandura, A. (1997). *Self-efficacy. The exercise of control.* New York: W.H. Freeman and Company.

Buckman, R., Korsch, B. & Baile, W. (1998). *A practical guide to communication skills in clinical practice.* Toronto: Medical Audio Visual Communications Inc.

Burke, L.E. & Dunbar-Jacob, J. (1995). Adherence to medication, diet, and activity recommendations: form assessment to maintenance. *Journal of Cardiovascular Nursing*, 9, 62–79.

Cabana, M.D., Rand, C.S., Powe, N.R., *et al.* (1999). Why don't physicians follow clinical practice guidelines? A framework for improvement. *Journal of the American Medical Association*, 282, 1453–1465.

Caplin, D.L. (1998). *Variables contributing to the relapse and long-term maintenance of self-management for individuals with asthma.* Unpublished doctoral dissertation, Ohio University, Athens, OH.

Clark, N.M. (1994). The influence of education on morbidity and mortality in asthma. *Mondaldi Archives of Chest Disease*, 49, 169–172.

Clark, N.M. & Nothwehr, F. (1997). Self-management of asthma by adult patients. *Patient Education & Counseling*, 32 (Suppl 1), S5–S20.

Clark, M.N. & Starr-Schneidkraut, N.J. (1994). Management of asthma by patients and families. *American Journal of Respiratory and Critical Care Medicine*, 149, 554-566.

Clark, N.M. & Zimmerman B.J., (1990). A social cognitive view of self-regulated learning about health. *Health Education Research*, 5, 371–379.

Creer, T.L. (1983). Self-management psychology and treatment of childhood asthma. *Journal of Allergy and Clinical Immunology*, 72, 607–610.

Creer, T.L. (1990). Strategies for judgment and decision-making in the management of childhood asthma. *Pediatric Asthma, Allergy & Immunology*, 4, 253–264.

Creer, T.L. (1993). Medication compliance and childhood asthma. In: N.A. Krasnegor, L. Epstein, S.B. Johnson & S.J. Yaffe (Eds), *Developmental aspects of health compliance behavior* (pp. 303–333). Hillsdale, NJ: Lawrence Erlbaum Associates.

Creer, T.L. (1997). *Psychology of adjustment. An applied approach.* Upper Saddle River, NJ: Prentice Hall.

Creer, T.L. (1998). The complexity of asthma. *Journal of Asthma*, 35, 451–454.

Creer, T.L. (2000). Self-management of chronic illness. In: M. Boekaerts, P.R. Pintrich & M. Zeidner (Eds), *Self-regulation: theory, research, applications.* San Diego, CA: Academic Press.

Creer, T.L. & Bender, B.B. (1993). Asthma. In: R.J. Gatchel & E.B. Blanchard (Eds), *Psychophysiological disorders* (pp. 151–208). Washington, DC: American Psychological Association.

Creer, T.L. & Christian, W.P. (1976). *Chronically-ill and handicapped children. Their management and rehabilitation.* Champaign, IL: Research Press.

Creer, T.L. & Holroyd, K.A. (1997). Self-management. In: A. Baum, S. Newman, J. Weinman, R. West & C. McManus (Eds), *Cambridge handbook of psychology, health, and medicine* (pp. 255–257). Cambridge: Cambridge University Press.

Creer, T.L. & Levstek, D.A. (1996). Medication compliance and asthma: overlooking the trees because of the forest. *Journal of Asthma*, 33, 203–211.

Creer, T.L., Backial, M., Burns, K.L., *et al.* (1988). Living with asthma. Part I. Genesis and development of a self-management program for childhood asthma. *Journal of Asthma*, 25, 335–362.

Creer, T.L. & Levstek, D.A. & Reynolds, D. (1998). History and conclusions. In: H. Kotses & A. Harver (Eds), *Self-management of asthma* (pp. 379–405). New York: Marcel Dekker.

Creer, T.L., Winder, J.A. & Tinkelman, D.A. (1999). Guidelines for the diagnosis and management of asthma: accepting the challenge. *Journal of Asthma*, 36, 391–407.

Ford, D.H. (1987). *Humans as self-constructing living systems. A developmental perspective on behavior and personality.* Hillsdale, NJ: Lawrence Erlbaum Associates.

Ford, D.H. & Urban, H.B. (1998). *Contemporary models of psychotherapy. A comparative analysis*, 2nd edn, New York: John Wiley & Sons.

Fritz, G.K., Yeung, A. & Taitel, M.S. (1994). Symptom perception and self-management in childhood asthma. *Current Opinion in Pediatrics*, 6, 423–427.

Gerards, F. (1993). Health counseling. In: V. Damoiseaux, H.T. van der Molen & G.J. Kok (Eds), *Gezondheidsvoorlichting en gedragsverandering* [Health education and behavior change] (pp. 353–363). Maastricht: Van Gorcum.

Glanz, K., Lewis, F.M. & Rimer, B.K. (Eds) (1997). *Health behavior and health education. Theory, research and practice*, 2nd edn. San Francisco: Jossey-Bass Publishers.

Harver, A. & Mahler, D.A. (1998). Perception of increased resistance to breathing. In: H. Kotses & A. Harver (Eds), *Self-management of asthma* (pp. 147–193). New York: Marcel Dekker, Inc.

Holroyd, K.A. & Creer, T.L. (Eds) (1986). *Self-management of chronic diseases. A handbook of interventions and research.* New York: Academic Press.

Horn, C.R., Essex, E., Hill, P. & Cochrane, C.M. (1989). Does urinary salbutamol reflect compliance with inhaled drug regimen by asthmatics? *Respiratory Medicine*, 83, 15–18.

Janis, I.L. & Mann, L. (1978). *Decision making: a psychological analysis of conflict, choice, and commitment.* New York: Free Press.

Janz, N.K. & Becker, M.H. (1984). The

health belief model: a decade later. *Health Education Quarterly*, 11, 1–47.

Joos, S.K. & Hickam, D.H. (1990). How health professionals influence health behavior: Patient–provider interaction and health care outcomes. In: K. Glanz, F.M. Lewis & B.K. Rimer (Eds), *Health behavior and health education, theory, research, and practice* (pp. 216–241). San Francisco: Jossey-Bass Publishers.

Karoly, P. (1993). Mechanisms of self-regulation: a systems approach. *Annual Review of Psychology*, 44, 23–52.

Kendrick, A.H., Higgs, C.M.B., Whitfield, M.J., Laszlo, G. (1993). Accuracy of perception of severity of asthma: patients treated in general practice. *British Medical Journal*, 307, 422–424.

Kok, G. (1992). Quality of planning as a decisive determinant of health education effectiveness. *Hygie*, 11, 5–9.

Kok, G., Van den Borne, B. & Mullen, P.D. (1997). Effectiveness of health education and health promotion: meta-analysis of effect studies and determinants of effectiveness. *Patient Education & Counseling*, 30, 19–27.

Kotses, H. (1998). Individualized asthma self-management. In: H. Kotses & A. Harver (Eds), *Self-management of asthma* (pp. 309–328). New York: Marcel Dekker.

Kotses, H. & Harver, A. (Eds) (1998). *Self-management of asthma.* New York: Marcel Dekker.

Kotses, H., Bernstein, I.L., Bernstein, D.I., *et al.* (1995). A self-management program for adult asthma. Part I. Development and evaluation. *Journal of Allergy and Clinical Immunology*, 95, 529–540.

Krutzch, C.B., Bellicha, T.C. & Parker, S.R. (1987). Making childhood asthma management education happen in the community: translating health behavioral research into local programs. *Health Education Quarterly*, 14, 357–373.

Larsen, J.S., Hahn, M., Ekholm, B. & Wick, K.A. (1994). Evaluation of conventional press-and-breathe metered dose inhaler technique in 501 patients. *Journal of Asthma*, 31, 193–199.

Lee, T.W., Locke, E.A. & Latham, G.P. (1989). Goal setting theory and job performance. In: L. Pervin (Ed.), *Goal concepts in personality and social psychology* (pp. 291–326). Hillsdale, NJ: Lawrence Erlbaum.

Ley, P. (1982). Giving information to patients. In: J.R. Eiser (Ed.), *Social psychology and behavioural science* (pp. 339–373). Chichester: John Wiley and Sons.

Lieu, T.A., Quesenberry, C.P., Jr., Capra, A.M., Sorel, M.E., Martin, K.E. & Mendoza, G.A. (1997). Outpatient management practices associated with reduced risk of pediatric asthma hospitalization and emergency department visits. *Pediatrics*, 100, 334–341.

Liljas, B. & Lahdensuo, A. (1997). Is asthma self-management cost-effective. *Patient Education & Counseling*, 32 (Suppl 1), S97–S104.

Lloyd, M. & Bor, R. (1996). *Communication skills for medicine.* New York: Churchill Livingstone.

Lorig, K. (1996). *Patient education. A practical approach.* Thousand Oaks, CA: Sage Publications.

Marlatt, G.A. & Gordon, J.R. (Eds), (1985). *Relapse prevention. Maintenance strategies in the treatment of addictive behaviors.* New York: The Guilford Press.

Mesters, I., Pieterse, M. & Meertens, R. (1991). Pediatric asthma, a qualitative and quantitative approach to needs assessment. *Patient Education & Counseling*, 17, 23–34.

Mesters, I., Meertens R., Kok, G., Parcel, G.S. (1994). Effectiveness of a multidisciplinary education protocol in children with asthma (0–4 years) in primary health care. *Journal of Asthma*, 31, 347–359.

Mesters, I., Van Nunen, M., Crebolder, H. & Meertens, R. (1995). Education of parents about pediatric asthma: effects of a protocol on medical consumption. *Patient Education & Counseling*, 25, 131–136.

Modeste, N.N. (1996). *Dictionary of public health promotion and education, terms and concepts.* (p. 106). Thousand Oaks: Sage Publications.

Moeller, K.A. (1998). In 16 years of providing consume information what have we learned: *Gratefully yours*. (pp. 1–3). Washington, DC: National Library of Medicine.

Monahan, J.L. (1995). Using positive affect when designing health messages. In: E. Maibach & R.L. Parrott (Eds), *Designing health messages, approaches from communication theory and public health care* (pp. 81–98). London: Academic Press.

Mullen, P.D., Douglas, A.M. & Velez, R. (1992). A meta-analysis of controlled trials of cardiac patient education. *Patient Education and Counseling*, 19, 129–142.

National Institutes of Health (1995). *Global initiative for asthma* (Publication No. 95–3659). Washington, DC: National Institutes of Health.

National Institutes of Health (1995). *Global initiative for asthma* (NIH Publication No. 95–3659). Bethesda, MD: National Institutes of Health.

National Institutes of Health (1997). *Highlights of the Expert Panel Report 2: Guidelines for the diagnosis and management of asthma* (Publication No. 97–4051A). Washington, DC: US Department of Health and Human Services.

Northhouse, L.L. & Northouse P.G. (1998). *Health communication. Strategies for health professionals.* Stanford: Appleton and Lange.

Overbye, D. (1999). Did God have a choice? *The New York Times Magazine*, April 18, p. 180.

Rietveld, S. (1998). Symptom perception in asthma: a multidisciplinary review. *Journal of Asthma*, 35, 137–146.

Rutten-Van Mölken, M.P.M.H., Van Doorslaer, E.K.A. & Rutten, F.F.H. (1992), Economic appraisal of asthma and COPD care: a literature review 1980–1991. *Social Science & Medicine*, 35, 161–175.

Silverman, J.D., Kurtz, S.M. & Draper, O.J. (1998). *Skills for communicating with patients.* Abingdon, UK: Radcliffe Medical Press.

Sontag, D. & Richardson, L. (1997). Doctors withhold HIV pill regimen from some. *The New York Times*, March 2, 1, 18.

Sontag, S. (1976). *Illness as metaphor.* New York: Farrar, Straus & Giroux.

Spector, S.L. (1985). Is your asthmatic patient really complying? *Annals of Allergy*, 55, 552–556.

Strecher, V.J., Seijts, G.H., Kok, G.J., *et al.* (1995). Goal setting as a strategy for health behavior change. *Health Education Quarterly*, 22, 190–200.

Sulzer-Azaroff, B. & Mayer, G.R. (1991). *Behavior analysis for lasting change.* Ft. Worth, TX: Holt, Rinehart & Winston.

Taitel, M.S., Kotses, H., Bernstein, I.L., Bernstein, D.I. & Creer, T.L. (1995). A self-management program for adult asthma. Part 2. Cost–benefit analysis. *Journal of Allergy and Clinical Immunology*, 94, 672–676.

Taplin, P.S. & Creer, T.L. (1978). A procedure for using peak expiratory flow-rate data to increase the predictability of asthma episodes. *Journal of Asthma Research*, 16, 15–19.

Thompson, J., Irvine, Th., Grathwohl, K. & Roth, B. (1994). Misuse of metered-dose inhalers in hospitalized patients. *Chest*, 105, 715–717.

Thoresen, C.E. & Kirmil-Gray, K. (1983). Self-management psychology and the treatment of childhood asthma. *Journal of Allergy and Clinical Immunology*, 72, 596–606.

Thoresen C.E. & Mahoney, J.J. (1974). *Behavioral self-control.* New York: Holt, Rinehart & Winston.

Tiep, B.L. (1997). Disease management of COPD with pulmonary rehabilitation. *Chest*, 112, 1630–1656.

Tobin, D.L., Reynolds, R.V.C., Holroyd, K.A. & Creer, T.L. (1986). Self-management and social learning theory. In: K.A. Holroyd & T.L. Creer (Eds), *Self-management of chronic diseases. A handbook of interventions and research* (pp. 29–55). New York: Academic Press.

Turner, M.O., Taylor, D., Bennett, R. & Fitzgerald, J.M. (1998). A randomized trial comparing peak expiratory flow and symptom self-management plans for patients with asthma attending a primary care clinic. *American Journal of Respiratory and Critical Care Medicine*, 157, 540–546.

van Beerendonk, I., Mesters, I., Mudde, A.N. & Tan, T.D. (1998). Assessment of the inhalation technique in outpatients with asthma or COPD using a MDI or dry powder device. *Journal of Asthma*, 35, 275–285.

van den Heuvel, C. (1994). *A matter of adherence, a study of adherence to exercise-prescriptions by patients with COPD.* Unpublished doctoral dissertation, Maastricht University.

van der Palen, J., Klein, J.J., Kerkhoff, A.H.M., Van Herwaarden, C.L.A. & Seydel, E.R., (1997). Evaluation of long-term effectiveness of three instructional models for inhaling medication. *Patient Education and Counseling*, 32, S87–S95.

van der Palen, J., Klein, J.J., Zielhuis, G.A. & Van Herwaarden, (1998). The role of self-management guidelines in self-management education for adult asthmatics. *Respiratory Medicine*, 92, 668–675.

Varni, J.W. (1983). *Clinical behavioral pediatrics: an interdisciplinary biobehavioral approach.* New York: Pergamon Press.

Vries de, H. & Mudde, A.N. (1998). Predicting stage transitions for smoking cessation applying the Attitude–Social influence–Efficacy model. *Psychology and Health*, 13, 369–385.

Weiner, B. (1986). *An attributional theory of motivation and emotion.* New York: Springer-Verlag.

Wigal, J.K., Creer, T.L., Kotses, H. & Lewis, P.D. (1990). A critique of 19 self-management programs for childhood asthma: part I. The development and evaluation of the programs. *Pediatric Asthma, Allergy & Immunology*, 4, 17–39.

Wigal, J.K., Stout, C., Brandon, M., *et al.* (1993). The knowledge, attitude and self efficacy asthma questionnaire. *Chest*, 104, 1144–1148.

Wilson-Pessano, S.R. & Mellins, R.B. (1987). Workshop on asthma self-management. Summary of workshop discussion. *Journal of Allergy & Clinical Immunology*, 80, 487–490.

Zimmerman, B.J. (1986). Development of self-regulated learning: which are the key subprocesses? *Contemporary Educational Psychology*, 16, 307–313.

7
Neuropsychological and psychiatric side effects of medications used to treat asthma and allergic rhinitis

Bruce G. Bender and Henry Milgrom

Editors' note—*The past three decades have seen an explosion of treatments – particularly those involving new medications – for respiratory disorders, including asthma, COPD, and tuberculosis. Many of these treatments are described throughout the book. The drugs have enhanced the ability of health care providers, in co-operation with patients, to establish control over respiratory diseases and conditions.*

The evolution of a new armamentarium of drugs for treating respiratory disorders has often thrust side effects of these medications into the limelight. While the drugs have improved control over asthma, COPD, and tuberculosis, they have also sparked debate about possible side effects of the compounds. Bruce Bender and Henry Milgrom describe the array of side effects reported with many of the medications used to treat respiratory disorders. In doing so, they describe pioneering research they have conducted to isolate and describe specific side effects. Their work is exemplary with respect to its scientific merit.

There are a number of other issues encountered by Bruce and Henry in their research. Of particular interest is their investigation and, in many instances, their dispelling of the lore or myths generated about certain drugs and preparations. Perhaps the best example is their research that allayed popular misconceptions surrounding the use of theophylline in the treatment of asthma. Concern over side effects of the drug, a medication that falls in the same class as caffeine, had been generated by a number of patient reports. When these concerns were widely disseminated through the popular media in the United States, the lore regarding theophylline was firmly established. It then became the task of Bender & Milgrom (1992) to conduct a scientifically solid investigation to dissipate the myths. The study stands out as an example of research that must be conducted if we are ever to know both the benefits and perceived costs of any medication. The body of research conducted by Bruce Bender and Henry Milgrom is equally of value to both medical and behavioral scientists.

Introduction

Physicians treat asthma and allergic rhinitis with a variety of medications intended to reduce bronchospasm, prevent pulmonary hyperresponsiveness, decrease inflammation, and suppress histamine production in response to allergens. It is not unusual for an asthmatic patient to be receiving several medications targeting all of these problems concurrently and chronically. Patients may additionally add to this regimen, with or without their physician's knowledge, over-the-counter (OTC) medications to relieve rhinitis symptoms. The reported side effects of these medications are frequently serious and include psychosis, disturbed affect, sedation, impaired attention and memory, and decreased school learning. The neuropsychological and psychiatric implications of many of these medications are not entirely known.

Neuropsychological side effects of some medications, such as antihistamines, corticosteroids, and theophylline, have been carefully studied, while others have not. Psychiatric side effects have primarily been documented through case reports. The combined effects of these medications on patients' emotional and cognitive functioning is little understood. This chapter reviews what has been learned about the neuropsychological and psychiatric side effects of medications used to treat asthma and allergic rhinitis, describes medication-specific changes, identifies erroneously attributed side effects, proposes additional areas requiring investigation, and makes recommendations about the clinical application of this information.

Asthma Medications

Psychological changes have been attributed to a number of the medications used to treat asthma, including theophylline, beta-agonists, and corticosteroids.

Theophylline

Once a leading medication in the treatment of asthma, theophylline has been largely replaced by inhaled anti-inflammatory medications. Theophylline is a bronchodilator which now serves primarily an adjunctive role to corticosteroids. The decline in theophylline prescription frequency has occurred for several reasons, including increasing recognition of the importance of anti-inflammatory drugs, its potential for toxicity requiring periodic blood work, and perceived behavioral side effects. These side effects included cognitive, behavioral, and attention problems in children (Furukawa *et al.*, 1984; Painter, 1986; Rachelefsky *et al.*, 1986). Theophylline was implicated in problems of impulse control (Firestone & Martin, 1979), fine motor control (Springer *et al.*, 1985), depression (Murphy *et al.*, 1980), stammering (McCarty, 1981), and psychosis (Wasser *et al.*, 1981). Many parents voice concerns about the effects of theophylline on their children's behavior. In a survey of parents of asthmatic children, half reported that taking theophylline caused their children to become restless, hyperactive, or both (*American asthma report*, 1989).

There is evidence that these widespread reports may be overstated. Some of the original observations of theophylline-induced psychological side effects consisted of single case studies, while other investigations have been criticized for measurement, design, or interpretive shortcomings (Creer & McLaughlin, 1989; Milgrom & Bender, 1993). Findings of theophylline-induced psychological change in these early reports are probably exaggerated. In most studies which reported theophylline-related behavior change, nonsignificant results greatly outnumbered significant findings. In some instances, investigators appear to have overemphasized a single outcome (Milgrom & Bender, 1993). In most cases, treatment-related differences were small, and there was little consistency across studies.

Subsequent studies provided more objective evaluation of theophylline's impact on children's behavior. Psychological side effects of theophylline were evaluated in two investigations: one open label (Bender *et al.*, 1991a) and one blinded (Bender & Milgrom, 1992). Both investigations included asthmatic children and employed identical parent questionnaires and tests measuring attention, impulsivity, activity level, hand steadiness, memory, and self-reported mood. Children in the open label study demonstrated improved attention on laboratory measures, but their parents noted conduct problems and hyperactivity, which were frequently attributed to theophylline (Bender *et al.*, 1991a). In the blinded, placebo-controlled, randomized study, asthmatic children again demonstrated improved attention, along with a trend toward increased hand tremor and anxiety during the active theophylline phase (Tables 7.1 and 7.2) (Bender & Milgrom, 1992). However, on this occasion the parents could not discriminate between placebo and theophylline treatment conditions, a striking finding inasmuch as only children with a history of theophylline-induced psychological side effects reported by their parents participated. Other studies have similarly demonstrated that parents cannot detect theophylline-related changes when blinded to the treatment condition (Rachelefsky *et al.*, 1986; Rappaport *et al.*, 1989; Schlieper *et al.*, 1991). In the study by Schlieper *et al.* (1991), of 21 psychological variables – tests of memory, maze tracing, logic and analysis, perceptual motor speed, self-reported mood, and parent reported behavior – none revealed significant theophylline or placebo treatment changes. Finally, a recent meta-analysis examined the collective results from 12 studies of theophylline's effect on cognition, behavior, or sleep representing more than 340 children and adolescents, concluding that there were no consistent or statistically significant differences between theophylline and placebo.

How do we explain the widespread belief that theophylline causes significant mood and behavior disruption given the negative results from

Table 7.1 Parent questionnaire problem scales from a blinded comparison of theophylline and placebo (From Bender & Milgrom, 1992.)

	Placebo		Theophylline		
	Mean	SE	Mean	SE	p*
Conduct	53.4	2.1	55.7	2.4	0.296
Learning	56.7	2.2	54.9	3.2	0.262
Psychosomatic	56.6	2.7	52.9	4.4	0.484
Impulsive	55.1	2.0	55.1	2.8	0.961
Anxiety	49.4	1.6	50.8	1.5	0.547
Hyperactivity	57.8	2.2	60.9	2.9	0.208

* p = two-tailed treatment effect from the repeated measures analysis of variance.

Table 7.2 Psychological test scores from a blinded comparison of theophylline and placebo (From Bender & Milgrom, 1992.)

	Placebo		Theophylline		
	Mean	SE	Mean	SE	p†
Selective Reminding Test					
Verbal memory‡	8.3	0.2	8.2	0.2	0.151
Children's Manifest Anxiety Scale					
Self-reported anxiety‡	9.9	1.2	11.2	1.3	0.060
Children's Depression Inventory					
Self-reported depression‡	10.1	1.4	11.5	1.5	0.206
CPT commissions					
Attention‡	83.9	23.1	55.6	10.5	0.092
CPD omissions					
Attention‡	22.9	3.0	23.6	3.3	0.486
Delayed Responding Test					
Impulsivity‡	67.2	4.0	66.2	4.4	0.847
Movement					
Physical activity‡	312.2	29.5	309.9	34.1	0.675
Hand steadiness					
Tremor‡					
Dominant hand contacts	68.7	8.6	83.7	9.0	0.034
Nondominant hand contacts	114.8	20.6	122.2	17.5	0.746

CPT = Continuous Performance Test.

† p = two-tailed treatment effect from the repeated measures analysis of variance.

‡ Trait measured.

these blinded studies? Two possible answers can be identified. The central nervous system (CNS) stimulant effects of theophylline may be present at the initial introduction of theophylline but decrease over time to insignificant levels. In one investigation, parents identified detrimental changes in behavior during the first week of theophylline therapy, but not the second, leaving the authors to conclude that these side effects were transient (Stein & Lerner, 1993).

Alternatively, a small subgroup of asthmatic children may experience heightened sensitivity to the CNS stimulatory effects of theophylline. Histories of 162 asthmatic children were reviewed in one investigation which estimated that actual behavioral side effects from theophylline therapy occurred in 5–6% of children (Nelson & Schwartz, 1987). Because most reported results from previous studies were based on group data, individual variability and response to theophylline may be obscured. Investigators have hypothesized that a theophylline-sensitive subgroup may include young children (Nelson & Schwartz, 1987) or those with low IQs (Springer *et al.*, 1985) or learning problems (Schlieper *et al.*, 1991). Most studies have included only children 8 years and older, and therefore the effects of theophylline on young children remain unknown. However, one study examined a younger and potentially more theophylline-sensitive subject population but did not detect any negative cognitive or behavioral sequelae (Stein & Lerner, 1993). Additionally, multivariate analyses in two separate studies failed to demonstrate any relationship between medication-related change and age, sex, socioeconomic status, intelligence, or psychiatric history (Bender *et al.*, 1991a; Bender & Milgrom, 1992). Thus, if a small subset of asthmatic children is particularly sensitive to the behavioral effects of theophylline, a defining picture which might be used by prescribing physicians to anticipate those children at risk is not yet available.

In summary, most studies reporting theophylline-related change include a far greater proportion of nonsignificant than significant findings. There is little objective evidence that theophylline has a widespread adverse effect on children's mood and behavior, although subtle changes such as enhanced attention or memory (Bender & Milgrom, 1992; Milgrom & Bender, 1993) and increased hand tremor and anxiety (Bender & Milgrom, 1992) have been documented. In each case mean differences were small and probably not of clinical importance. The report that standardized scholastic achievement test scores of children taking theophylline for treatment of asthma are not different from those of their sibling controls provides further evidence against theophylline's effects on school performance (Lindgren *et al.*, 1992).

Although there are few studies of behavioral side effects of theophylline in adults, results from such studies are similar to those of the larger body of research conducted in children. Theophylline has been associated with improved verbal learning but decreased motor steadiness in both adults and adolescents with asthma (Joad *et al.*, 1986). A study of normal adults, which avoided the potentially confounding effects of bronchodilation, reported no significant differences between theophylline and placebo on subjective or objective assessment of cognitive function (Fitzpatrick *et al.*, 1992).

In summary, the following conclusions are drawn regarding theophylline's neuropsychological side effects:

1 Theophylline's neuropsychological side effects in children are much like those of caffeine, a related methylxanthine.
2 The CNS stimulatory effects of theophylline cause mildly increased anxiety and hand tremor.
3 The stimulatory effects of theophylline may be transient for many children, abating with time.
4 Theophylline may enhance attention and/or memory in some asthmatic children.
5 Theophylline does not cause learning disabilities.
6 Parents may inaccurately report theophylline side effects.
7 A theophylline-sensitive subgroup of asthmatic children who are more likely to show significant behavioural change may exist but has not yet been clearly identified.
8 Large, controlled studies of children under the age of 8 remain to be conducted.

Beta-agonists

Beta-agonists are bronchodilators, usually inhaled and, in the case of moderate to severe asthma, used together with anti-inflammatory medications. Early case reports indicated an association between beta-agonists and psychotic episodes (Gluckman, 1974; Feline & Jouvent, 1977; Ray & Evans, 1978; Jacquot & Bouttari, 1981; Whitehouse & Novosel, 1989). More commonly, oral and inhaled forms of these drugs have been associated with short-term CNS stimulation, increased pulse rate (Lonnerholm *et al.*, 1984), and skeletal muscle tremor (Mazer *et al.*, 1990). More serious psychological side effects have generally been ruled out. A blinded study of 20 asthmatic children indicated that treatment with inhaled beta-agonists resulted in a fine motor tremor but did not compromise performance on more complex perceptual–motor tasks involving response speed, visual–motor control, and dexterity (Mazer *et al.*, 1990). A study of 18 adolescent and adult asthmatics similarly reported that inhaled albuterol did not result in impaired verbal learning, verbal perception, mental speed and efficiency, or attention (Joad *et al.*, 1986).

Corticosteroids

Corticosteroids represent the most potent class of anti-inflammatory medications used to treat asthma. As with theophylline, the psychological side effects of corticosteroids have been a source of confusion and controversy. A large case report and case review literature with adult patients indicates that a small percentage of hospitalized patients treated with prednisone experience psychoses. The largest of these studies is the Boston Collaborative Drug Surveillance Program, which reviewed records of 676 hospitalizations involving corticosteroids. Of these, 3.1% demonstrated acute psychiatric reactions. Further, a dose–response relationship was revealed; patients receiving more than 40 mg/day of prednisone were significantly more likely to develop serious psychiatric symptoms than those on lower dosages (Boston Collaborative Drug Surveillance Program, 1972; Ling *et al.*, 1981). Only 1.3% of patients receiving less than 40 mg/day prednisone had such reactions compared with 18.4% of patients receiving more than 80 mg. This and other studies led to the conclusion by Ling *et al.* (1981) that

1 prednisone doses lower than 40 mg/day reduce the risk of psychiatric reactions;
2 patients with a significant psychiatric history are not necessarily predisposed to steroid-induced disturbance; and
3 women have an apparent increased risk relative to men.

A clear and scientific analysis of the relationship between oral corticosteroids and psychiatric disturbance cannot be produced from the literature comprised exclusively of case reports. While a large number of case reports can establish that a relationship exists between the use of corticosteroids and psychiatric disorder, the nature of that relationship and, in particular, the causal sequence cannot be proven outside of a blinded and scientifically controlled experimental design. Unfortunately, few such studies of the neuropsychological consequences of corticosteroids exist, particularly in adults. Three prospective studies employed a quasi-experimental design (Campbell & Stanley, 1966), in which patients who were already receiving the medication and who remained unblinded were studied; all three concluded that psychological change did not result from corticosteroid therapy (Lewis & Fleminger, 1954; Cordess *et al.*, 1981; Joffe *et al.*, 1988). A single study included an experimental design in which 15 patients with proliferative glomerulonephritis caused by SLE were randomly assigned to one of four treatment groups: (1) prednisone; (2) azathioprine; (3) prednisone and azathioprine; and (4) azathioprine and heparin (Cade *et al.*, 1973). Thirty-two percent of the patients receiving 60–100 mg/day of prednisone developed psychotic symptoms, in contrast to none of the patients in the other three groups. Interpretation of these findings is complicated by the fact that systemic lupus erythematosus (SLE) patients are prone to psychiatric disturbance and by the absence of psychiatric disturbance in renal transplant patients receiving higher doses of corticosteroids (Cade *et al.*, 1973). Most probably, the psychiatric effect of oral corticosteroids is enhanced by the chronic illness being treated.

The pediatric literature examining corticosteroid-induced neuropsychological side effects depends less upon case reports and more on scientifically objective assessment. While there is little evidence from these studies of serious psychiatric disturbance resulting from corticosteroid use in children, they have been shown to produce detrimental effects on cognition and mood in asthmatic children. In one study, visual and verbal memory test scores were reduced in a steroid-treated group of asthmatic children on the day of treatment, but not 24 or 48 hours later (Suess *et al.*, 1986). Two studies examined the effects of before, during, and after brief prednisone burst therapy. In one study, 27 hospitalized children were contrasted at peak prednisone burst (61.5 mg/day on average) and low dose (3.33 mg/day on average) (Bender *et al.*, 1988). The order of low- and high-dose evaluation was mixed. No changes occurred between the two dose levels on tests of attention, impulsivity, hyperactivity, or fine motor control. In contrast, memory scores were reduced during high-steroid days. In a second report, 32 hospitalized children again demonstrated impaired memory on high-steroid days, with no associated change on tests of hyperactivity, attention, impulsivity, or fine motor control (Bender *et al.*, 1991b). These changes had no relationship to age, IQ, socioeconomic status, or asthma severity, although girls were somewhat more affected than boys. Measures of psychological functioning in the child and the family were significantly associated with the memory deficit, indicating that psychosocial dysfunction predisposes the asthmatic children toward the neuropsychological side effects of corticosteroids.

Children's affect is also significantly influenced by corticosteroids. Patients with cancer in remission demonstrated increased irritability, fatigue, argumentativeness, sleep disturbance, and excessive talking and crying during a 4-month steroid-treatment phase (Harris *et al.*, 1986). The investigators further observed a trend toward more severe changes in children under 6 years of age. An increase in negative and anxious feelings at high-steroid dose was also found in the two studies by Bender and colleagues (Bender *et al.*, 1988, 1991b).

Inhaled corticosteroids have become increasingly the treatment of choice for significant asthma. Although free of some of the more serious systemic side effects of oral corticosteroids, inhaled corticosteroids can be absorbed systemically and may produce some significant side effects such as delayed growth acceleration (Tinkelman *et al.*, 1993). Hyperactive, aggressive, and oppositional behavior have been reported in six cases of children treated with inhaled corticosteroids (Lewis & Cochrane, 1983; Meyboom & de Graaf-Breederveld, 1988; Connett & Lenney, 1991). Once again, however, the inability of case reports to establish a causal relationship requires that reports of such behavioral reactions be greeted with caution. In the only controlled investigation of neuropsychological side effects of inhaled corticosteroids, 102 asthmatic children were randomly assigned to one of two treatments, inhaled steroid (beclomethasone) or theophylline. Neuropsychological evaluations conducted at baseline, 1 month, and 1 year into treatment included measures of attention, concentration, memory and learning, and problem solving. Test scores in the two groups did not differ significantly from each other or from baseline scores, leading the authors to conclude that neither medication should be avoided out of concern for significant neuropsychological side effects (Bender *et al.*, 1997).

In conclusion:

1 Serious side effects related to the use of oral corticosteroids have been established only in adults, primarily in those receiving over 40 mg/day of prednisone or its equivalent. The causal relationship between steroids and psychosis has not been clearly established by blinded, experimental studies and may be mediated by the illness itself.
2 In children, oral corticosteroids may produce mild mood and memory decline. In most cases these are serious enough to prevent use of the medication but do require judicious monitoring.
3 As is the case with theophylline, studies of side effects in young children are lacking but needed; and
4 At the present time, no evidence exists of significant neuropsychological side effects related to treatment with inhaled corticosteroids, although evidence is limited and more studies are needed.

Other Asthma Medications

Other drugs, including the nonsteroidal anti-inflammatory agents cromolyn sodium and nedocromil, and the newer leukotriene modifiers zafirlukast and zileuton, have gained an increasing role in the treatment of asthma. Little is known of their neuropsychological or psychiatric potential. Children taking cromolyn sodium were found to have less impairment in visual–spatial planning (Springer *et al.*, 1985) and better memory and concentration (Furukawa *et al.*, 1988) than children treated with theophylline, although a third study found no cognitive differences between the two drugs (Furukawa *et al.*, 1984).

Medications Used to Treat Allergic Rhinitis

Seasonal allergic rhinitis affects up to 10% of school-age children and over 20% of adolescents. A variety of medications are used to treat symptoms of seasonal allergies. Medications for cough, colds, and allergic rhinitis comprise the largest group of drugs consumed (Wertheimer, 1985). These include antihistamines, decongestants, and anticholinergic agents. Many are available OTC, and in many cases are offered in combinations that can include antihistamines and adrenergic agents for the simultaneous control of sneezing, rhinorrhea, and nasal obstruction.

Information about the side effects of this group of medications includes a relatively large body of research with antihistamines, a limited number of case reports involving sympathomimetics and anticholinergics, and little information about the combined medications.

Antihistamines

Histamine receptors are increased in patients with nasal allergy, causing sneezing, itching, rhinorrhea, and congestion. Treatment with antihistamines suppresses these responses and, consequently, the troublesome symptoms of allergic rhinitis. First-generation H_1 (sedating) antihistamines are highly lipophilic and readily cross the blood–brain barrier, with the consequence that they can both stimulate and suppress the CNS. Drowsiness resulting from the use of these medications is reported to affect 25% of adults (Simons & Simons, 1988).

Much more research into the sedating effects of antihistamines has focused on adults than on children. This has occurred largely because of the recognition that adults perform functions that affect their safety and that of others, including driving a car or other vehicles, or operating heavy machinery. Second-generation H_1 (nonsedating) antihistamines are lipophilic, and in most studies have been shown to be less likely to produce sedation or psychomotor impairment than sedating antihistamines (Milgrom & Bender, 1997). A large portion of research devoted to the examination of performance differences produced by sedating versus nonsedating antihistamine utilizes evaluation of the relative effects of these medications on driving skills through a variety of means that include driving simulators, closed-track tests, and open-road driving testing, and employ various innovative technologies which measure driving accuracy. These studies have demonstrated that adults taking sedating antihistamines are likely to have more driving errors, longer response times, more erratic steering, more lane weaving, and less speed and accuracy in covering a driving course (Betts *et al.*, 1984; Riedel *et al.*, 1987; Moskowitz & Burns, 1988; Aso & Sakai, 1989). Nonsedating antihistamines are not completely free of any potential for sedation. When given at twice the therapeutic dose, one nonsedating antihistamine was found to produce significant driving impairment (O'Hanlon & Ramaekers, 1995).

Adults frequently are unable to detect the point at which sedating effects of antihistamines take hold. This is of particular importance because it suggests that many people cannot adequately judge when their driving performance may be impaired. Subjects in two studies reported that they perceived sedation after taking antihistamines, while tests of psychomotor performance indicated no change (Kulshrestha *et al.*, 1978; Moser *et al.*, 1978); in contrast, subjects in another study reported the experience of no sedation, although laboratory testing revealed performance impairment (Seidel *et al.*, 1987). In another study, sustained-release triprolidine (10 mg twice a day) resulted in sedation similar to that caused by the consumption of alcohol, resulting in blood alcohol concentrations of 0.05 mg/dl (O'Hanlon & Ramaekers, 1995). One hour after ingestion of triprolidine, testing revealed that driving was impaired; at 3 hours, however, testing revealed continued impairment that was no longer recognized by the drivers. When first-generation antihistamines are combined with alcohol, the result is even greater driving impairment (Roehrs *et al.*, 1993). However, the sedating effects of antihistamines may be apparent only upon initial use of the drug. Evidence of the temporary nature of the sedative effects of classic antihistamines was found in a study showing that reaction time was slowed on day 1, but no different from placebo by day 3 of drug treatment (Fig. 7.1) (Schweitzer *et al.*, 1994).

Much less is understood about the effects of antihistamines upon children. Nonetheless, antihistamines are widely used with school-age children, raising concern about their potential impact on school learning and performance. One controlled, double-blind study examined the relative effects of loratadine, a nonsedating antihistamine, and diphenhydramine, a sedating antihistamine. Twenty-one children with no history of allergy and 52 children with active seasonal allergic rhinitis were trained in the use of a computer-simulation learning task. In the program, the student is taught to make decisions as a farmer about the use of available land, livestock, and money. Allergic children were randomly assigned to either diphenhydramine (25 mg), loratadine (10 mg), or placebo during the training. The diphenhydramine group received another 25 mg dose after training. Two weeks later, all children underwent a paper and pencil examination, testing their knowledge of the simulation. The examination measured factual knowledge, conceptual knowledge, and knowledge

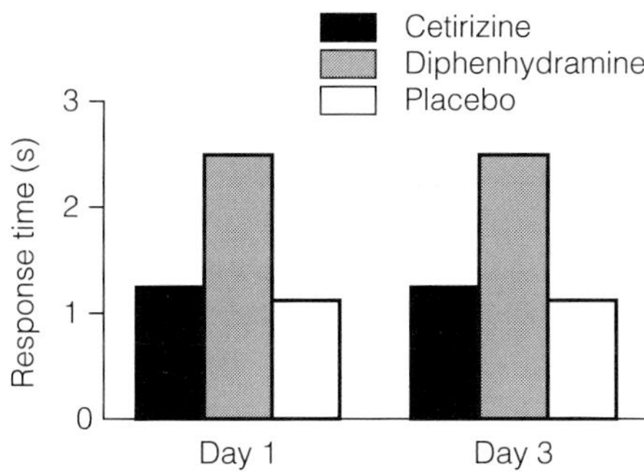

Figure 7.1

Simulated assembly line task (SALT). Mean response time (in seconds) to alarms for days 1 and 3 of treatment period. (Reprinted with permission from Schweitzer *et al.*, 1994.)

application, along with a composite score (Vuurman *et al.*, 1993). Scores for the allergic children in all three treatment groups were significantly lower than those of the nonallergic control children. Children in the placebo and diphenhydramine groups had significantly lower mean composite learning scores than the normal control children, indicating that symptomatic atopic children learn significantly less than their healthy counterparts. On all tests, loratadine-treated children performed lower than the normal controls but better than the placebo group, while diphenhydramine-treated subjects performed worse than the placebo group. Thus, children treated with the nonsedating antihistamine showed an improvement in learning, while those treated with the sedating antihistamine experienced a decrease in learning relative to the untreated group.

A second study explored the effects of an antihistamine/decongestant combination in adolescents and young adults. Sixty-seven allergic patients were randomly assigned to diphenhydramine (15 mg) or a combination produce (8 mg acrivastine plus 60 mg pseudoephedrine) or placebo and learned to use the same computer-simulation program employed in the pediatric study by Vuurman *et al.* (1993). All atopic subjects performed significantly less well than a group of 28 nonallergic control subjects. However, atopic individuals receiving the combination product during training learned as well as healthy subjects. Diphenhydramine-treated subjects performed significantly worse than controls and worse than the allergic individuals receiving the combined product (Fig. 7.2). The authors concluded that these results, as was the case in the pediatric study, indicate that allergy impairs learning, and that learning is further impaired by sedating antihistamines (Vuurman *et al.*, 1996).

Other studies offer further evidence of the relative benefits of nonsedating antihistamines in children. In a study involving the direct measurement of brain functions, P300-evoked potentials were evaluated in children treated with antihistamines, and it was found that chlorpheniramine increased latency relative to placebo and terfenadine (Simons *et al.*, 1996). Other case reports have indicated more serious behavioral changes in children treated with antihistamines, including uncontrollable behavior or hallucinations documented in three children who had received triprolidine–pseudoephedrine (Bain, 1983; Ackland, 1984; Sankey, Nunn, & Sills, 1984). It is difficult to determine whether these reports indicate a greater psychiatric susceptibility in children to antihistamines, or whether the source of behavior change in these children is due to an unidentified cause. As with neuropsychological investigations of other medications, the causal relationship implied by these case reports must be examined with caution.

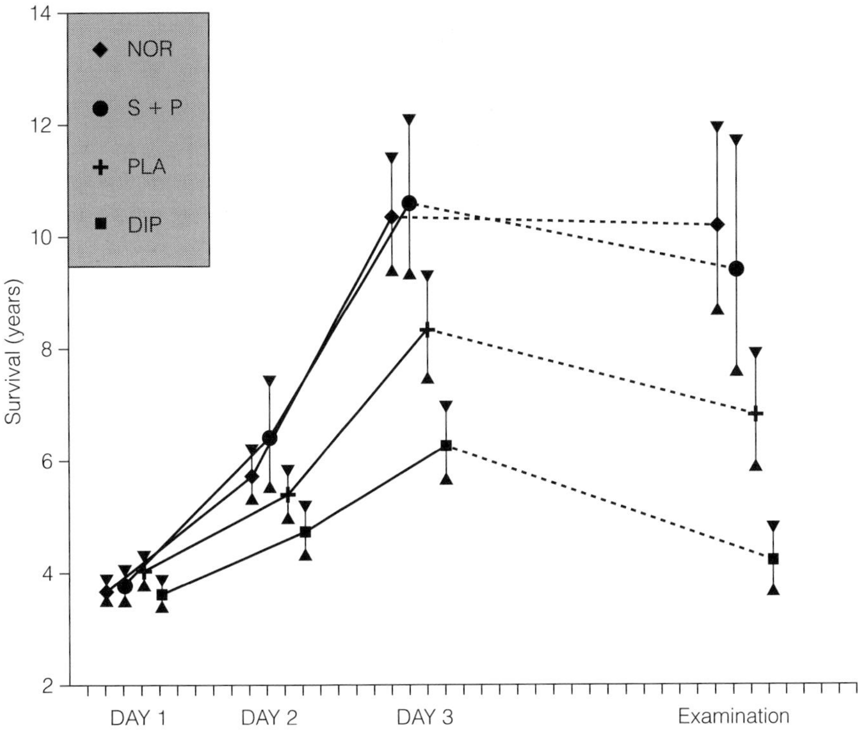

Figure 7.2

Mean (SE) years of survival on the simulation for patient groups receiving diphenhydramine (DIP), acrivastine + pseudoephedrine (A + P), placebo (PLA), and nontreated normal controls (NOR) during training and examination sessions. There was a 2-week period between day 3 of the training and the examination. Higher scores indicate better learning acquisition. (Reprinted with permission from Vuurman *et al.*, 1996.)

In conclusion:

1 Second-generation, nonsedating antihistamines have been shown in numerous investigations to have distinct advantages over first-generation antihistamines, controlling histamine production while not producing untoward side effects.
2 While much more is understood about these effects in adults than in children, it is clear that there are advantages also for the later group, particularly as they appear to learn better when treated with second-generation antihistamines.
3 Because investigations of children's school learning are limited to one European study, these results must be duplicated with other groups of children in other learning situations.

4 Little is known of the relative effects of nonsedating antihistamine use in children under the age of 10 who may be more susceptible to the side effects of sedating antihistamines (Feldman *et al.*, 1992).
5 Most investigations have focused upon the administration of single medications, usually antihistamines.

Because of the widespread use of antihistamine–decongestants drugs, investigation of the neuropsychological effects of such combination drugs is essential.

Sympathomimetics

Phenylpropanolamine, ephedrine, and pseudoephedrine are all drugs closely related to amphetamine. All are sympathomimetics, stimulate the sympathetic nervous system, and are used as decongestants. Phenylpropanolamine has been additionally packaged and sold as an appetite suppressant.

Report of psychiatric side effects in this group of sympathomimetics has been most frequent and dramatic in the case of phenylpropanolamine, which is a component of more than 150 OTC preparations. Lake *et al.* (1988, 1990) reviewed 30 case reports of individuals who developed psychiatric symptoms, including paranoid schizophrenia, acute mania, anxiety, hallucinations, and confusion, following ingestion of phenylpropanolamine. Groups at increased risk appeared to be those with a past personal or family psychiatric history, children under the age of 6, and postpartum women (Lake *et al.*, 1988, 1990). In most of these cases, the psychiatric symptoms resolved completely within several weeks of cessation of the drug. Psychiatric reactions were more likely to occur following the ingestion of combination products than preparations containing phenylpropanolamine alone. Ingestion of coffee together with phenylpropanolamine may also increase the risk of psychiatric side effects (Lake, 1991).

Forty-eight out of 61 cases of adverse reactions to phenylpropanolamine reported to the Swedish Adverse Drug Reaction Committee involved patients under 15 years of age (Norvenius *et al.*, 1979). Five patients, four of whom were children, manifested acute psychosis, including profound confusion and visual hallucination; the remainder experienced irritability, restlessness, and sleep disturbance. Aggressiveness was reported in some patients, particularly younger children. A 17-year-old boy was hospitalized three times within a few months with psychosis typified by mania which was subsequently attributed to high doses of phenylpropanolamine alone and with brompheniramine (Norvenius *et al.*, 1979).

Psychiatric reactions have also been linked to ephedrine and pseudoephedrine, although more so to the latter. Reported ephedrine side effects included psychosis (Herridge & A'Brook, 1968), mania, auditory hallucinations, and delusions (Whitehouse & Duncan, 1987), and electroencephalographic (EEG) abnormalities (Shucard *et al.*, 1985). In a series of case reports, pseudoephedrine has been associated with serious psychiatric disturbance in young children. In particular, visual hallucinations, often involving spiders and other insects, were reported in a series of reports appearing in the *British Medical Journal* (Ackland, 1984; Sankey *et al.*, 1984; Sills *et al.*, 1984). All five preschool-age children included in these reports had ingested an OTC combination drug consisting of pseudoephedrine and triprolidine. In a follow-up letter to the editor, one group noted that they had received over 50 communications in response to an initial article reporting side effects to the same medication that included visual hallucinations, behavioral disturbances, or both in children (Sills *et al.*, 1984).

While all of these case reports involving sympathomimetic drugs, and in particular those involving children, are serious, the need to exercise caution in attributing clear causal pathways is again emphasized. Only prospective, controlled, blinded studies can establish the causal sequence. One controlled study examined the effects of pseudoephedrine, triprolidine, or placebo in 218 children. Twelve children taking pseudoephedrine withdrew from the study because of side effects that included irritability, dizziness, poor sleeping, and general malaise (Bain, 1983). However, this set of symptoms does not resemble significant psychiatric reactions included in numerous case reports. Recent clinical trials involving the use of ephedrine (Tokola, 1984; Fuller *et al.*, 1996) and pseudoephedrine (Empey *et al.*, 1975; Janssens & Lins, 1995; Horak *et al.*, 1996; Stanley *et al.*, 1996; Varan *et al.*, 1996) with adults consistently reported no significant neuropsychological or psychiatric side effects to these medications. A review of 985 hospitalizations among some 100,000 pseudoephedrine users in one self-contained health care group revealed that 929 were not related to the drug. The incidence of hospitalizations for myocardial infarction, seizures, or psychiatric disorders, which have been associated with pseudoephedrine use, was no greater than that found in the general population (Porta *et al.*, 1986). While these findings do not rule out the possibility of significant adverse reactions in a very small proportion of people using ephedrine or pseudoephedrine, they highlight the absence of any scientifically established causal relationship.

In conclusion:

1 three sympathomimetic decongestants – phenylpropanolamine, ephedrine, and pseudoephedrine – have been associated with significant psychiatric side effects in adults and children;
2 phenylpropanolamine accounts for the largest number of such case reports, although this finding alone does not establish true incidence in the general population;

3 mania in adults and visual hallucinations in children have been most frequently reported following ingestion of ephedrine and pseudoephedrine;
4 no causal mechanism has been scientifically established; and
5 the frequent reporting of neuropsychological and psychiatric changes observed in children underscores the need to study effects of OTC antihistamines and decongestants in this age group.

Anticholinergic Drugs

Anticholinergic agents are frequently used as therapy for rhinorrhea; they diminish the excessive secretion of the serous glands, resulting in nasal mucosa. Inhalation of quaternary salts of atropine, such as ipratropium bromide, is not associated with neuropsychological or psychiatric side effects. However, a number of case reports describe psychiatric reactions to the oral or ophthalmic use of other anticholinergic agents. Additionally, several controlled studies have evaluated specific behavioral changes following the administration of atropine in the laboratory. Visual perception, reaction time, verbal memory, coordination, and motor steadiness improved following atropine inhalation in normal male volunteers, with a greater deficit at higher dose (1.7 mg) than at lower dose (0.85 mg) (Seppala & Visakorpi, 1983). In a second study, dose-related side effects were again documented. Impairment in visual discrimination, calculation, and memory was most marked at 6.0 mg, less so at 3.0 mg, and nonexistent at 1.5 mg. Subjects in this study additionally reported dose-related symptoms including nausea, restlessness, sleepiness, confusion, blurred vision, and feeling 'high' that began 90 min after ingestion and abated 7–9 hours later (Higgins *et al.*, 1989).

Psychiatric side effects have been reported at doses of atropine that exceed recommended levels (Brizer & Maning, 1982). In a group of 212 cases of stramonium overdose, visual hallucinations were present in 50% of the cases, and hyperactivity, competitiveness, amnesia, and disorientation in 10–21% (Gowdy, 1972). Auditory and visual hallucinations and amnesia have also been reported in the use of anticholinergic eye drops, even at recommended doses (Freund & Merin, 1970; Shihab, 1980; Khurana *et al.*, 1988).

In conclusion:

1 serious psychiatric reactions have been described in case reports involving anticholinergic agents;
2 in contrast to several other categories of drugs described in this report, controlled studies involving anticholinergic drugs have been conducted and have found neuropsychological impairment but no significant psychiatric reactions/ and
3 serious adverse psychiatric reactions have been described by case

report but not by controlled studies in the use of anticholinergic eye drops.

Conclusion

A wide variety of neuropsychological and psychiatric side effects have been attributed to numerous medications used to treat asthma and allergic rhinitis. The published literature supporting these attributions is inconsistent and controversial. In particular, the tendency to associate these medications with serious psychiatric reactions must be greeted with exercised objectivity. Despite the proliferation of case reports to the contrary, there is little scientific evidence that theophylline, sympathomimetics, inhaled corticosteroids, or anticholinergics cause insanity. Case reports are frequently retrospective accounts of circumstances involving the development of serious psychiatric and neuropsychological problems. The attribution of causation is based upon the questionable assumption that because the medication was ingested in a time frame prior to the behavioral changes it is therefore responsible for them. Among other problems, the case report identification of a correlate, in this case a medication, may be spurious and unrelated to the psychiatric event, or related to yet a third variable. For instance, the illness which resulted in the patient's use of a decongestant may be a more significant factor contributing to the psychiatric disorder than the medication.

In some cases, the number of case reports may be so overwhelming that the cause-and-effect relationship between the drug and side effect gradually gains widespread acceptance. This appears to be the situation with regard to oral corticosteroids, aided by one very large, retrospective, chart-review study which attempted to control for numerous circumstantial variables (Boston Collaborative Drug Surveillance Program, 1972). For other medications discussed in this chapter, however, a causal relationship between medication and psychiatric disorder has not been proven. Inhaled corticosteroids, pseudoephedrine, sympathomimetics, and anticholinergics may be the source of reasonable suspicions but have no firmly established capacity to cause potent psychological changes.

In those instances where controlled studies have included psychological measures, which is true for theophylline, inhaled corticosteroids, and anticholinergic eye drops, subtle neuropsychological or mood changes have sometimes been documented, but never major psychiatric changes. This finding does not rule out the possibility that the proportion of patients experiencing a specific side effect may be so small that the event may emerge in a study of only 30 patients. However, when the total, cumulative patient sample grows to several hundred participants over numerous clinical trials with no reporting of an adverse psychiatric event, the association weakens.

In many cases, the clinician's best choice may be to simply advise against future use of the medication in question and move toward a different medication to treat the target symptoms. Even without clear cause-and-effect information, this choice may be the most efficient, particularly if the psychological symptoms were transient and occurred only at the time of medication use and no further symptoms persist. The situation is more problematic, however, if a patient assigns culpability for a recurrent, chronic psychiatric condition to a medication ingested for treatment of asthma or allergic rhinitis. Although at least one case report has suggested that use of pseudoephedrine precipitated a bipolar disorder requiring long-term lithium treatment (Dalton, 1990), evidence that asthma and allergy medications can produce psychiatric conditions that continue long after cessation of the drugs is particularly threadbare. The conditions surrounding onset of any serious psychiatric condition are invariably complex, frequently multifactorial, and in many instances do not alter the required intervention. In short, preoccupation with placing blame on a medication that appeared to induce a psychiatric illness, but for which no causal basis can be scientifically proven, may serve only to distract all parties involved from planning the optimal treatment strategy.

For the clinician faced with a patient or a patient's family who are convinced that a particular medication caused untoward psychological changes, the task of disentangling cause and effect may be difficult. In most instances, providing a respectful audience to these complaints, followed by a careful examination of the evidence, will be more successful than quick dismissal of the complaint. Once having established a belief that behavioral problems are caused by a drug, many patients are reluctant to relinquish that belief and search for another cause. In a few instances, patients and families may suspect other reasons for the psychiatric symptoms, but avoided pursuing them, choosing instead to identify an external factor to blame rather than to examine personal and family dynamics which may have contributed. Referral to a mental health professional is frequently appropriate to further assess and treat the source of psychological difficulty. However, the success of that referral may depend upon the physician first helping the patient and family to begin to relinquish the hypothesis of medication-induced changes and to accept the possibility of psychological difficulty arising for other reasons.

References

Ackland, F.M. (1984). Hallucinations in a child after drinking triprolidine/pseudoephedrine linctus. *Lancet*, 1, 1180.

American asthma report (1989). New York: Research and Forecasts.

Aso, T. & Sakai, Y. (1989). Effect of terfenadine, a novel antihistamine, on actual driving performance. *Annals of Allergy*, 62, 250.

Bain, D.J.G. (1983). Can the clinical course of acute otitis media be modified by systemic decongestant or antihistamine treatment? *British Medical Journal*, 287, 654–656.

Bender, B., Lerner, J., & Kollasch, E. (1988). Mood and memory changes in asthmatic children receiving corticosteroids. *Journal of the American Academy of Child and Adolescent Psychiatry*, 6, 720–725.

Bender, B.G., Milgrom, H., Calvin, J., & Ackerson, L. (1991a). A double-blind crossover study of behavior change in asthmatic children treated with theophylline and placebo. *Annals of Allergy*, 66, 65.

Bender, B.G., Lerner, J.A., & Polland, J.E. (1991b). Association between corticosteroids and psychologic change in hospitalized asthmatic children. *Annals of Allergy*, 66, 414–419.

Bender, B., & Milgrom, H. (1992). Theophylline-induced behavior change in children: an objective evaluation of parents' perceptions. *Journal of the American Medical Association*, 267, 2621–2624.

Bender, B., Iklé, D., DuHamel, T., & Tinkelman, D. (1998). Neuropsychological and behavioral changes in asthmatic children treated with beclomethasone dipropionate versus theophylline. *Pediatrics*, 101(3): 355–360.

Betts, T., Markman, D., Debenham, S., Mortiboy, D., & McKevitt, T. (1984). Effect of two antihistamine drugs on actual driving performance. *British Medical Journal (Clin. Res.)*, 288, 281–282.

Boston Collaborative Drug Surveillance Program (1972). Acute adverse reactions in relation to dosage. *Clinical Pharmacology*, 13, 694–698.

Brizer, D.A. & Maning, D.W. (1982). Delirium induced by poisoning with anticholinergic agents. *American Journal of Psychiatry*, 139, 1343–1344.

Cade, R., Spooner, G., & Schlein, E. (1973). Comparison of azathioprine, prednisone, and heparin alone or combined in treated lupus nephritis. *Nephron*, 10, 37–56.

Campbell, D.T. & Stanley, J.C. (1966). *Experimental and quasi-experimental designs for research.* Chicago: Rand McNally College Publishing Co.

Connett, G. & Lenney, W. (1991). Inhaled budensonide and behavioral disturbances. *Lancet*, 338, 634–635.

Cordess, C., Folstein, M., & Drachman, D. (1981). Psychiatric effects of alternate day steroid therapy. *British Journal of Psychiatry*, 138, 504–506.

Creer, T.L. & McLaughlin, J.A. (1989). The effects of theophylline on cognitive and behavioral performance. *Journal of Allergy and Clinical Immunology*, 83, 1027–1029.

Dalton, R. (1990). Mixed bipolar disorder precipitated by pseudophedrine hydrochloride. *Southern Medical Journal*, 83, 64–65.

Empey, D.W., Bye, C., Hodder, M., & Hughes, D.T. (1975). A double-blind crossover trial of pseudoephedrine and triprolidine, alone and in combination, for treatment of allergic rhinitis. *Annals of Allergy*, 34(1), 41–46.

Feldman, W., Shanon, A., Leiken, L., Hampong, A., & Peterson, R. (1992). Central nervous system side effects of antihistamines in schoolchildren. *Rhinology*, 13, 13–19.

Feline, A. & Jouvent, R. (1977). Manifestations psychosensorielles observees chez des psychotiques soumises a des medications beta-mimetiques. *Encephale*, 3, 149–158.

Firestone, P. & Martin, J. (1979). An analysis of the hyperactive syndrome: a comparison of hyperactive, behavior problem, asthmatic, and normal children. *Journal of Abnormal Child Psychology*, 7(5), 261–273.

Fitzpatrick, M.F., Engleman, H.M., Boellert, F., *et al.* (1992). Effect of therapeutic theophylline levels on the sleep quality and daytime cognitive performance of normal subjects. *American Review of Respiratory Disorders*, 145, 1355–1358.

Freund, M. & Merin, S. (1970). Toxic effects of scopolamine eye drops. *American Journal of Ophthalmology*, 70, 637–639.

Fuller, M.A., Borovicka, M.C., Jaskiw, G.E., Simon, M.R., Kevon, K., & Konicki, P.E. (1996). Clozapine-induced urinary incontinence: incidence and treatment with ephedrine. *Journal of Clinical Psychiatry*, 57(11), 514–518.

Furukawa, C.T., Shapiro, G.G., Bierman, C.W., Kraemer, M.J., Ward, D.J., & Pierson, W.E. (1984). A double-blind study comparing the effectiveness of cromolyn sodium and sustained-release theophylline in childhood asthma. *Pediatrics*, 74, 453–459.

Furukawa C.T., DuHamel T.R., Weimer L, Shapiro, G.G., Pierson, W.E., & Bierman C.W. (1988). Cognitive and behavioral findings in children taking theophylline. *Journal of Allergy and Clinical Immunology*, 81, 83–88.

Gluckman, L. (1974). Ventolin psychosis. *New Zealand Medical Journal*, 80, 411.

Gowdy, J.M. (1972). Stramonium intoxication: review of symptomatology in 212 cases. *Journal of the American Medical Association*, 221, 585–587.

Harris, J.C., Carel, C.A., Rosenberg, L.A., Joshi, P., & Leventhal, B.G. (1986). Intermittent high dose corticosteroid treatment in childhood cancer. *Journal of the American Academy of Child Psychiatry*, 25, 120–124.

Herridge, C. & A'Brook, M. (1968). Ephedrine psychosis (Abstract). *British Medical Journal*, 2, 160.

Higgins, S., Lamb, R., & Henningfield, J. (1989). Dose-dependent effects of atropine on behavioral and physiologic responses in humans. *Pharmacology, Biochemistry and Behavior*, 34, 303–311.

Horak, F., Jager, S., Toth, J., & Berger, V. (1996). Efficacy and tolerability of astemizole-D and loratadine-D during prolonged, controlled allergen challenge in the Vienna Challenge Chamber. *Arzneimittelforschung*, 46(11), 1077–1081.

Jacquot, M. & Bottari, R. (1981). Etat maniaque ayant ete declenche par la prise orale de salbutamol. *Encephale*, 7, 45–49.

Janssens, M.M. & Lins, R.L. (1995). Astemizole-D causes less sleep impairment than loratadine-D. *Journal of International Medical Research*, 23(3), 167–174.

Joad, J., Ahrens, R.C., Lindgren, S.D., & Weinberger, M.M. (1986). Extrapulmonary effects of maintenance therapy with theophylline and inhaled albuterol in patients with chronic asthma. *Journal of Allergy and Clinical Immunology*, 78(6), 1147–1153.

Khurana, A.K., Ahluwalia, B.K., Rajan, C., & Vohra, A.K. (1988). Acute psychosis associated with topical cyclopentolate hydrochloride. *American Journal of Ophthalmology*, 105, 91.

Kulshrestha, V.K., Gupta, P.P., Turner, P., & Wadsworth, J. (1978). Some clinical pharmacological studies with terfenadine, a new antihistaminic drug. *British Journal of Clinical Pharmacology*, 6, 25–29.

Lake, C.R. (1991). Manic psychosis after coffee and phenylpropanolamine. *Biological Psychiatry*, 30, 401–404.

Lake, C.R., Masson, E.B., & Quirk, R.S. (1988). Psychiatric side effects attributed to phenylpropanolamine. *Pharmacopsychiatry*, 21, 171–181.

Lake, C.R., Gallant, S., Masson, E., & Miller, P. (1990). Adverse drug effects attributed to phenylpropanolamine: a review of 142 case reports. *American Journal of Medicine*, 89, 195–208.

Lewis, A. & Fleminger, J.J. (1954). The psychiatric risk from corticotrophin and cortisone. *Lancet*, 1, 383–386.

Lewis, L.D. & Cochrane, G.M. (1983). Psychosis in a child inhaling budesonide. *Lancet*, 2, 634.

Lindgren, S., Lokshin, B., Stromquist, A., *et al.* (1992). Does asthma or treatment with theophylline limit children's academic performance? *New England Journal of Medicine*, 327, 926–930.

Ling, M.H.M., Perry, P.J., & Tsuang, M.T. (1981). Side effects of corticosteroid therapy. *Archives of General Psychiatry*, 38, 471–477.

Lonnerholm, G., Foucard, T., & Lindstrom, B. (1984). Dose, plasma concentration, and effect of oral terbutaline in long-term treatment of childhood asthma. *Journal of Allergy and Clinical Immunology*, 73, 508–515.

McCarthy, M.M. (1981). Speech effects of theophylline. *Pediatrics*, 68, 749.

Mazer, B., Figueroa-Rosario, W., Bender, B. (1990). The effect of albuterol aerosol on fine-motor performance in children with chronic asthma. *Journal of Allergy and Clinical Immunology*, 86, 243–248.

Meyboom, R.H. & de Graaf-Breederveld, N. (1988). Budesonide and psychic side effects. *Annals of Internal Medicine*, 109(8), 683.

Milgrom, H. & Bender, B.G. (1993). Psychologic side effects of therapy with corticosteroids. *American Review of Respiratory Disease*, 147, 471–473.

Milgrom, H. & Bender, B. (1997). Adverse effects of medications for rhinitis. *Annals of Allergy, Asthma, and Immunology*, 78, 439–446.

Moser, L., Huther, K.J., Koch-Weser, J. & Lundt, P.V. (1978). Effects of terfenadine and diphenhydramine alone or in combination with diazepam or alcohol on psychomotor performance and subjective feelings. *European Journal of Clinical Pharmacology*, 14, 417–423.

Moskowitz, H. & Burns, M. (1988). Effects of terfenadine, diphenhydramine, and placebo on skills performance. *Cutis*, 42, 14–18.

Murphy, M., Dillon, A., & Fitzgerald, M. (1980). Theophylline and depression. *British Medical Journal*, 15, 281.

Nelson, L. & Schwartz, J. (1987). Theophylline-induced age-related CNS stimulation. *Pediatric Asthma, Allergy and Immunology*, 1, 175–183.

Norvenius, G., Wilderlov, E., & Lonnerholm, G. (1979). Phenylpropanolamine and mental disturbances (letter). *Lancet*, 2, 1367–1368.

O'Hanlon, J.F. & Ramaekers, J.G. (1995). Antihistamine effects on actual driving performance in a standard test: a summary of Dutch experience, 1989–94. *Allergy*, 50, 234–242.

Painter, K. (1986). Asthma drug hard on kids. *USA Today*, Dec. 2, 1.

Porta, M., Jick, H., & Habakangas, J.A.S. (1986). Follow-up study of pseudoephedrine users. *Annals of Allergy*, 57, 340–342.

Rachelefsky, G., Wo, J., Adelson, J., *et al.* (1986). Behavior abnormalities and poor school performance due to oral theophylline use. *Pediatrics*, 78, 1133–1138.

Rappaport, L., Coffman, H., Guare, R., Fenton, T., DeGraw, C., & Twarog F. (1989). Effects of theophylline on behavior and learning in children with asthma. *American Journal of Diseases of Children*, 143, 368–372.

Ray, I. & Evans, C.J. (1978). Paranoid psychosis with Ventolin (salbutamol tablets). *Canadian Psychiatric Association Journal*, 23, 417.

Riedel, W.J., Schoenmakers, E.A.J.M., & O'Hanlon, J.F. (1987). The effects of loratadine alone and in combination with alcohol on actual driving performance. Maastricht, The Netherlands: Institute for Drugs, Safety and Behavior (University of Limburg), Tech. Rep. 87-01.

Roehrs, T., Zwyghuizen-Doorenbos, A., & Roth, T. (1993). Sedative effects and plasma concentrations following single dose of triazolam, diphenhydramine, ethanol, and placebo. *Sleep*, 16, 301–305.

Sankey, R.J., Nunn, A.J., & Sills, J.A. (1984). Visual hallucinations in children receiving decongestants. *British Medical Journal*, 288, 1369.

Schlieper, A., Adcock, D., Beaudry, P., Feldman, W., & Leikin, L. (1991). Effect of therapeutic plasma concentrations of theophylline on behavior, cognitive processing, and affect in children with asthma. *Journal of Pediatrics*, 118, 449–455.

Schweitzer, P.K., Muehlback, M.J., & Walsh, J.K. (1994). Sleepiness and performance during three-day administration of cetirizine or diphenhydramine. *Journal of Allergy and Clinical Immunology*, 94, 716–724.

Seidel, W.F., Cohen, S., Bliwise, N.G., & Dement, W.C. (1987). Cetirizine effects on objective measures of daytime sleepiness and performance. *Annals of Allergy*, 59, 58–62.

Seppala, T. & Visakorpi, R. (1983). Psychophysiological measurements after oral atropine in man. *Acta Pharmacologica et Toxicologica (Copenhagen)*, 52, 68–74.

Shihab, Z.M. (1980). Psychotic reaction in an adult after topical cyclopentolate. *Ophthalmologica*, 181, 228–230.

Shucard, D.W., Spector, S.L., Euwer, R.L., Cummins, K.R., Shucard, J.L., & Friedman, A. (1985). Central nervous system effects of antiasthma medication – an EEG study. *Annals of Allergy*, 54(3), 177–184.

Sills, J.A., Nunn, A.J., & Sankey, R.J. (1984). Visual hallucinations in children receiving decongestants (Letter). *British Medical Journal (Clinical Research Ed.)*, 288, 1912–1913.

Simons, F.E.R. & Simons, K.J. (1988). H_1-receptor antagonist treatment of chronic rhinitis. *Journal of Allergy and Clinical Immunology*, 81, 975–980.

Simons, F.E.R., Fraser, T., Regin, J., Roberts, J.R., & Simons, K.J. (1996). Adverse central nervous system effects of the older antihistamine in children. *Pediatric Allergy and Immunology*, 7, 22–27.

Springer, C., Goldenberg, B., Ben Dov, I., & Godfrey, S. (1985). Clinical, physiologic and psychologic comparison of treatment by cromolyn or theophylline in childhood asthma. *Journal of Allergy and Clinical Immunology*, 76, 64–49.

Stanley, N., Alford, C.A., Rombaut, N.E., & Hindmarch, I. (1996). Comparison of the effects of astemizole/pseudoephedrine and triprolidine/pseudoephedrine on CNS activity and psychomotor function. *International Clinical Psychopharmacology*, 11(1), 31–36.

Stein, M.A. & Lerner, C.A. (1993). Behavioral and cognitive effect of theophylline: a dose–response study. *Annals of Allergy*, 70, 135–140.

Suess, W.M., Stump, N., Chai, H., & Kalisker, A. (1986). Mnemonic effects of asthma medication in children. *Journal of Asthma*, 23, 291–296.

Tinklelman, D.G., Reed, C.E., Nelson, H.S., & Offord, K.P. (1993). Aerosol beclomethasone diproprionate compared with theophylline as primary treatment of chronic, mild to moderately severe asthma in children. *Pediatrics*, 92, 64–77.

Tokola, O. (1984). Drug treatment of motion sickness: scopolamine alone and combined with ephedrine in real and simulated situations. *Aviation Space and Environmental Medicine*, 55(7), 636–641.

Varan, B., Saata, U., Ozen, S., Bakkalogu, A., & Besbas, N. (1996). Efficacy of oxybutynin, pseudoephedrine and indomethacin in the treatment of primary nocturnal enuresis. *Turkish Journal of Pediatrics*, 38(2), 155–159.

Vuurman, E.F., Veggel, V.L., Uiterwijk, M.M., Leutner, D., O'Hanlon, J.F. (1993). Seasonal allergic rhinitis and antihistamine effects on children's learning. *Annals of Allergy*, 71, 121–126.

Vuurman, E.F.P.M., van Veggel, L.M.A., Sanders, R.L., Muntjewerff, N.D., & O'Hanlon, J.F. (1996). Effects of Semprex-D and diphenhydramine on learning in young adults with seasonal allergic rhinitis. *Annals of Allergy, Asthma, and Immunology*, 6, 247–252.

Wasser, W.G., Bronheim, H.E., Richardson, B.K. (1981). Theophylline madness. *Annals of Internal Medicine*, 95, 191.

Wertheimer, A. (1985). Phenylalklamines: preparations, marketing, and economics: U.S. and abroad. In J. Morgan, D. Kagan, & J. Brody (Eds), *Phenylpropanolamine* (pp. 37–52). New York: Praeger.

Whitehouse, A.M. & Duncan, J.M. (1987). Ephedrine psychosis rediscovered. *British Journal of Psychiatry*, 150, 258–261.

Whitehouse, A. & Novosel, S. (1989). Salbutamol psychosis. *Biological Psychiatry*, 26, 631–633.

8
Compliance and respiratory disorders

Deirdre A. Levstek Caplin

Editors' note—*Although the issue of compliance has been around since the first health care provider suggested how a fellow caveman treat a physical problem, interest in its role in the management of respiratory disorders is relatively recent. In fact, interest in the topic of compliance was virtually nonexistent until the widespread prescribing of oral corticosteroids and, in particular, theophylline occurred (Creer, 1993). As theophylline medications are effective only within narrow ranges – and as potentially serious side effects could occur in taking the drugs – interest in the topic of medications compliance or adherence was generated.*

In this chapter, Deirdre Caplin describes research on medication compliance. It is, as she notes, a significant problem in the management of respiratory problems. Ways that the problem can be assessed, as well as proven techniques for improving adherent behavior, are described. Alas, the problem is nowhere near a solution. Besides the reasons, many of which are valid, that patients cite for not taking a drug, three recent trends present caveats to both medical and behavioral scientists.

First, newer inhaled respiratory medications are effective only when taken as directed. This point is emphasized in every set of treatment guidelines for respiratory disorders, particularly those for asthma (e.g., National Heart, Lung and Blood Institute, 1995). Yet, patients are not always taught how to use their inhalers correctly (Creer & Levstek, 1996). Consequently, they fail to receive full benefit from any inhaled drug. In addition, monitoring of the patient's medication-taking behaviors rarely occurs. This results in a sequence of behaviors that, beginning with failure to use an inhaler correctly, results in inadequate control of a respiratory disorder. The consequence is taken by a patient to mean that the drug does not work; he may cease using the drug. Meanwhile, the patient's health care provider lays the blame for noncompliance on the shoulders of the patient and fails to recognize her role in the emergence or avoidance of the problem.

Secondly, a recent philosophy regarding medication use seems to be that 'more and more is better.' As described by Creer et al. (1999), the trend is characterized by asthma patients being asked to follow a regimen that includes a quick-relief short-acting β-agonist medication taken as needed, and up to four preventive or controller drugs – inhaled corticosteroids, a long-lasting β-agonist, cromolyn sodium, and an anti-leukotriene drug – taken on a daily basis. This approach is fraught with danger to both medical and behavioral scientists. Health care providers, for example, have no idea of the interactive or cumulative effect of prescribing four controller drugs, nor the burden placed on patients in attempting to coordinate and perform such a medication-taking schedule. Health care providers also fail to consider the financial burden placed on patients in prescribing such a complex regimen. Behavioral scientists, on the other hand, can be placed in harm's way by being asked to improve compliance to complex regimens when they, along with medical scientists and patients, have no idea of the long-term consequences resulting from patient adherence to such treatment plans.

Finally, as stressed by Deirdre throughout her chapter, medication compliance is but one part of the cooperative strategy of management encompassed by self-management. Adherence to any regimen first requires that health care providers and patients sit down and, working together, decide upon and write the best action plan that can be followed to control a respiratory disorder. Focusing only on medication compliance is an example of micromanagement; it focuses on only one part of the overall strategy for disease management. It would be analogous to a health care provider focusing on one symptom, such as a cough, without considering the underlying mechanism that produces the cough. While the latter would be unlikely to occur, it has not deterred medical and behavioral scientists from considering only medication compliance and not the overall strategy taken by tandems of health care providers and patients to treat a respiratory disorder. For this reason, it is important to consider these trends in considering how the research described by Deirdre Caplin can be best used to control respiratory disorders.

Introduction

Compliance is a multifaceted, complex construct that has a critical impact on medical research and treatment of respiratory disorders. Compliance is a concept that affects all members of the health care community, including physicians, therapists, nurses, pharmacists, and patients. This chapter outlines the core issues and problems surrounding the significance, definition, measurement, and factors influencing patient decisions about treatment. In addition, the issue of physician compliance is discussed in terms of its impact on quality of treatment and on addressing patient noncompliance. Finally, suggestions are made to enhance patient–physician efforts to improve treatment acceptance.

Significance of the Problem

Poor compliance to medical regimens is a continuing source of frustration for health professionals who study and treat chronic respiratory disorders. Diseases such as asthma, cystic fibrosis, and chronic obstructive pulmonary disease (COPD) demand considerable patient effort to be effectively controlled; yet practitioners frequently find it difficult to get patients to adopt and maintain recommended treatments. A healthy body of literature has been accumulated on the topic. Numerous investigations have delineated factors thought to influence compliance, ways to measure compliance, and methods for improving compliance; however, the problem of patient adherence remains. Models of decision making and behavior change have been used in an attempt to explain the complex process of patient disease management. These models have helped us understand that the issue of compliance is not as simple as patients forgetting or ignoring physician orders (Powell & Hudson, 1997; Rand & Sevick, 2000).

In a recent article, Creer (1998) noted that some of the difficulties with medication compliance originate with the nature of the diseases being studied. The respiratory diseases of gravest concern are those that are long term and incurable, often requiring lifelong treatment. Treatment regimens for cystic fibrosis, COPD, and asthma are characterized by complex medical, behavioral, and environmental demands placed on patients. The acceptance of a regimen that can achieve complex treatment goals requires considerable time, effort, and attention that may last a lifetime. To fully understand patient compliance, we not only need to examine why patients have difficulty achieving the targets set for their treatment but also the expectations and responsibilities that practitioners have with respect to this process.

Bender *et al.* (1997) reviewed the existing literature on adherence to asthma treatment. They noted that the consequences of patient noncompliance result in significant costs at the personal, financial, and research level. Poor adherence to treatment may have several implications for patients, the most serious being side effects from medication misuse, life-threatening illness exacerbations, and even death (Bender *et al.*, 1997). Physicians may misinterpret the effectiveness of a particular regimen based on an inadequate medication trial. Financially, the chronic nature of most respiratory diseases requires continuous, costly treatment. For asthma the cost associated with treatment was estimated at $10.7 billion in the United States (Weiss *et al.*, 2000). Even more significant is the finding that about 5% of patients with respiratory diseases incurred the majority of health care costs (Bender *et al.*, 1997). The financial costs of noncompliance include direct costs of unused medication, additional diagnostic and treatment evaluation, frequent hospitalizations, and an increase in overall cost of health care (Creer & Levstek, 1998). Research problems associated with poor patient adherence originate from a variety of sources, including failure to take medications, failure to perform other therapies (e.g., chest physiotherapy, oxygen therapy), failure to adequately record data, failure to show up for scheduled appointments, and even fabricating data. In clinical medication trials, the degree of adherence to treatment has a significant impact on the cost, duration, and potential outcomes of the study. If it is not monitored or corrected, patient noncompliance may result in inaccurate conclusions, which eventually interfere with appropriate patient treatment (Bender *et al.*, 1997; Vitolins *et al.*, 2000).

Definition and Description

Compliance is a term that denotes how successfully patients behave in accordance with the various components of the medical advice they receive. Professionals have interpreted patient decisions in a variety of ways, including denial, procrastination, forgetfulness, refusal, and reasoned decision making (Lask, 1997). Many authors (e.g., Wills & Moore, 1994) have voiced concern about the term 'compliance' in discussions of patient practices, suggesting that it categorizes patients as passive and places the patient in a subordinate role in the treatment process. Realistically, the term compliance involves patients' active, more realistic acceptance and adaptation of their behaviors to conform with the regimens developed under the guidance of their health care providers. Compliance tends to connote the idea of patient action and patient responsibility; ultimately, patients are responsible for their own behavior (Cesar-Ramos, 1997). Some researchers have offered the terms 'adherence,' 'concordance,' 'acceptance,' and 'commitment' as substitutes for the connotative discomfort associated with the term 'compliance' (Mullen, 1997; Anderson & Funnell, 2000; Creer, 1998). It appears that practitioners and researchers have difficulty acknowledging that their interest lies in patient conformity to prescribed treatments. However, as Creer (1998, p. 5) notes, 'discussion and coining of terms [to describe compliance] serves to dance around the issue.' Semantically, there is no real difference between a nonadherent, an uncommitted, or a noncompliant patient. Each term implies an equally undesirable state, characterized by patients not performing the actions prescribed for them. In this chapter, the terms are used interchangeably.

The labels that health professionals use to define patient behaviors are likely to have little impact or significance for patients. According to some authors, compliance is a value-laden construct that was developed and promoted by practitioners, but one that is meaningless to patients (Anderson & Funnell, 2000; Huss *et al.*, 1997). Patients do not assess their own behaviors by how closely they agree with medical advice. Rather, they weigh the costs and benefits of adherence within the constraints of their everyday lives. In doing so, patients balance their physical state with the economic, social, and psychological impact of treatment options. Although physicians are the primary source by which patients receive knowledge and treatment, prescriptive advice requires patient action. It is the patient who must perform the daily actions necessary to successfully manage a chronic respiratory disease. It is patients who decide to accept or reject what is offered to them (Sockrider & Wolle, 1996).

Problems with Definitions of Compliance

Reported patient noncompliance among asthma, cystic fibrosis, and COPD populations is highly variable, and often inaccurate or incomplete

Table 8.1 Four major problems with current definitions of compliance

- No standardized definition of compliance
- Inadequate attention to multiple components of treatment
- Inadequate use of continuous approach for determining compliance
- Inadequate attention to within-patient variability in compliance behaviors

Adapted from Lask, 1997.

(Rand & Sevick, 2000; Lask, 1997). Four major difficulties arise with our ability to standardize our definitions for what constitutes a compliant patient, and they are summarized in Table 8.1 (Lask, 1997).

First, few comparisons are possible across studies because patients are deemed noncompliant based on a variety of inconsistent factors and criteria. These include the population studied, the setting, the medication or regimen investigated, and the level of patient action that determines compliance. Clinical researchers define adherence by arbitrarily assigning some percentage of medication use, time of use, or levels of medication in the body at the time of assessment. Often, compliance is considered adequate if the patient received at least 50% of the medication prescribed (e.g., Vitolins *et al.*, 2000). In other investigations, compliance is consumption of greater than 60–70% of medication doses (Corden *et al.*, 1997); others suggest that 80–100% compliance be a standard for complete compliance (Bosley *et al.*, 1994). Some workers assert that patients should be differentiated by levels of noncompliance based on actual behavior. For example, Dowell and Hudson (1997) separated patients into three groups: those who never adhered, those who adhered passively, and those who actively decided to take more or less medication than prescribed. In one study of asthma patients, about one-third of patients took medications as prescribed, another one-third took medications occasionally, and the final one-third did not comply at all. However, for other areas of compliance, there are no accurate and reliable measures to assess patient performance (Vitolins *et al.*, 2000). As a result, compliance and the factors influencing it are rarely consistent across studies. In clinical settings, patient perceptions of symptoms and overall health outcomes are commonly used as criteria for adequate compliance; these perceptions showed even greater variability and less specificity than other measures. However, it has been suggested that it is more important for practitioners to develop minimum standards necessary to achieve treatment goals, and base determinations of compliance on the goals of treatment rather than on 100% adherence (Rand & Sevick, 2000). The multifaceted nature of compliance is frequently ignored in favor of assessing compliance with one aspect of treatment, usually medication use.

A second reason for difficulties in defining adherence focuses on the multifaceted nature of treatment for respiratory diseases. In the treatment of respiratory disease, medication is only one component of a comprehensive treatment regimen. Cystic fibrosis treatment, for example, is extremely complex, and includes medication, diet, exercise, chest therapy, and daily monitoring as a part of a regular regimen. COPD patients are frequently required to make a number of difficult lifestyle changes, such as smoking cessation, limiting some activities, and initiating regular exercise monitoring; they may also receive oxygen therapy supplemental to medications. Patients with asthma are often required to take specific medications for acute symptom relief in addition to daily controller medications. They are often asked to monitor symptoms and lung functioning, and to participate in establishing environmental control. For each respiratory disorder, compliance for each dimension of treatment is a separate issue that needs to be independently defined and measured in order to be useful. Lask (1997) reported that with cystic fibrosis patients, rates of adherence vary according to which dimension of treatment is studied. Similar findings were reported with COPD (Vitolins *et al.*, 2000) and asthma (Caplin, 1998). A comprehensive approach is more likely to facilitate an accurate understanding of patient behaviors (Sockrider & Wolle, 1996; Lask, 1997; Creer, 1998).

Another concern with current definitions of compliance is the tendency of researchers and practitioners to label patients as either 'adherent' or 'nonadherent' (Lask, 1997). Lask describes what he labels 'incomplete adherence' to account for the vast majority of patients, who are neither 100% compliant nor 100% noncompliant. Similarly, Hindi-Alexander *et al.* (1987) have suggested that patients range from a blind adherence to all instructions of their caregivers, to total nonadherence of any recommendations. They note that neither end of the spectrum is necessarily a desirable state, and that it is important to identify where patients fall in their approach to treatment. In studies of adherence to medical regimens for respiratory disorders, patients have rarely been found 100% compliant; in general, as suggested by Hindi-Alexander *et al.* (1987), patients fall along a continuum anchored at one end by a complete rejection of the treatment regimen, to what has been referred to as 'obsessive-compulsive self-regulation' (e.g., Kirschenbaum & Tomarken, 1982). This appears true for patients with asthma (Dunbar-Jacobs, 1993; Creer & Levstek, 1996), cystic fibrosis (Lask, 1997), and COPD (Simmons *et al.*, 2000).

Finally, Creer (1998) emphasized that assessments of adherence are limited by within-patient variability in behavior. Frequently, studies of compliance track behavior over short periods of time, which may not be an accurate picture for a given patient. Changes in regimen, environment, or symptom presentation may influence rates of compliance in any specific time period, without influencing overall rates.

Measurement of Compliance

Despite the problems faced in the definition and measurement of compliance, a variety of techniques are used to assess patient behaviors. Each method of assessment has its own set of advantages and drawbacks. Bender *et al.* (1997), and Vitolins and colleagues (2000) have provided comprehensive reviews of contemporary methods for assessing adherence of patients with respiratory disease. These techniques are summarized in Table 8.2, and are briefly described below.

Drug Assays

These include saliva and serum assays that detect the amount of medication remaining in the patient's system at the time of the assessment. Drug assays provide objective, quantifiable data. However, for many of the medications and treatments used by patients with chronic respiratory diseases, a specific assay test is either unavailable or too expensive for

Table 8.2 Typical methods of compliance measurement

Technique	Primary advantages	Primary disadvantages
Drug assays	• Objective, quantifiable information	• Limited availability • Expensive
Observation	• Able to ensure proper techniques	• Relies on patient commitment and persistence • Can be inconvenient
Clinical judgment	• Easy, inexpensive • Can be a positive adjunct to other measures	• Relies on positive patient–clinician relations • Subject to clinician bias
Self-report	• Able to observe trends in symptoms and behaviors • Simple, inexpensive, easy to administer	• Subject to patient bias, demand characteristics and recall
Medication measurement	• Accurate measure of medication practices • Can be direct or indirect	• Relies on patient and practitioner commitment • No guarantee of medication use
Electronic monitoring	• Objective information about patterns of use	• Expensive, impractical • Subject to mechanical failures

everyday use. In addition, the assessment only provides information about a specific moment in time rather than adherence over time.

Observation of Performance

Observational methods include observation of inhaler technique, or requiring parents and other family members to observe and record patients ingesting medication, exercising, or performing therapeutic tasks. These methods require time and commitment by parents and may be more indicative of family compliance than patient treatment adherence. However, many parents are able to accurately monitor their child's progress; in particular, positive results have been shown when families make weekly telephone reports to physicians (Simmons *et al.*, 2000). Observing inhaler technique, percussion technique, and other behavioral skills are helpful as an adjunct to clinical treatment to ensure the proper delivery of treatment.

Clinical Judgment

Clinician estimates of patient adherence occur commonly in practice, and are frequently the basis for treatment decisions. However, it has been noted that many physicians frequently overestimate the degree to which their patients follow prescribed regimens (Bender *et al.*, 1997). Rand & Wise (1994) suggest that the validity and reliability of physician estimates of compliance can be enhanced when used in combination with other measures. Rather than relying on intuition or stereotypes of what the compliant patient does, Bender *et al.* (1997) suggested that emphasizing quality in patient–clinical communications is likely to result in better estimates of compliance with treatment.

Self-Report

Self-reported compliance is another common form of compliance assessment. Assessments of performance for illness-related behaviors other than medication use, such as compliance with exercise and dietary control, rely heavily on patient or family recording and self-report. Assessments can be completed in an interview format, whereby the patient is asked to recall patterns of performance, difficulties with treatment, and appropriate treatment and medication delivery. More commonly, patients are asked to keep daily recordings (diaries) of their medication use, symptoms, and illness-related behaviors. Self-reports are simple, easy-to-administer, and inexpensive methods of tracking patients' experiences with their disease. In addition, self-reports are able to identify patterns of use with medications that are not prescribed by the practitioner. It is frequently the case that, unless asked, patients fail to supply information about over-the-counter (OTC) or other prescribed medications. However, it is well noted that self-reports are subject to bias, particularly memory problems and demand characteristics. In studies comparing self-reports with other objective measures of adherence, patients tend to overestimate their adherence to treatment (Bender *et al.*, 1997).

Brooks *et al.* (1994) validated two self-report scales for measuring adult adherence to medication regimens for asthma. They found that the measures exhibited adequate reliability and were useful at distinguishing variations in patient adherence to treatment. Similarly, Vitolins and colleagues (2000) recommend that all self-report measures be validated with other reports of behavior and have demonstrated reliability. They further suggest that measures should assess daily behavior patterns and trends in prn (as required) medication use for acute symptom relief. Patient self-reports may have the added advantage of facilitating practitioner insight into patient attitudes, barriers, and beliefs about their treatment regimens.

Medication Measurement

Some measures are designed specifically to assess medication compliance. Frequently, in clinical drug studies, various methods are employed that assess the amount of medication acquired and used by patients. Medications can be measured by the amount dispensed (either by study personnel or by perusing pharmacy records), or by measuring the amount of medication remaining in canisters and pill bottles during follow-up visits (Vitolins *et al.*, 2000; Bender *et al.*, 1997). Although these measures can be used as a comparison to self-reports, Bender *et al.* (1997) identified a number of potential limitations:

1 Medication measurement requires an effort both from the practitioner, who must record exact amounts of medication dispensed and returned at each visit, and from the patient, who must return all medication containers at every visit.
2 Medication 'dumping' (whereby patients discard medications prior to follow-up) has been identified in some studies as a problem (Simmons *et al.*, 2000).
3 Medications may be shared within a household, especially if more than one family member is prescribed a particular treatment.
4. When relying on pharmacy databases for medication measurements, the assumption is that patients are exclusively acquiring medications from one dispensary.
5. The measurement of medications does not confirm that patients used the medication, nor does it detect anything about patterns in medication usage (Bender *et al.*, 1997).

Electronic Monitoring

Of particular interest to the study of respiratory disease, electronic devices that monitor and record container usage have been developed for pill bottles (e.g., the Medication Event Monitoring System) and inhalation devices (the Nebulizer Chronolog and the Doser). These instruments are designed to record the date and number of actuations of the medication dispenser. Used in conjunction with patient reports, electronic devices have been a valuable tool in contemporary studies of medication compliance (Spector *et al.*, 1986; Vitolins *et al.*, 2000). They provide objective information about specific patterns of daily use over time. However, the method is costly, and may not be practical for use in a primary care office. They are subject to bias by patient misuse, device failure, and mechanical difficulties (Bender *et al.*, 1997). In addition, the method relies on the transfer of data from the patient to health care personnel.

Patient Compliance

Medication Compliance

There exists a large database of rates for patient adherence to medication regimens across acute and chronic medical problems. For patients with chronic respiratory illnesses, rates of adherence are highly variable. Compliance in pediatric asthma populations has ranged from 2–100% (Creer, 1993), and 30–70% for those with adult asthma (Lemanek, 1990). Most recent reports document compliance with asthma medications at around 30%–50% overall (Van Sciver *et al.*, 1995; Bender *et al.*, 1997). In a study of emergency department follow-up, where asthma was a presenting diagnosis, 12% of patients did not get their prescription filled upon discharge. Furthermore, asthma as a diagnosis was independently predictive of noncompliance.

For patients with cystic fibrosis, rates of compliance vary according to the medication regimen that is studied. Patient adherence rates appear to be highest with daily enzymes, and are reported to be 83%. However, compliance rates are only between 40% and 50% with vitamin therapies and acute antibiotic regimens. Hains *et al.* (1997) reported that about 35% of children with cystic fibrosis are nonadherent, a figure that tends to increase in adolescents. Other studies report that overall rates of compliance with cystic fibrosis treatment hover between 50% and 65% (Drotar, 1995; Abbott *et al.*, 1996; Conway *et al.*, 1996). Adherence estimates for persons with COPD are estimated around 50% for inhaled medications (Simmons *et al.*, 2000); patient compliance with nebulized treatments was slightly higher, at around 57% (Corden *et al.*, 1997).

Behavioral Compliance

The prevalence of nonadherence to the various behavioral aspects of respiratory care is largely undocumented. As previously noted, most studies of adherence have failed to address within-patient variability in adherence to different aspects of treatment (Abbott *et al.*, 1996). Most treatment regimens for respiratory diseases require compliance with a variety of behaviors and therapies in addition to medication use. These include lifestyle and activity restrictions, medical appointments, and environmental and behavioral prescriptions (Creer & Levstek, 1998).

Lifestyle and Activity Restrictions

Some studies of quality of life have attempted to measure the degree of interference of treatment with the expected roles of patients (McSweeny & Creer, 1995; Newacheck & Halfon, 1998). Alterations in lifestyle required by patients with respiratory diseases can range from no changes to being bedridden and unable to function independently. Many of the studies looking at behavioral compliance with lifestyle changes have focused on work- and home-related role functioning. Patients with mild asthma, for example, do not miss school or work days because of their symptoms. However, a study by Taylor & Newacheck (1992) reported that, overall, children with asthma missed an average of 10.1 million days of school annually over children with other chronic conditions. In a recent profile of children with chronic health conditions, Newacheck & Halfon (1998) reported that respiratory disease was one of the most common sources of childhood disability, accounting for about one-quarter of all cases of activity-limiting problems. In addition, they found that 47% of children with a respiratory disorder were significantly limited in their school attendance.

Medical Appointments

Most of the information available on patient compliance with medical appointments has been accumulated from patients with asthma. One study reported that respiratory disorders accounted for an average of 887 hospital days per 100 children per year (Newacheck & Halfon, 1998). Similarly, Brenner & Kohn (1998) reported that a significant percentage of emergency department visits (3–10%) were for acute asthma episodes, and that many of these patients were return visitors. Relapse in emergency room occurs about 30% of the time for patients with asthma, and usually within 10 days (Ducharme & Kramer, 1993). Emergency medicine departments often make follow-up appointments for patients who present at the emergency room in an attempt to reduce relapse. Thomas *et al.* (1996) found that of the asthma patients identified in one emergency department study, 42% patients admitted to having missed their scheduled follow-up appointment. Similarly, Levy (1997) reported that only 68% of patients with high rates of asthma morbidity regularly attend follow-up appointments. Turk & Meichenbaum (1991) reported 50–60% of patients did not attend scheduled appointments, and between 20 and 80% of patients drop out of self-care training programs designed to improve their disease management.

Environmental and Behavioral Prescriptions
Information about noncompliance with behavioral prescriptions has predominantly been studied with cystic fibrosis patients, but is thought to be prevalent among patients with most respiratory diseases. Lask (1997) noted that patient performance varies from task to task for patients with cystic fibrosis; the performance is known as treatment-specific adherence. Defining and describing the specific task demands for patients with cystic fibrosis is, therefore, an important element of adherence measurement. In one study, Abbott *et al.* (1996) found that 53% of patients were compliant with chest physiotherapy, compared with 75% who were exercising adequately. Similarly, patients reported the greatest noncompliance with chest physiotherapy, using dietary supplements, and adding pancreatic enzymes to snacks (Abbott *et al.*, 1996; Conway *et al.*, 1996).

Factors Influencing Patient Compliance

Many patients do not achieve complete symptom relief even if they are 100% adherent to their treatment protocol. In studies of treatment effects, adherence was often unrelated to medical outcome (Simmons *et al.*, 2000; Abbott *et al.*, 2001; Bender *et al.*, 1997). However, medication compliance for patients with chronic respiratory diseases is a well-studied issue. As a result, a variety of factors have been found that are statistically related to adherence (Creer & Kotses, 1990). Some of the factors are unique to pediatric compliance, other variables are more problematic for adult patients with respiratory disease. The illness-related variables, personal variables, and family variables that influence patient compliance are summarized in Table 8.3, and are discussed in greater detail below.

Illness-Related Influences of Compliance

Illness-related variables include the symptoms and characteristics of the illness, the direct effects of treatment, and the morbidity associated with disease and its treatment.

Illness Characteristics
Clinical wisdom predicts that patients with respiratory disorders are more likely to adhere to treatment regimens when their illness is characterized as severe in terms of symptoms and overall disability. In clinical trials,

Table 8.3 Factors reported to affect compliance for patients with respiratory diseases

Illness factors
Illness characteristics
- disease severity
- morbidity (e.g., missed work/school, hospitalizations/clinical visits, activity limitations)
- patient-perceived disability
- disease duration and rhythm
- time since diagnosis

Treatment complexity
- frequency of treatment
- timing of treatment
- number and dosages of medications
- difficulty of task requirements
- patient error
- route of medication delivery

Attitudes toward medications
- perceptions of medication effectiveness
- concerns about side effects
- dissatisfaction with regimen
- delayed effect of medications

Personal and family factors
Demographic factors
- age trends
- developmental trends
- marital status
- race
- language of origin
- gender

Patient and family functioning
- patient or family psychopathology
- quality of familial relationships
- family caregiving abilities
- family conflict
- family acceptance of treatment

Cognitive factors
- motivation
- social stigma
- cognitive or memory abilities
- attributions
- self-efficacy beliefs

patients with COPD who experienced more severe airway obstruction and shortness of breath showed greater compliance to treatment protocols. In addition, morbidity factors, such as activity limitation and frequent hospitalization, were related to patient adherence (Simmons *et al.*, 2000). However, with some patients, the level of perceived severity was associated with reduced compliance. Abbott *et al.* (1996) suggested that there may be a threshold for perceived severity; if it becomes too great, some individuals may respond by avoiding treatment. Conversely, Spector (1985) reported that pediatric studies of compliance associated noncompliance with mild perceptions of respiratory disease. Patients who had never been hospitalized for asthma and had fewer activity restrictions were less likely to be compliant. It has been hypothesized that the relationship between adherence and perceived disease severity is nonlinear, but curvilinear in nature. Evidence supports the notion that patients with either mild or severe respiratory illness were less likely to adhere than patients with moderate disease (Abbott *et al.*, 1996; Bender *et al.*, 1997).

Creer & Kotses (1990) noted that the duration and rhythm of chronic disease influence patient adherence. Patients with chronic respiratory disorders are required, by the very nature of their disease, to respond to the long-term variations in symptoms. Most respiratory diseases have periods of exacerbation that require additional attention to treatment, but also periods of reduced symptomatology where treatment requirements are less intense. They suggested that extended periods of reduced symptomatology may increase nonadherence because treatment behaviors are not practiced or reinforced.

Across chronic respiratory disorders, patients are less adherent over time. In fact, length of time since patient diagnosis has frequently been negatively associated with adherence (e.g., Creer, 1998). Some patients with asthma reported what has been coined 'perennial noncompliance' (Cesar-Ramos, 1997). When patients with asthma are asymptomatic, some consciously make a decision with their practitioner to forego treatments until symptoms return. Cesar-Ramos (1997) suggests that perennial noncompliance is helpful for both patients and practitioners in that it allows for breaks from the daily treatment, while allowing the physician and patient to see the effects of treatments versus no treatments over a long period of time.

Treatment Complexity

Complexity refers to the frequency, duration, and task requirements of the treatment regimen. Related to disease severity, it has been noted that more complex treatment regimens are likely to result in reduced adherence. This finding has been demonstrated in patients with asthma (Creer & Kotses, 1990; Bender *et al.*, 1997), COPD (Simmons *et al.* 2000), and cystic fibrosis (Abbott *et al.*, 1996).

Regarding frequency and timing of treatment, correlates of nonadherence have included the number of medications, the number of doses required, the side effects of medications, and the side effects of lifestyle restrictions associated with treatment. Numerous investigations and clinical examples have provided support for the notion that less frequent administrations of medications led to improvements with compliance (Vitolins *et al.*, 2000; Creer & Kotses, 1990; Creer, 1993; Lask, 1997). Other investigators have shown that inconvenience and timing of treatment was a major determinant of compliance (e.g., Cohn & Pizzi, 1993). Generally, increased duration of prescriptions and the requirement of prophylactic treatments have resulted in reduced compliance across disorders (Kelloway *et al.*, 1994).

The task requirements of respiratory treatment can be demanding and difficult. For example, many patients are required to use metered dose inhalers as a primary source of medication delivery. When used properly, inhaled medications have the advantages of direct medication delivery to the needed site, a rapid onset of action, and the need for smaller amounts of a drug to produce the desired effect (McFadden, 1995). However, optimal medication delivery is only achieved when actuations are inhaled at a large volume, at a slow rate, and with a long end-expiratory breathhold. In contrast, McFadden (1995) noted that patient inhalation technique is rarely adequate due to the tendency for untrained patients to inhale rapidly and omit breathholding after inhalation. It is well established that patient adherence rates are linked with poor inhaler technique (Pedersen *et al.*, 1986; McFadden, 1995; Bender *et al.*, 1997). Nonadherence with inhaled medications primarily occurs in two ways:

1 patient errors often result in suboptimal medication delivery, which influences disease control and is usually interpreted as poor adherence;
2 compliance with inhaled medications is significantly lower than with prescribed oral medications, suggesting that the route of delivery is a primary influence on patient use (Kelloway *et al.*, 1994).

For patients who are prescribed behavioral regimens, such as exercise and physiotherapy, time commitment and physical effort are the most commonly cited reasons for noncompliance (Conway *et al.*, 1996; Caplin, 1998).

Attitudes Towards Medications

Patients with chronic respiratory diseases require long-term treatment. It is not always easy for patients to determine the positive effects of adherence on a daily basis. Adherence may not prevent all illness exacerbations; conversely, the consequences of nonadherence are often delayed or unclear. Creer & Kotses (1990) identified that characteristics of medications have been shown to increase the likelihood of adherence difficulties. Medications may be expensive, difficult to administer, have uncomfortable side effects, or be incompletely understood by patients. As a result, medications may be misused, which can be dangerous and ineffective. In fact, reported rates of medication compliance vary according to the medication studied.

Generally, patients report higher use of medications used to alleviate acute symptoms of their illness (e.g., oral steroid bursts, beta-agonists, antibiotics) than daily preventative medications (e.g., inhaled corticosteroids, theophylline, enzymes, cromolyn) (Hand & Bradley, 1996; Bender *et al.*, 1997). A number of studies have surveyed patient attitudes toward their medications, and have shown that patients tend to have a general dislike of using daily and relief type medications (Osman *et al.*, 1993). However, dissatisfaction, delayed effects, and concerns about side effects were cited as primary reasons why patients are more likely to use relief medications over long-term maintenance drugs (Osman *et al.*, 1993; Bosley *et al.*, 1994).

Personal and Family Factors Influencing Compliance

A number of studies have attempted to link various demographic and personal characteristics of patients to noncompliance in an attempt to develop a profile of the prototypical nonadherent patient.

Demographic Factors

For patients with cystic fibrosis, investigations of potential demographic predictors of nonadherence, such as gender and age, have been inconclusive (Abbott *et al.*, 1996). For patients with other respiratory diseases, age trends were noted in compliant behavior. There are variations in rates of compliance for pediatric, adolescent, and adult groups of patients. For example, in a study of preschool asthma patients and their caregivers, Gibson *et al.* (1995) found that families demonstrated variable and suboptimal compliance with inhaled prophylactic asthma therapy. Interestingly, they found that individual patients received anywhere from 15 to 99% of their prescribed medication, and that medication decisions appeared to be independent of the presence of daily symptoms. Creer (1998) emphasizes that patient compliance for younger children is largely an issue of parent compliance. Another study of adolescent asthma patients reported average compliance rates of only 10%, a phenomenon frequently reported in adolescent patients across chronic illnesses (Miller, 1987; Creer, 1998). Across studies, there is a tendency for older patients to be more adherent to treatment than other groups; adolescence appears to be a period of increased noncompliance for most patient groups (Spector, 1985; Creer & Kotses, 1990; Rand *et al.*, 1995; Lask, 1997). For adolescents, the natural process of individuation and the development of autonomy can be complicated by a chronic disease. The physical, emotional, and cognitive changes that occur during adolescence are often incompatible with the requirements of a chronic disease. Adolescents may make a conscious effort to be noncompliant as one way of exerting their newfound independence from their parents and caregivers.

Other demographic factors that have had a notable effect on compliance include marital status, race, and language of origin (Manson, 1988; Rand *et al.*, 1995). Gender differences in compliance have been noted for patients with COPD, such that females typically adhere to treatment regimens more frequently and diligently than males (Rand *et al.*, 1995).

Patient and Family Functioning

Patient and family psychopathology are probably the most well-addressed correlates of patient adherence. Familial caregivers can contribute to noncompliance in a number of ways, including failing to have medications available, failing to read medical instructions, apathetic or indifferent attitude toward treatment, and poor social support for treatment (Creer & Kotses, 1990; Lask, 1997). Patterns of inconsistent care can result from such factors as patient depression and perceived helplessness, parent–child conflict, and family instability. For example, in a study of theophylline use by asthma patients, Christiaanse *et al.* (1989) found that the single best predictor of medication adherence was the interaction between psychological adjustment of patients and family conflict. Similarly, Drotar (1995) reported that a family's ability to balance the needs of the ill family member with the needs of the rest of the family predicted treatment success. In some cases, inappropriate attention is given to the care of the respiratory disorder because of poor organization within the family unit, parent or child pathology, or emotional resistance towards the illness (Spector, 1985; Drotar, 1995; Lask, 1997). In more severe cases, a pattern of poor management and significant parent psychopathology has been linked to mortality from pediatric asthma (Bender *et al.*, 1997).

Patient depression, anxiety, and overall psychological functioning have notably been linked with reduced adherence (Miller, 1987; Christiaanse *et al.*, 1989; Conway *et al.*, 1996; Hains *et al.*, 1997; Weinstein & Faust, 1997). In one study, pediatric compliance was notably higher in patients who showed high levels of psychological organization and low emotional distress. Results further indicated that children who were clinically impaired (e.g., had poor psychological functioning) were largely noncompliant with treatment (Weinstein & Faust, 1997). It has been suggested that psychological dysfunction can result in increased denial and negative outlook about the future, and frequent inconsistencies in care (Conway *et al.*, 1996; Bender *et al.*, 1997). Patients with cystic fibrosis are reported to have increased anxiety and depression during their transition from pediatric- to adult-based health care, which corresponds to a period of increased noncompliance with treatment (Hains *et al.*, 1997).

Cognitive Correlates of Adherence

Patient perceptions about their medical regimens are strong determinants of adherent behavior. Cognitive factors such as motivation, social stigma, past experiences, cognitive ability, reinforcement, memory, attribution, and self-efficacy are important influences in the context of patient adherence. However, our understanding of the cognitive and motivational factors associated with patient acceptance of treatment remains incomplete (Wills & Moore, 1994). Patients with asthma reported that they want to comply with treatment, and 'know they should' perform the tasks prescribed by their caregivers. However, many patients report that other facets of their lives often take precedence, that they forget, or that they feel that they are not in a position to do what is necessary to control their disease (Caplin, 1998).

Patient Attitudes

A number of other studies found that compliance of patients was related to their attitudes and beliefs. Patients who chose not to comply often did so as a way to express personal control over their disease, as a way to fight against the medical system, or as a way to fight against mistreatment by a practitioner (Donovan & Blake, 1992). Osman *et al.* (1993) found evidence of a strong and consistent negative attitude by patients about their medications and disease. Negative attitudes were clustered into four broad areas:

- dislike of inhaled daily and relief medications;
- dislike of interference in public life;
- concern about disease and future; and
- dislike of physical limitations.

Self-Efficacy Beliefs

Self-efficacy is a term that denotes a specific belief system about the expectations for performing particular actions. The two primary components of self-efficacy involve:

- a belief that one is able to perform the skills necessary to complete a particular action
- a belief that if a particular action is performed, it will have the desired outcome (Bandura, 1997).

A breakdown in one or both of these components can easily lead to poor patient adherence. First, patients must believe that they are able to perform the skills necessary for treatment, and that the treatment will work to control their disease. Many patients report feeling inadequate or unprepared for problems with their illness, and that this feeling leads to reduced action (Caplin, 1998). Secondly, it was found across disorders that patients or their families often hold the belief that their prescribed treatments will not make a difference (Creer & Kotses, 1990; Lask, 1997). VanSciver *et al.* (1995) found that – compared with other chronic conditions – young asthma patients who had inconsistent treatment practices expressed neutral attitudes toward treatment and health outcomes, and did not believe that treatment would improve outcome. Bandura (1997) suggests that treatment-specific self-efficacy is imperative to adequate adherence to any regimen. Indeed, cognitive influences are most apparent when viewed in the context of the processes associated with patient decision making. It has been suggested that – beyond initial performance – self-efficacy is a primary determinant for long-term adherence to any treatment regimen (Maddux *et al.*, 1995; Caplin, 1998).

The Impact of Patient Decision Making

Donovan & Blake (1992) found that of the patients who were noncompliant with a medical regimen, a large majority were 'active' in their nonadherence to prescriptive advice. Rather than forgetting or misinterpreting what was presented to them, these patients chose to ignore or modify their regimen. Their decisions were based on information received from their physician, as well as information from pharmacists, friends, and their own beliefs and experiences. Similarly, research on decision making points to the importance of configurality, or the complexity of the context within which a decision is made. According to Wills & Moore (1994), the use of configural information implies that patient decisions about specific treatments are based on three factors:

- information they receive about the specified treatment,
- other information they receive, and
- which pieces of information the patient perceives as most important.

Kaplan & Simon (1990) view compliance as a simple formula of patient decision making. They suggest that patients are rational and tend to comply when they perceive health benefits outweigh the consequences of noncompliance. Patients do not appear to make decisions regarding their medical treatment randomly or lightly. Nonadherence reflects appropriate decision making in many cases when patients observe changes in their disease status. Some authors have termed this behavior 'educated noncompliance' (Koocher *et al.*, 1990; Sockrider & Wolle, 1996). In a study of patient noncompliance with asthma medications, Tettersell (1993) reported that many patients were less likely to comply when they felt their medications were unnecessary, or when they felt able to adjust their medications according to their symptoms and without their physicians' assistance.

A review of medical decisions made by COPD patients noted that most patients base decisions on such factors as perceived risks and benefits of treatment, duration of treatment, complexity of regimen, and frequency (Rand *et al.*, 1995). Deaton (1985) studied the nature of parent decision making about their children's asthma. Results supported the notion that parents view themselves as equal in expertise to their child's physician. They tend to weigh the positive and negative consequences of adherence, and base their decisions on the process. Lask (1997) reported similar processes involved in the decision making of patients with cystic fibrosis. He suggested that patients are less likely to comply with treatments when they do not see any immediate benefits and they decide that the symptoms of the disease are less bothersome than complying with treatment.

It may be that patients make their decisions based on misinformation or inadequate information. Informed consent is required for patients to participate in research, but clinically, the process may be lagging behind. Gibson *et al.* (1995) suggested that parents of young children with asthma may misunderstand the rationale behind certain components of their medical regimen. Thus, they may be inadequately aware of the benefits of taking, for example, maintenance medications. A similar phenomenon was noted with cystic fibrosis patients (Drotar, 1995).

Putnam *et al.* (1994) developed a model for understanding patient decisions in terms of commitment to adherence. They suggested that commitment to adherence is a function of three primary domains:

1 satisfaction, which is defined as the difference between the physical rewards and the costs of treatment adherence;
2 investment, which includes the time and energy expended by the patient in order to be compliant; and
3 alternatives, which is seen as the other choices weighed by a patient in his decision to accept one treatment regimen over another.

According to their model, patient commitment or adherence is an aggregate of these factors (Putnam *et al.*, 1994).

The Health Belief Model of behavior has frequently been applied to the patient decision-making process regarding medical adherence. This model defines compliance as an aggregate of the following factors: perceived susceptibility, severity estimation, perceived treatment effectiveness, and perceived physical, psychological, and financial costs of treatment (Maddux *et al.*, 1995). Abbott *et al.* (1996) evaluated patient decisions about perceived control in the context of the Health Belief Model. Specifically, they determined the relationship between medical adherence and patient beliefs about their own disease severity, their concern about having cystic fibrosis, and their perceptions about vulnerability to infection. They found that concern about having cystic fibrosis increased perceptions of personal control, and a belief in the benefits of treatment each discriminated patients who were or were not compliant with physiotherapy, enzyme medication, and vitamin regimens. Some investigators attempted to apply the Health Belief Model to treatment issues in asthma. However, evidence suggests that the relationship is not a simple linear link between health beliefs and patient actions (VanSciver *et al.*, 1995).

As with other decision-making processes, patients' decisions about their medical regimens are subject to biases (Redelmeier *et al.*, 1993). For example, framing effects, or the manner in which an option is represented, can significantly influence the acceptance of a treatment. Patients with COPD who are told to quit smoking are likely to respond to the request differently if it is framed in terms of the positive health benefits rather than the negative health risks. On the other hand, patients with cystic fibrosis showed increased adherence to medication and chest physical therapy when they were worried or fearful about their disease (Abbott *et al.*, 1996). Hindsight bias also influences patient compliance with respiratory treatment: it involves relying heavily on past experience to determine current behavior, such as smokers who conclude that they have not gotten sick in the past from smoking and are, therefore, unlikely to get sick from it in the future.

Patient decisions appear illogical at times, especially when they do not agree with what clinical wisdom defines as optimal treatment. According to Redelmeier *et al.* (1993), the source of this discrepancy may lie in the goals and expected outcomes that patients have regarding treatment compared with the goals of their care providers. Patient expectations for treatment are frequently assumed, but rarely explored with patients. As pointed out by some authors, patients tend to look for an acceptable treatment for their disease whereas practitioners desire the best treatment for their patients (Kaplan & Simon, 1990; Redelmeier *et al.*, 1993). Poor compliance frequently stems from trying to achieve success without relinquishing certain routines. Judgment research has found that people are often reluctant to lose some aspects of their lives in order to regain control of other aspects. Kaplan & Simon (1990) have termed this reaction 'environment-centered noncompliance.'

Physician Compliance

Practitioner adherence has surfaced as a significant concern in the treatment of chronic respiratory diseases, especially in the treatment of asthma (Creer & Levstek, 1996) and COPD (Rand *et al.*, 1995). Creer (1998) makes the point that compliance does not just involve the patient, but also involves the people who are responsible for that patient's care.

Providing Adequate Information to Patients

There have been indications that current rates of compliance may be in part due to patients receiving inadequate instruction from their practitioners. In many cases, it has been suggested that patients are often prescribed treatments that require certain skills and information to be successful. To this end, systematic evaluations of physician behaviors in the treatment of chronic respiratory disease are discouraging. Notably, results have repeatedly identified that physicians are often neglectful in reviewing with patients the correct use of medications, the importance of adherence, and newly prescribed regimen changes (Creer & Kotses, 1990; Rand & Wise, 1994).

McFadden (1995) reviewed a healthy body of literature suggesting that patient incompetence with inhaled medication was largely due to inadequate instruction in the use of devices such as metered dose inhalers and nebulizers. When left to learn proper inhaler technique without formal instruction, most patients are unable to master the skills necessary to use their inhaled medications appropriately. In one study of 256 pediatric asthma patients, Pedersen *et al.* (1986) found that 52% of children were ineffectively using their metered dose inhalers; similar difficulties were noted in younger patients with cystic fibrosis (O'Donohue, 1996). These authors concluded that patient incompetence was primarily due to ignorance. Practitioners in both studies were either incompetent or making inadequate efforts to instruct patients on proper inhalation technique.

Creer & Levstek (1996) suggest that poor inhalation technique is a notable skill deficit for many physicians, nurses, and other medical staff treating patients with respiratory diseases. Studies have shown that a significant percentage of health care professionals responsible for the inpatient care of asthma patients are deficient in the proper use of metered dose inhalers (e.g., Interiano *et al.*, 1993). In one particularly disturbing study of physician knowledge of nebulizers, it was noted that only four of the 55 participants demonstrated correct inhalation technique, and three of those four physicians suffered from asthma (Kelling *et al.*, 1984).

In addition to inhalation technique, nebulizers are prone to unique difficulties that need to be described to patients. These pitfalls include the potential for inconsistent medication delivery and bacterial contamination (Corden *et al.*, 1997; Rosenfeld *et al.*, 1998). Rosenfeld *et al.* (1998) noted that there are no standard guidelines for patient use of nebulizers in the treatment of respiratory disease. They found that many patients were using nebulizers to co-deliver multiple medications and to deliver medications that were not recommended by FDA (Food and Drug Administration) guidelines for inhaled use. In addition, cleaning of the equipment by patients was not in accordance with recommended manufacturer guidelines.

Communication with patients is the mainstay for adequate adherence.

Patients have reported a misunderstanding of medications and side effects, benefits of adherence, and concerns about the efficacy of prescribed regimens (Creer & Kotses, 1990). Patients sometimes confuse the proper use of inhalers when different medications for preventive and relief use are prescribed (Hand & Bradley, 1996). Ultimately, it is the responsibility of the health care practitioner to insure that patients completely understand and accept their treatment regimens. Additionally, adequate follow-up to respond to questions, concerns, and inconsistencies in behaviors should be part of any treatment plan by practitioners. Most authors argue for a cooperative approach to treatment that includes patients as an integral part of the treatment planning.

Compliance with Published Guidelines for Treatment

Some of the responsibility for physician adherence with treating respiratory disorders lies in the poor distribution and training of standards for care. A significant number of investigations have shown that treatment guidelines *do* improve clinical practice (Gibson & Wilson, 1996). However, many hospitals and health care facilities support their own standardized procedures that may or may not agree with consensus groups that have convened to improve the consistency of care. For example, despite the publication and distribution of national and international guidelines for the treatment of asthma, COPD, and cystic fibrosis (Woolcock *et al.*, 1989; British Thoracic Society, 1993; O'Donohue, 1996; National Asthma Education and Prevention Program Expert Panel, 1997; Neville *et al.*, 1997), medical practice is plagued with poor physician compliance to preferred treatments. Although there has been some increase in compliance with management guidelines in the past several years, a significant gap was noted between recommended and actual management of respiratory disorders by general practitioners (Gibson & Wilson, 1996; Jackevicius & Chapman, 1997; Neville *et al.*, 1997). Gibson & Wilson (1996) audited the practices of physicians in primary and emergency care treating asthma. They found that initial treatment of asthma episodes was adequate, but that patients went home with very little follow-up; only 28% of patients had a written plan for how to respond to their asthma in the future.

Turk & Meichenbaum (1991) reported that physicians are frequently ignorant of new treatment recommendations and guidelines, and tend to use only a few of the resources at their disposal when making treatment decisions with patients. However, a recent publication by Gibson & Wilson (1996) found that – even with training in applying published treatment guidelines – many of the patients physicians assessed were inadequately treated or showed poor asthma management skills; in fact, only 28% of the patients in this study exhibited correct inhaler technique 3 months after their physicians were trained in the use of the instrument.

Some authors argue for specialist treatment as one way of improving patient care of asthma (e.g., Pearson & Harrison, 1996). They note that general practitioners have shown poor practice in prescribing anti-inflammatory agents and provide insufficient long-term care and follow-up to their patients. Indeed, patients with chronic respiratory diseases require considerable time, effort, and expertise to be managed adequately. Other researchers have found that physicians assume that patients are responsible for the success or failure of a particular treatment regimen.

According to Turk & Meichenbaum (1991), health care professionals need to change their perceptions about their role in the treatment of chronic disease. They suggest that clinicians should understand that patients are their own primary provider, and others, such as their physician, are there to assist, support, and teach.

One of the major causes of treatment failure is that patients are receiving inappropriate medications and inadequate dosages of those medications (Sublett *et al.*, 1979; Jackevicius & Chapman, 1997). It is well known, for example, that many patients overuse reliever medications and underuse maintenance medications. Ignorance about the purpose and effect of different medications can be a common source for noncompliance, poor response, and medical complications. For example, it has been noted that the use of oral steroid therapy can be problematic and even dangerous for many patients. Educating patients on the effects and side effects of steroids should be of primary concern to physicians, as patient compliance is a requirement for their safe use (The National Lung Health Education Program (NLHEP), 1998). The expected benefit of inhaled corticosteroids by COPD patients is as low as 5%; as a result, their use is not endorsed in contemporary guidelines for treatment. Despite this finding, a recent study found that physicians tended to treat COPD in a manner similar to their treatment practices for asthma by prescribing inhaled corticosteroids at the same rates for asthma and COPD (Jackevicius & Chapman, 1997). The authors make the point that needless prescription of inhaled corticosteroids contributes to both patient costs and patient noncompliance with treatment.

An Issue of Time

Levy (1997, p. 578) points out that adequate caregiving, such as is recommended by current treatment guidelines, is 'clearly impractical during an average six-minute consultation', allowed in most contemporary primary care practices. Other studies also reported that time constraints were a significant predictor of physician noncompliance (Gibson & Wilson, 1996). Generally, patients are required to wait longer in an office reception area for a shorter visit with their provider (Rapoff & Christophersen, 1982). Indeed, without the support of health organizations, it is unlikely that physician compliance, and therefore patient compliance, will significantly improve. Bender *et al.* (1997) suggest that health care organizations might be more effective at providing care if time and efforts were placed on improving patient education, allowing for additional time and frequency of visits when adherence is a concern, referring for mental health services when needed, and providing specialized trainers to assist in developing individualized treatment programming for difficult-to-treat patients.

Improving Compliance with Medical Regimens

What Practitioners Can Do to Improve Compliance

When fostered, the patient-practitioner relationship is a valuable tool for improving compliance. As Bender *et al.* (1997, p. 182) point out, 'other attempts to improve adherence are unlikely to succeed if the patient does not like and trust his or her doctor.' Lask (1997) recommends that practitioners develop a therapeutic alliance with patients – a relationship that implies a mutual empathetic, supportive, and working relationship based on trust and common goals. The subtle nonverbal cues that are presented to patients – including eye contact, body language, and active listening – reinforce a genuine interest in the patient and his needs. In a study of 202 patient–provider interactions, Stewart (1984) reported that the accuracy of physician estimates of compliance was about 75% overall when the visits were patient-centered.

Basic skill in effective communication is essential to successful treatment of respiratory diseases. However, many physicians fail when it comes to communicating their expertise and advice to patients. Schraa & Dirks (1982) outlined a number of basic steps that physicians could take to improve their communication skill. Presenting important facts and instructions first, and then again at the end of an interview, will take advantage of such cognitive effects as primacy, recency, and repetition. Overtly emphasizing key points in a repetitive fashion and organizing information into logical categories also facilitates recall. Providing written and verbal instruction, and asking patients to repeat information are further steps that increase comprehension and recall. Although these tasks may appear simple, they are required for adequate communication of necessary information and are frequently ignored in the average office visit (Schraa & Dirks, 1982; Spector, 1985; Hand & Bradley, 1996; Cesar-Ramos, 1997).

Practitioners can work with patients to reduce the complexity of treatment requirements that may interfere with adherence. Decreasing complexity should include taking a stepwise approach to treatment, beginning with the easiest-to-administer tasks of treatment, and adding components that are more complex, as needed, to achieve optimal control of symptoms (Creer, 1993). Sensitivity to possible side effects of prescribed treatments is an additional way that providers can facilitate compliance. This includes choosing medications that have minimal physical side effects, as well as those that require the fewest number of lifestyle changes or have minimal interference into the patients' daily schedule (Creer, 1998). It is important that this process be based on input from both the providers and the patients. Practitioners must decide what is sufficient for adequate care. Especially for diseases such as cystic fibrosis, where the regimen is demanding and complex, it is necessary that clinicians learn to accept and reinforce reasonable degrees of compliant behavior from patients.

Negotiation is a key process for improving patient commitment to and compliance with their medical regimens. Patient involvement in treatment planning is not a new concept: patient–practitioner negotiation has been adopted as an integral part of the *Guidelines for the Diagnosis and Management of Asthma* (National Asthma Education and Prevention Program Expert Panel, 1997). It is well known that written contracts, developed and signed by both the practitioner and the patient, increase patient commitment to treatment (Turk & Meichenbaum, 1991). The process of negotiation provides an atmosphere whereby patients can express what they are willing and able to contribute to the treatment process. Physicians and other health care personnel can also describe their bottom line, or the minimum that they need from patients to adequately treat their illness.

Adherence to treatment appears to improve with a comprehensive multidisciplinary approach to treatment. As with most chronic conditions, medical issues are only part of respiratory disease treatment: consideration for psychological, behavioral, social, and environmental issues is integral to therapeutic success (Lask, 1997).

Formal Interventions for Increasing Patient Compliance

Bender *et al.* (1997) note that individualized and intensive treatment is sometimes necessary for the particularly difficult patient. As with most disorders, there exists a subgroup of patients with respiratory disorders who are inconsistent, ambivalent, or even hostile about treatment. This is especially true for patient populations dealing with multiple survival issues, such as poverty, family dysfunction, or environmental chaos. For such patients, daily survival tends to outweigh health maintenance, and a crisis management approach to treatment results in missed appointments, poor adherence, and overutilization of hospitals and emergency centers. In such instances, specialized outreach care programs have been successful at providing individualized education and treatment programming to decrease use of crisis services, i.e., hospitalizations and emergency room use (Greineder *et al.*, 1995).

Effective behavioral techniques have been adapted for use in medical settings to increase the level of adherence by patients with respiratory diseases: most well-recognized are programs designed to improve education and skill in the self-management of asthma (Bender *et al.*, 1997; Creer, 1998). Many clinics that treat respiratory diseases already make adequate attempts to provide education and information to their patients. However, it has been emphasized that education is not enough for improved management (Creer & Levstek, 1996; Bender *et al.*, 1997; Caplin, 1998; Creer, 1998). The behavioral and attitudinal changes that come from learning to perform the necessary skills for successful management are required for lasting and lifelong change.

Patient Education

Providing educational information, at the comprehension level of the patient, has become an integral part of disease management. It is important that patients are informed consumers of medical care. For patients with a chronic disease, it is a necessary condition. The day-to-day responsibility that rests on patients with chronic respiratory diseases requires that they understand the characteristics of their disease, the necessary steps in treatment, and the expected positive and negative effects of adhering to treatment. Providing education to patients requires clinician time, effort, and skill. It is notable that effective physicians interact with their patients rather than reciting and lecturing to them; they realize that their patients are the experts when it comes to their own treatment needs (Creer, 1990; Sockrider & Wolle, 1996).

For physicians, strategies have been suggested that can increase the educational value of a follow-up visit with patients (Spector, 1985). These include:

- asking patients to repeat instructions to clinicians after learning their regimen;
- talking to patients about recording medications, behaviors, and symptoms;
- talking to patients about specific problems and concerns with their regimens; and
- reinforcing patients for positive efforts toward compliance.

Brock (1995) suggests that pharmacists are a valuable resource in patient education, especially with regard to proper medication administration. He suggests four steps, summarized in Table 8.4, based on

Table 8.4 Suggestions for health care professionals to assist patients with respiratory care

- Assess patients' current asthma status and medication knowledge
- Determine patients' expectations for their asthma care
- Verify with patients that they can name the different components of their treatment regimens
- Review and demonstrate appropriate use of medications and delivery devices

recently published guidelines, that other health care professionals, such as a pharmacy staff, can take to provide comprehensive care to their respiratory patients.

Formal education programs that use such resources as videos, computer programs, and printed materials continue to provide successful media for teaching patients about their illness and treatments. However, clinical personnel need to follow-up formal education with personalized inquiry and discussion. Some physicians have voiced concerns about patient education, suggesting that it increases litigation and unreasonable patient demands for care (Sockrider & Wolle, 1996). However, when provided within an appropriate context, education is helpful.

Behavioral Techniques

Creer (1998) reviewed the behavioral techniques that have been useful for improving compliance with chronic disease regimens. These techniques include shaping, reinforcement, modeling, self-monitoring, and self-management.

Shaping is a procedure that involves training patients to perform a targeted task by reinforcing successive approximations to the desired behavior in a stepwise fashion. For example, shaping proper inhalation technique may begin by teaching a patient to first hold their inhaler correctly, then proceed with the steps of proper preparation and actuation.

Reinforcement has been successfully employed to improve pediatric compliance in a variety of settings. Providing patients with incentives and rewards for desired behavioral performance is a technique that is commonly recognized by most parents and teachers, but one that has rarely been employed to improve adherence to medical regimens. Reinforcement can take the form of giving points that can be used to 'buy' privileges or treats, praise, or other desired consequences. Some authors have reported positive effects of such an approach in the clinical management of pediatric asthma (DaCosta *et al.*, 1997).

Modeling involves having the patient witness the appropriate behaviors being performed by the trainer, such as taking medications, using a nebulizer, or performing percussion therapies.

Self-monitoring is yet another behavioral technique that involves training patients to monitor the daily symptoms and activities associated with their treatment. Self-monitoring improves compliance in two ways: first, the process increases patient awareness of the effects of their illness and the associated effects of treatment; secondly, monitoring records can be used by practitioners to evaluate trends in a patient's symptoms, to assess the effects of different aspects of treatment, and to adjust treatments as deemed necessary.

Finally, self-management is an approach that trains patients to become responsible for their illness care. It combines cognitive and behavioral elements of behavior change to facilitate independent care by patients.

The positive effects of self-management training are well recognized. Wigal *et al.* (1990) found that children as young as 5 years old were able to learn the skills necessary to participate in their treatment using self-management. In addition, a recent investigation found that most adults continued to use self-management principles in their treatment up to 10 years after their training (Caplin, 1998).

Creer (1998) noted that self-management has evolved over the past 30 years, and highlighted five recent advancements, summarized in Table 8.5, that have been strengthened in traditional self-management paradigms.

Improving Health-Promoting Behaviors

Smoking Cessation

Cigarette smoke is a known cause and antagonist for respiratory disease. It is especially significant for patients with progressive respiratory conditions such as COPD. According to the NLHEP (1998), most individuals who successfully quit smoking do so without outside assistance. However, a significant minority of smokers struggle with numerous unsuccessful attempts to stop. To assist these patients, the NLHEP report identifies a number of helpful strategies to increase the likelihood that attempts to quit will be successful. The report suggests contracting with patients to formalize their intentions goes a long way toward increasing patient commitment. In addition, reinforcement of new behaviors and support throughout the process has been shown to lead to a higher rate of quitting. Finally, for those patients who require extra help, nicotine replacement therapy might be a helpful adjunct (NLHEP, 1998).

Rand *et al.* (1995) added an 'adherence-promotion' program to their clinical study of smoking cessation and bronchodilator therapy for early intervention with COPD patients. Strategies for improving adherence in patients where it was suboptimal were individualized and based on continuing assessment of difficulties experienced by individual patients.

Table 8.5 Improvements to traditional self-management training

- Introduction and persistent delivery of education from a team of health professionals
- Negotiation and joint development of patient treatment plans
- Empirical evidence for the efficacy of the basic self-management processes
- Finding that cognitive influences (e.g., self-efficacy) underlie successful self-management
- Development of efficacy-enhancing strategies to promote mastery of self-management

Their results indicated, however, that while compliance rates initially improved, they declined toward baseline behaviors over time (Rand *et al.*, 1995). Changing smoking behavior requires significant patient skill and motivation. Generally, patients are aware of the risks associated with smoking. However, many are not ready to change their behavior, or have tried to change with little success (Sockrider & Wolle, 1996). Some patients are physically addicted to nicotine and may require assistance in dealing with the negative withdrawal effects. Others may require a behavioral approach to treatment that encourages the development of new habits to replace unhealthy behaviors. Regardless of the method, most patients will require a great deal of support, understanding, and encouragement from their practitioner, and an organized plan with specific goals for quitting.

Exercise Programs

The development and implementation of standardized exercise regimens are commonly part of a comprehensive treatment regimen, especially for patients with progressive lung disease. Maddux *et al.* (1995) suggest that exercise often starts as a prevention regimen to reduce the progression of disease. However, if successfully adopted, many exercise regimens evolve into promotion behaviors, and patient perception of exercise goals shifts to improving good health. Beliefs about exercise, similar to other health beliefs, are largely influenced by expectations for action and for outcome and are known collectively as self-efficacy (Maddux *et al.*, 1995). Exercise regimens require consistent, long-standing performance to produce noticeable and lasting benefits. Implementing exercise into patients' daily routine requires that they are able to schedule exercise into their day, and that they are able to overcome the barriers to exercising (Maddux *et al.*, 1995).

General guidelines for exercise were outlined by Creer & Levstek (1998), and include prescribing an individually tailored regimen, consisting of simple, useful, and inexpensive exercises that improve both tolerance and endurance. More specific approaches have been postulated for patients with cystic fibrosis, as exercise tends to have positive influences on both lung function and nutritional status (Boas, 1997). In a recent article, Boas (1997) outlines five health-related categories of physical fitness that are important for patients with cystic fibrosis, including cardiorespiratory fitness, muscular endurance, muscular strength, body composition, and flexibility. Exercise regimens that attend to these areas of functioning tend to produce improvement in pulmonary function, mucus clearance, oxygen consumption, and quality of life. Although the benefits of regular exercise are well-documented, it appears that only 22% of comprehensive care centers for cystic fibrosis in the United States include an organized exercise program (Boas, 1997). Boas suggests that collaborative efforts are required by patients, parents, and health care personnel to establish realistic goals and expectations for patient exercise. The instillation of formal programs might be useful in training patients to improve their adherence to exercise recommendations.

Conclusions and Future Directions

The primary goal of any treatment regimen is good medical outcomes. Patients and practitioners, however, do not always agree on what constitutes adequate care or optimal outcomes. The process of patient decision making is extremely complicated and often appears illogical to health care providers. The vast number of influences that can affect patient action present one of the enigmas to treating chronic respiratory diseases: How do we get patients to voluntarily perform whatever behaviors are necessary for as long as necessary, to manage their disease? (Creer *et al.*, 1998). It is important for health care practitioners to decide what they can accept as adequate performance by patients, and to alter their expectations for patients according to realistic standards. As Creer *et al.* (1998) noted, most clinicians have patients who do everything they are told. However, the vast majority do not want to make their illness the center of their lives. The challenge is to strike a balance between making treatment compliance a priority in the patient's mind and providing realistic treatment. This requires a partnership between the patient and the physician. With partnership comes responsibility; noncompliance is not simply a patient problem, and changing patient attitudes and behaviors is not the only solution. Clinicians need to begin looking inward for solutions to the problems of adherence.

Foremost, the field of compliance is in dire need of a comprehensive definition of compliant behavior. Developing standardized procedures for measuring and determining rates of compliance across disciplines would greatly advance our understanding of the true nature of this issue. Research in the area of patient compliance has shown that the process of patient disease management is dependent upon a multitude of factors that are not all under the patient's control. It may be that the process of patient decision making is largely a factor of cognitive, situational, and interactional factors that do not fit easily into traditional theories of compliance. A great deal of insight might be gained from trying to understand patient perceptions about their health, their treatment, and their health care professionals. In addition, exploring the relationship between clinician knowledge and patient compliance may provide another avenue of effective intervention.

References

Abbott, J., Dodd, M. & Webb, A.K. (1996). Health perceptions and treatment adherence in adults with cystic fibrosis. *Thorax*, 51, 1233–1238.

Abbott, J. Dodd, M., Gee L., & Webb, K. (2001) Ways of coping with cystic fibrosis: Implications for treatment adherence. *Disability and Rehabilitation*, 23, 315–324.

Anderson, R.M., & Funnell, M.M. (2000). Compliance and adherence are dysfunctional concepts in diabetes care. *Diabetes Education*, 26, 597–604.

Bandura, A. (1997). *Self-efficacy: the exercise of control.* New York: Freeman.

Bender, B., Milgrom, H. & Rand, C. (1997). Nonadherence in asthmatic patients: is there a solution to the problem? *Annals of Allergy, Asthma & Immunology*, 79, 177–186.

Boas, S.R. (1997). Exercise recommendations for individuals with cystic fibrosis. *Sports Medicine*, 24, 28–32.

Brenner, B. & Kohn, M.S. (1998). The acute asthma patient in the ED: to admit or discharge. *American Journal of Emergency Medicine*, 16, 69–75.

British Thoracic Society (1993). Guidelines for the management of asthma: a summary. *British Medical Journal*, 306, 776–782.

Brock, P. (1995). Helping patients manage asthma. *American Journal of Health System Pharmacy*, 52, 2662–2666.

Brooks, C.M., Richards, J.M., Kohler, C.L., *et al.* (1994). Assessing adherence to asthma medication and inhaler regimens; a psychometric analysis of adult self-report scales. *Medical Care*, 32, 298–307.

Caplin, D.L. (1998). *Variables contributing to the relapse and long-term maintenance of self-management for individuals with asthma.* Ann Arbor, MI: UMI.

Cesar-Ramos, J.M. (1997). Evaluation of compliance with prescribed treatment in asthmatic children and adolescents: a Portuguese problem. *Journal of Investigational Allergology & Clinical Immunology*, 7, 290–291.

Cicutto, L.C., Llewellyn-Thomas, H.A., & Geerts, W.H. (2000). The management of asthma: A case-scenario-based survey of family physicians and pulmonary specialists. *Journal of Asthma*, 37, 235–246.

Cohn, J.R. & Pizzi, A. (1993). Determinants of patients compliance with allergen immunotherapy. *Journal of Allergy & Clinical Immunology*, 91, 734–737.

Conway, S.P., Pond, M.N., Hamnett, T. & Watson, A. (1996). Compliance with treatment in adult patients with cystic fibrosis. *Thorax*, 51, 29–33.

Corden, Z.M., Bosley, C.M., Rees, P.J. & Cochrane, G.M. (1997). Home nebulized therapy for patients with COPD: patient compliance with treatment and its relation to quality of life. *Chest*, 112, 1278–1282.

Creer, T.L. (1993). Medication compliance and childhood asthma. In: N.A. Krasnegor, L. Epstein, S.B. Johnson & S.J. Yaffe (Eds), *Handbook of health behavior research* (pp. 303–333). Hillsdale, NJ: Lawrence Erlbaum Associates.

Creer, T.L. (1998). Medication compliance in chronically-ill children. *Tijdschr Kindergeneeskd*, 66, 142–145.

Creer, T.L. & Kotses, H. (1990). An extension of the Reed and Townley conception of the pathogenesis of asthma: the role of behavioral and psychological stimuli and responses. *Pediatric Asthma, Allergy, and Immunology*, 2, 169–184.

Creer, T.L. & Levstek, D.A. (1996). Medication compliance and asthma: overlooking the trees because of the forest. *Journal of Asthma*, 33, 203–211.

Creer, T.L. & Levstek, D.A. (1998). Respiratory disorders. In: A. Bellack & M. Hersen (Eds), *Comprehensive clinical psychology* (pp. 335–359). New York: Pergamon Press.

Creer, T.L., Levstek, D.A. & Reynolds, R.V.C. (1998). History and evaluation. In: H. Kotses & A. Harver (Eds), *Self-management of asthma* (pp. 379–406). New York: Marcel Dekker.

Creer, T.L., Winder, J.A. & Tinkelman, D. (1999). Guidelines for the diagnosis and management of asthma: accepting the challenge. *Journal of Asthma*, 36, 391–407.

DaCosta, I.G., Rapoff, M.A., Lemanek, K. & Goldstein, G.L. (1997). Improving adherence to medication regimens for children with asthma and its effect on clinical outcome. *Journal of Applied Behavior Analysis*, 30, 687–691.

Dowell, J. & Hudson, H. (1997). A qualitative study of medication-taking behaviour in primary care, *Family Practice*, 14, 369–375.

Drotar, D. (1995). Commentary: cystic fibrosis. *Journal of Pediatric Psychology*, 20, 413–416.

Ducharme, F.M. & Kramer, M.S. (1993). Relapse following emergency treatment for acute asthma: can it be predicted or prevented? *Journal of Clinical Epidemiology*, 46, 1395–1402.

Dunbar-Jacobs, J. (1993). Contributions to patient adherence: is it time to share the blame? *Health Psychology*, 12, 91.

Gibson, N.A & Wilson, A.J. (1996). The use of continuous quality improvement methods to implement practice guidelines in asthma. *Journal of Quality Clinical Practice*, 16, 87–102.

Gibson, N.A., Ferguson, A.E., Aitchison, T.C., Paton, J.Y. (1995). Compliance with inhaled asthma medication in preschool children. *Thorax*, 50, 1274–1279.

Greineder, D.K., Loane, K.C. & Parks, P. (1995). Reduction in resource utilization by an asthma outreach program. *Archives of Pediatric and Adolescent Medicine*, 149, 415–420.

Hains, A.A., Davies, W.H., Behrens, D. & Biller, J.A. (1997). Cognitive behavioral interventions for adolescents with cystic fibrosis. *Journal of Pediatric Psychology*, 22, 669–687.

Hand, C.H. & Bradley, C. (1996). Health beliefs of adults with asthma: towards an understanding of the difference between symptomatic and preventive use of inhaler treatment. *Journal of Asthma*, 33, 331–338.

Hindi-Alexander, M.C., Throm, J. & Middleton, E. (1987). Collaborative asthma self-management: evaluation designs. *Clinical Review in Allergy*, 5, 249–258.

Huss, K., Travis, P. & Huss, R.W. (1997). Adherence issues in clinical practice. *Allergic Disorders*, 1, 199–206.

Interiano, B., Kalpalatha, K. & Guntupalli, K.K. (1993). Metered dose inhalers: do health care providers know what to teach? *Archives of Internal Medicine*, 153, 81–85.

Ievers, C.E., Brown, R.T., Drotar, D., Caplan, D., Pishevar, B.S., & Lambert, R.G. (1999). Knowledge of physician prescriptions and adherence to treatment among children with cystic fibrosis and their mothers. *Journal of Developmental and Behavioural Pediatrics*, 20, 335–343.

Jackevicius, C.A. & Chapman, K.R. (1997). Prevalence of inhaled corticosteroid use among patients with chronic obstructive pulmonary disease: a survey. *The Annals of Pharmacotherapy*, 31, 160–164.

Kaplan, R.M. & Simon, H.J. (1990). Compliance in medical care: reconsideration of self predictions. *Annals of Behavioral Medicine*, 12, 66–71.

Kelling, J.S., Strohl, K.P, Smith, R.L. & Altose, M.D. (1983). Physician knowledge in the use of canister nebulizers. *Chest*, 83, 612–614.

Kelloway, J.S., Wyatt, R.A. & Aldis, S.A. (1994). Comparison of patients' compliance with prescribed oral and inhaled asthma medications. *Archives of Internal Medicine*, 154, 1349–1352.

Kirschenbaum, D.S. & Tomarken, A.J. (1982). On facing the generalization problem: the study of self-regulatory failure. In: P.C. Kendall (Ed.), *Advances in cognitive-behavioral research and therapy* (pp. 119–200). Hillsdale, NJ: Lawrence Erlbaum Associates.

Koocher, G.P., McGrath, M.L. & Gudas, L.J. (1990). Typologies of nonadherence in cystic fibrosis. *Journal of Developmental and Behavioral Pediatrics*, 11, 353–358.

Langer, N. (1999) Culturally competent professionals in therapeutic alliances enhance patient compliance. *Journal of Health Care for the Poor and Underserved*. 10, 19–26.

Lask, B. (1997). Understanding and managing poor adherence in cystic fibrosis. *Pediatric Pulmonology*, S16, 260–261.

Lemanek, K. (1990). Adherence issues in the medical management of asthma. *Journal of Pediatric Psychology*, 15, 437–458.

Levy, M.L. (1997). Organized care in general practice: structure and evaluation. *Respiratory Medicine*, 91, 578–580.

McFadden, E.R. (1995). Improper patient techniques with metered dose inhalers: Clinical consequences and solutions to misuse. *Journal of Allergy and Clinical Immunology*, 96, 278–283.

McSweeny, A.J. & Creer, T.L. (1995). Health-related quality of life assessment in medical care. *Disease-A-Month*, 41, 1–72.

Maddux, J.E., Brawley, L. & Boykin, A. (1995). Self-efficacy and healthy behavior. In: J.E. Maddux (Ed.), *Self-efficacy, adaptation, and adjustment: theory, research, and application.* (pp. 173–201). New York: Plenum Press.

Mullen, P.D. (1997). Compliance becomes concordance. *British Medical Journal*, 314, 691–692.

National Asthma Education and Prevention Program, Expert Panel (1997). *Highlights of the Expert Panel Report 2: Guidelines for the diagnosis and management of asthma.*

National Institutes of Health (1995). *Global strategy for asthma management and prevention* (NIH Publication No. 96-3659). Bethesda MD: National Heart, Lung and Blood Institute.

National Lung Health Education Program (NLHEP) Executive Committee (1998). Strategies for preserving lung health and preventing COPD and associated diseases. *Chest*, 113S, 123S–153S.

Neville, R.G., Hoskins, G., Smith, B. & Clark, R.A. (1997). How general practitioners manage acute asthma attacks. *Thorax*, 52, 153–156.

Newacheck, P.W. & Halfon, N. (1998). Prevalence and impact of disabling chronic conditions in childhood. *American Journal of Public Health*, 88, 610–617.

O'Donohue, W.J. (1996). National Association for the Medical Direction of Respiratory Care Consensus Group: guidelines for the use of nebulizers in the home and at domiciliary sites. *Chest*, 109, 814–820.

Osman, L.M., Russell, I.T., Friend, J.A.R., Legge, J.S. & Douglas, J.G. (1993). Predicting patient attitudes to asthma medication. *Thorax*, 48, 827–830.

Pearson, M.G. & Harrison, B.D.W. (1996). Who should look after asthma? *Thorax*, 51, 967–968.

Pedersen, S., Frost, L. & Arafred, T. (1986). Errors in inhalation technique and efficiency in inhaler use in asthmatic children. *Allergy*, 41, 118–124.

Putnam, D.E., Finney, J.W., Barkley, P.L. & Bonner, M.L. (1994). Enhancing commitment improves adherence to a medical regimen. *Journal of Consulting and Clinical Psychology*, 62, 191–194.

Rand, C.S., & Sevick, M.A. (2000). Ethics in adherence promotion and monitoring. *Controlled Clinical Trials*, 21, 241S–247S.

Redelmeier, D.A., Rozin, P. & Kahneman, D. (1993). Understanding patients' decisions: Cognitive and emotional perspectives. *Journal of the American Medical Association*, 270, 72–76.

Rosenfeld, M., Emerson, J., Astley, S., *et al.* (1998). Home nebulizer use among patients with cystic fibrosis. *Journal of Pediatrics*, 132, 125–131.

Schraa, J.C. & Dirks, J.F. (1982). Improving patient recall and comprehension of the treatment regimen. *Journal of Asthma*, 19, 159–162.

Simmons, M.S., Nides, M.A., Rand, C.S., Wise, R.A., & Tashkin, D.P. (2000). Unpredictability of deception in compliance with physician-prescribed bronchodilator inhaler use in a clinical trial. *Chest*, 118, 290–295.

Sockrider, M.M. & Wolle, J.W. (1996). Helping patients better adhere to treatment regimens. *The Journal of Respiratory Diseases*, 17, 204–216.

Spector, S.L. (1985). Is your asthmatic patient really complying? *Annals of Allergy*, 55, 552–556.

Spector, S.L., Kinsman, R., Mawhinney, H., *et al.* (1986). Compliance of patients with asthma with an experimental aerosolized medication: implications for controlled clinical trials. *Journal of Allergy and Clinical Immunology*, 77, 65–70.

Stewart, M. (1984). What is a successful doctor–patient interview? *Social Science and Medicine*, 19, 167–175.

Sublett, J.L., Pollard, S.J., Kadlec, G.J. & Karibo, J.M. (1979). Non-compliance in asthmatic children: a study of theophylline levels in pediatric emergency room populations. *Annals of Allergy*, 43, 95–97.

Taylor, W.R. & Newacheck, P.W. (1992). Impact of childhood asthma on health. *Pediatrics*, 90, 657–662.

Tettersell, M.J. (1993). Asthma patients' knowledge in relation to compliance with drug therapy. *Journal of Advanced Nursing*, 18, 103–113.

Thomas, E.J., Burstin, H.R., O'Neil, A.C., Orav, E.J. & Brennan, T.A. (1996). Patient noncompliance with medical advice after the emergency department visit. *Annals of Emergency Medicine*, 27, 49–55.

Turk, D.C. & Meichenbaum, D. (1991). Adherence to self-care regimens. In: J.J. Sweet, R.H. Rozensky & S.M. Tovian (Eds), *Handbook of clinical psychology in medical settings* (pp. 249–266). New York: Plenum Press.

VanSciver, M.M., D'Angelo, E.J., Rappaport, L. & Woolf, A.D. (1995). Pediatric compliance and the roles of distinct treatment characteristics, treatment attitudes, and family stress: A preliminary report. *Developmental and Behavioral Pediatrics*, 16, 350–358.

Vitolins, M.Z., Rand, C.S., Rapp, S.R., Ribisl, P.M., & Sevick, M.A. (2000). Measuring adherence to behavioral and medical interventions. *Controlled Clinical Trials*, 21, 188S–194S.

Weinstein, A.G. & Faust, D. (1997). Maintaining theophylline compliance/ adherence in severely asthmatic children: the role of psychological functioning of the child and family. *Annals of Allergy, Asthma & Immunology*, 99, 40–43.

Weiss, K.B., Sullivan, S.D., & Lyttle, C.S. (2000). Trends in the cost of illness for asthma in the United States, 1985–1994. *Journal of Allergy and Clinical Immunology*, 106, 493–499.

Wigal, J.K., Creer, T.L., Kotses, H. & Lewis, P. (1990). A critique of 19 self-management programs for childhood asthma: Part I. The development and evaluation of the programs. *Pediatric Asthma, Allergy & Immunology*, 4, 17–39.

Woolcock, A., Rubinfeld, A.R., Seale, J.P., *et al.* (1989). Thoracic Society of Australia and New Zealand. Asthma management plan. *Medical Journal of Australia*, 151, 650–653.

9
Quality of life in respiratory disease

Michael E. Hyland

Editors' note—*It has been increasingly accepted that control of a chronic respiratory disorder is not enough: a major consequence of establishing such control must be improved quality of life for patients and their families. The concept of health-related quality of life has a rich and vibrant history (McSweeney & Creer, 1995): there not only remains a great deal of ambiguity surrounding a definition of the concept but also in considering the ways in which the concept can be measured.*

Michael Hyland is one of the early innovators in the assessment of quality of life in patients with a respiratory disorder, particularly asthma. He suggests that quality of life must represent a causal interaction between psychological and morbidity factors and that the perception of symptoms, problems, and evaluations is causally related but the relationship is moderated by different variables. A dynamic scheme, consisting of a three-stage causal model, has been proposed for assessing quality of life in asthma (Hyland, 1992). The first and initial stage consists of morbidity that produces symptoms and anticipated symptoms. Hyland points out that patients tend to report not the objective symptomatology of their conditions, but the subjective symptoms they experience. The latter symptoms, in turn, are influenced by contextual factors such as depression and anxiety. The second stage in the causal consequence is for symptoms or anticipated symptoms to cause problems. The exact types and degree of problems, in turn, are moderated by psychological factors, particularly the coping skills that a patient knows and can perform. The third and final stage in the causal sequence concerns the evaluations of patients regarding symptoms and related problems. These evaluations are moderated by a variety of cognitive factors, including the perceived cause and outcomes of the illness.

What Michael has proposed is a dynamic system of perceived quality of life that involves the simultaneous interactions of a number of cognitive, behavioral, environmental, and physical variables. His work, as readers will discover in the chapter that follows, is often akin to the research of Bandura (1997). That's not bad company.

Introduction

The term 'quality of life' (QOL) is commonly used to refer to the patient's perception of the effect of illness and its treatment on his life. Before 1979, there were less than 200 articles per year in which the term 'quality of life' appeared in titles or abstracts searched by MEDLINE. Since 1992 there have been in excess of 2000 articles per year with quality of life in the title, key words, or abstract. The increased interest in this topic reflects several factors:

1 Greater demands on limited health resources has led to increased recognition that the patients' views, as consumers of health care, are important.
2 Where physiologically beneficial treatments have negative side effects (e.g. chemotherapy, antihypertensive therapy), the patient's own views need to be taken into account in order to balance the positive and negative consequences of treatment.
3 Where health care systems are cash constrained, evaluation of QOL gained for treatments for different diseases helps in the allocation of scarce resources.

Although physiological measures of respiratory function remain central to the management of patients with respiratory disease, the increased emphasis on quality of life reflects the relevance of this topic in respiratory medicine. This chapter focuses on the QOL of two kinds of patient: those with asthma and those with chronic pulmonary disease (COPD). The aim is to show how an understanding of QOL and, if appropriate, its formal assessment can be useful in clinical practice.

The Nature of Quality of Life Deficit in Asthma

The impact of asthma on QOL is highly variable, at least in part because asthma varies in severity: it is minimal in the case of mild asthmatics who need a bronchodilator infrequently at certain times of the year or when developing a cold. Acute self-management of very mild asthma fits into a 'normal' pattern of acute treatment for minor health complaints (i.e., self-limiting health complaints), and so, from the patient's perspective, he has only an additional minor health complaint which is easily managed. However, as asthma severity increases, five characteristics distinguish the lives of those with asthma from those without. Each of these characteristics can be described as a deficit of QOL.

1. The burden of treatment increases. The patient may need to take regular prophylactic medicine or reliever medicine, and to make regular visits to the health professional responsible for his care. At the very least, the patient spends time engaged in health care. In addition, he may be embarrassed by using an inhaler in public. Also, the cost of medicines places a burden on those patients who pay for their medicine, and these costs can be considerable, particularly for patients who require multiple or more effective treatments. The burden of treatment can also include concerns about future health, often associated with concerns about the long-term use of steroids.

2. Despite effective treatment, the patient may experience symptoms, sometimes on a regular basis, that can interfere with ongoing activities. In some cases, symptoms lead to the patient needing to slow down on ongoing activity, but in other instances the patient may need to stop completely or not initiate a planned activity. In the case of enjoyable activities (e.g., sexual activity), the occurrence of symptoms reduces enjoyment; in the case of activities requiring concentration (for example, work), it can reduce concentration. Symptoms at night lead to sleep disturbance. Thus, in one way or another, symptoms can interfere with the asthmatic's daily activities, although the degree of activity restriction varies considerably between patients as a function of asthma severity and the degree of asthma control provided by medication. In addition, the degree of activity restriction depends on patient preference for activity. A patient who is an active sportsperson will notice more disruption from equivalent symptoms compared with a person who spends leisure time watching television. However, health education for patients often stresses the need to maintain good health, particularly through exercise. A sedentary lifestyle, coupled with increased exposure to indoor allergens, may lead to a worsening of asthma.

3. As interference with activity often results from exposure to a trigger (airborne particles, exercise, psychological upset, etc.), patients can learn to avoid exacerbations of asthma by avoiding those situations in which precipitating triggers are present. For example, the patient may avoid visiting friends who have pets, avoid holidays, or avoid social situations where others smoke. The pattern of avoidance can mean that the patient misses out on activities enjoyed by others.

4. Because of the interruption and avoidance of activities, the patient's emotional well-being is affected. Patients can feel frustrated or angry with their bodies; there may be a general feeling of dysphoria. This dysphoria can be associated with preoccupation and anxiety associated with asthma and asthma attacks.

5. The patient may experience asthma attacks which not only are very frightening but may require hospital treatment. Although asthma attacks are rare, anxiety associated with them can have a substantial impact on the patient's QOL.

The QOL deficit in children to some extent parallels that of adults, but with some important differences. In particular, the impact of asthma on children depends crucially on the response of others, including parents, teachers, friends, and parents of friends. For example, if teachers insist on inhalers being locked up in a cupboard in the school office (which is contrary to recommended practice) then the impact of asthma is likely to be very much greater, because the child is unable to take a prophylactic dose of bronchodilator prior to exercise, and is unable to access a bronchodilator quickly in the event of increasing symptoms. Apart from the greater contribution that others have to the quality of life of the child who has asthma, there are several other differences between adults and children which arise because adults and children engage in different kinds of activity. In addition, adults and older children self-manage their asthma medication, whereas in the case of younger children asthma medication may be controlled by a parent.

Quality of Life Deficit in COPD

Chronic obstructive pulmonary disease occurs in older patients but many of its symptoms are similar to those of asthma. In addition, although COPD is defined in terms of chronic airways obstruction, the degree of breathlessness varies on a daily basis, much as it can with asthmatic patients. Consequently, the five deficits described above apply as much to COPD patients as they do to patients with asthma. However, patients with more severe COPD experience breathlessness with minimal (and sometimes no) activity, and so the QOL deficits of these patients are similar to only the severest of asthma patients. Apart from this effect of severity, differences in QOL deficit between asthma and COPD patients reflect the comparatively older age of the latter, and the concerns of older people. In addition, as COPD is associated with smoking, issues surrounding smoking cessation may be important. Smoking is highly addictive; therefore, either cessation or an inability to quit in conflict with the physician's advice can affect the QOL.

The above review shows that in both asthma and COPD there are several, distinctly different ways in which QOL is affected by disease. An important conclusion to draw is that QOL is not a single entity; instead it comprises a series of judgments that patients make about the different kinds of impact the disease has on their lives. Quality of life is multifaceted, and the different kinds of judgments patients make about their lives have different kinds of consequence for management.

The Interaction between Morbidity and Psychology in Quality of Life Deficit

The judgments that are labeled quality of life judgments are psychological events. Where do they come from? What are their antecedents? Because disease involves physiological disturbance, QOL judgments result from an interaction between physiology and psychology (Hyland, 1992). One way of representing these different judgments is in terms of a causal sequence of different kinds of judgments, such as symptoms, activity interference and avoidance, and emotional evaluations. Figure 9.1 shows how morbidity leads to symptoms, which then lead to activity interference or avoidance, which then leads to emotional evaluations.

However, psychological factors contribute at each stage of this causal sequence. The relative impact of psychological factors depends on which kind of QOL judgment is involved. Those at the distal end of the causal sequence will be comparatively more affected by physiology, whereas those at the proximal end by psychology. So, for example, emotional evaluation of asthma may be more determined by psychology than by morbidity (see Figure 9.1).

Symptoms are affected by *attention* and also by *mood* (Pennebaker, 1982). The recognition of symptoms is reduced if attention is focused on other environmental cues but enhanced if the patient has little external stimulation. A good example of this phenomenon is the amount of coughing that occurs at cinemas. Although 'tickliness' of the throat is physiologically caused, whether a person notices the tickle and coughs is affected by the interest value of the film. People cough more in the boring sequences, and less during the more dramatic sequences. Another example of the effect of attention on symptoms is the effect of the environment on exercise tolerance. If exercise tolerance (e.g., 6-min walk, shuttle walking test) is assessed in a stimulating environment, then patients should be less aware of their symptoms and so walk further than in a nonstimulating environment.

Mood also affects symptom perception. Patients who have chronically poor mood tend to perceive and recall symptoms more readily than those with a more positive mood (Watson & Pennebaker, 1989). In fact,

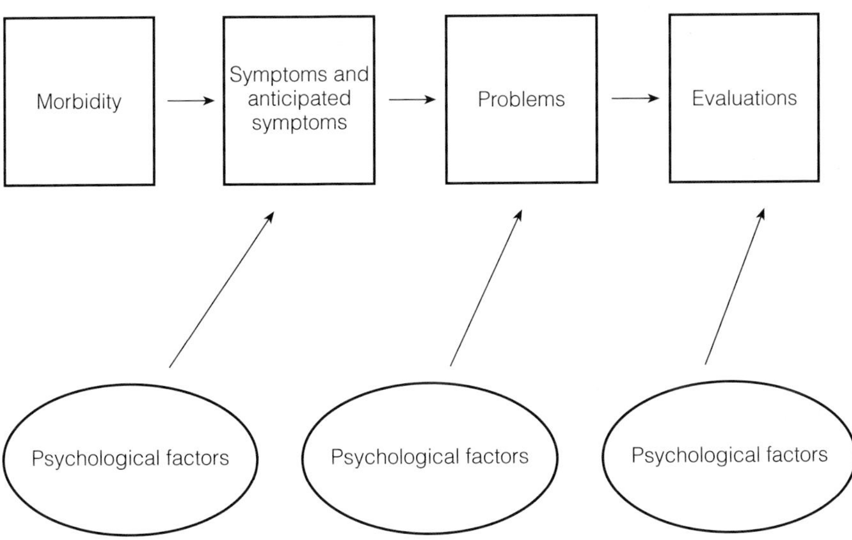

Figure 9.1

The causal sequence model of quality of life. (Adapted from Hyland, 1992.)

research on the relationship between symptoms and peak expiratory flow (PEF) shows that the relationship can be poor for some, but not all, patients (Kendrick *et al.*, 1993). The reason for the poor relationship between PEF and symptoms, where it occurs, is because the recognition of symptoms is affected not only by lung function but also by events which occur in the patient's life. The latter have a psychological impact on symptom recognition.

The effect of morbidity or symptoms on activity is affected by *coping strategies* and *motivation*. A good example of a coping strategy is the use of a bronchodilator prior to exercise, or the increased use of prophylactic medicine prior to going on holiday. Each of these strategies is an example of *planning* (Carver *et al.*, 1989) and, by that and other problem-focused coping strategies, patients can often find ways of preventing symptomatology interrupting their lives. In addition, if patients are highly motivated to engage in an activity, they are less likely to allow symptoms to interfere with that activity than if they are less motivated to carry out that activity. An analogy in everyday life will be familiar: some people struggle in to work despite having a cold while others stay at home and go to bed.

Finally, the emotional reaction that patients have to asthma will be affected by their general mood level. For reasons which are not fully understood, some people are happier than others; people have a personality disposition to experience the world in a comparatively positive or negative way (Costa & McCrae, 1980). In fact, the impact of events on life satisfaction is comparatively small – Suh *et al.* (1996) found that only recent life events influence subjective well-being. Andrews & Withey (1976) identified demographic factors as accounting for only 10% of the variance in subjective well-being. Winning the lottery may not bring happiness to people who are chronically depressed, and many people are happy despite not winning the lottery. The implication is that some patients are happy with their lives despite severe asthma, and others are unhappy with their lives even though their asthma is well controlled.

Figure 9.1 shows that 'problems' are closer to morbidity in the causal sequence than 'evaluations.' An implication of this arrangement is that problems should correlate more strongly with morbidity, and evaluations with psychological factors. Table 9.1 shows the relationship between a measure of exercise tolerance, the shuttle walking test, the personality scale of neuroticism, and QOL measures of problems and evaluations in a sample of COPD patients. The data show that the shuttle walking test is more strongly correlated with problems, and that neuroticism is more strongly correlated with evaluations (Hyland *et al.*, 1994). Other data confirm this general principle, e.g., lung function is more closely associated with problems compared with evaluations (Hyland & Crocker, 1995). Table 9.2 shows the stronger relation between PEF and QOL deficits associated with activity problems (Hyland *et al.*, 1996).

Table 9.1 Relationship of two components of quality of life – problems and evaluations – with the shuttle walking test and neuroticism in COPD patients

	Problems	Evaluations
Shuttle walking test	−0.60*	−0.24
Neuroticism	0.04	0.37*

Data first published in Hyland *et al.* (1994)
* $p < 0.05$

Table 9.2 Correlations between four different quality of life construct scores from the Living with Asthma Questionnaire and mean PEF (peak expiratory flow) taken at different times of the day

	Morning PEF	Evening PEF	Night time PEF
Avoidance	−0.21*	−0.24*	−0.21*
Distress	−0.17	−0.18	−0.19
Preoccupation	0.07	−0.04	0.03
Activities	−0.33***	−0.34***	−0.34***

Data first published in Hyland *et al.* (1997).
* $p < 0.05$
** $p < 0.01$
*** $p < 0.001$

Thus, although QOL results from an interaction between physiology and psychology, different aspects of QOL are affected to a greater or lesser extent by physiology and psychology. The relative contribution of physiology and psychology to a particular aspect of QOL has important implications for management.

First, the effect of improved drug treatment is greater on activity interference than on emotional evaluation of those problems (Hyland, 1994; Hyland *et al.*, 1997); i.e., when drugs are evaluated in a double-blind, placebo trial, improvement is more noticeable on activity interference. However, if an open-label phase of the trial is included after the double-blind phase (Hyland *et al.*, 1997) – i.e., patients know that they are on the superior treatment – then both problems and evaluations show improvement. Thus, the drug effect under double-blind conditions may not be the same when the drug plus placebo effects are combined, as often happens in real life. In clinical practice patients may be given new treatments that carry the expectation of improvement.

Secondly, although QOL can be enhanced by improved asthma control, it can also be improved simply by clinical contact particularly where such contact takes into account the psychological needs of the patient. That is, when improving QOL, the health professional not only has the opportunity to influence the physiology of the patient but also the psychology of the patient, which can also be changed in a way that leads to enhanced QOL. This focus on psychological management can be achieved in many different ways:

1 Focusing on the level of self-empowerment provided to the patient in the self-management plan. Plans which provide the patient with the degree of control preferred by the patient lead to greater satisfaction (and compliance) with the treatment given. Some patients prefer simple plans where they are told what to do by the doctor: others prefer more complex plans in which they initiate stepping down or up of treatment on their own.
2 Focusing on the device (e.g., dry powder inhaler versus metered dose inhaler) and frequency of dosing. Treatment using a prophylactic once per day (budesonide for mild and moderate asthma patients) may be preferred to twice or four times (e.g., cromolyns) per day treatment. In addition, patients develop their own idiosyncratic preferences for different kinds of inhaler, and feel that 'their' inhaler does them more good than others.
3 Focusing on the psychological distress and anxiety experienced by some patients, particularly with regard to asthma attacks. Cognitive–behavioural therapy may reduce unnecessary anxieties, coupled with clear and unambiguous guidelines about what to do in the event of an asthma attack.
4 Focusing on the relationship between the clinician and patient. A good, trusting, nonjudgmental relationship between patient and clinician can improve the quality of communication and hence enable the clinician to manage the patient's psychological needs more effectively.

The practical message to the health professional is that when the patient attends for a clinic appointment, the health professional *may* be able to have an impact on the physiology of asthma, but *will always* have some kind of impact on the patient's psychology. Quality of life can be enhanced by good clinical skills, i.e., the communication skill traditionally described as the bedside manner.

Interactions between Deficits of Quality of Life

Five different QOL deficits were listed above. Although each tends to increase with asthma severity, there are interactions which allow the patient to 'tradeoff' one deficit for another.

One important tradeoff is the burden of medicine versus other forms of

QOL deficit. A patient can choose to take less prophylactic medicine than advised and, consequently, experience more activity interruption and indeed more asthma attacks than would occur if regular prophylactic medicine was taken. From the health professional's perspective, the patient may be exhibiting noncompliance, but for the patient it may be a rational choice between different kinds of QOL deficit.

The decision not to take medicines as recommended may be motivated by a variety of QOL gains. For some patients, better self-esteem is achieved by denying that they have asthma. The statement: 'I haven't got asthma, I just sometimes have asthma attacks' summarizes this belief of asthma as some external agent that affects the patient, rather than some internal state of the patient for which the patient is responsible. Some patients believe that time invested in self-care is not profitably spent, given the demands of other activities; others believe that the cost of asthma medicines cannot be justified against other demands for resources; yet others believe (probably erroneously) that the long-term effect of steroids is worse than the short-term inconvenience of poor asthma control. In each case, the advantage of having well-controlled asthma in contrast to poorly controlled asthma is considered less than other types of QOL gain. It is worth reflecting that although all patients want to improve their QOL, they do not necessarily want to do it in the way that health professionals think advisable.

A second form of tradeoff is between activity interference and avoidance of activities. Consider, for example, a patient who is deciding whether or not to go to a party where others will be smoking. If the patient avoids going to the party, then there is the QOL deficit consisting of a restriction of life activities. The patient will have the experience of 'missing out' on things other people enjoy. However, if the patient goes to the party, then there is the possibility of the QOL deficit of interrupted activity. The patient will have to go home early, experience an asthma attack, or may even end up in hospital. More severe patients are faced with this kind of choice on a regular basis. Either choice has a probability of one kind of QOL deficit or another, but patients are able to choose the balance between these two kinds of QOL deficit.

The tradeoff between activity interference and avoidance of activities will be affected by preferences and coping strategies of individual patients. Some patients prefer a life of contentment that is devoid of emotional upset; others prefer an exciting life, and emotional upset – which may include an asthma attack – is part and parcel of that exciting life. Whether it is better to 'challenge asthma and take risks' or 'accept my limitations' is very much a value judgment that different patients will respond to differently. Health professionals may consider to what extent they should impose their own value judgments when providing recommendations of this kind to patients.

These two examples illustrate a general principle about the concept of

QOL. The meaning of 'good quality of life' is idiographic or person-specific. What is a good QOL for one person may not be good for another. Idiographic QOL is the term used to describe the specificity of QOL judgments to a particular patient. If patients are asked 'what aspects of life are important to its quality?' patients will provide a variety of different responses (O'Boyle *et al.*, 1992). Interestingly, the importance of good health as a contributor to QOL depends to some extent on the level of health of the person in question (Rijken *et al.*, 1995). For people who are healthy, good health is less important than other aspects of life, such as family or a good standard of living. Health becomes more important when it is under threat.

Measurement by Questionnaire

Insight into a patient's QOL can be obtained by talking to patients, but more formal assessment can be achieved through the use of questionnaires. The early QOL questionnaires were designed to be used for any disease. Such *generic* instruments had the advantage that they could be used to compare between different diseases states. However, in order to achieve a general perspective on health, such scales lack the specificity that would be achieved by designing a scale that is exclusive to a particular type of disease. For example, a well-validated generic scale such as the SF-36 (Ware & Sherbourne, 1992) contains items relating to pain, which is not normally relevant to asthma, but omits items about sleep. Although the SF-36 does have items which are relevant to asthma (e.g., social problems), the fact that it is not exclusive to the kind of QOL deficits that occur with asthma will have an impact on sensitivity. Consequently, *disease-specific* QOL questionnaires have been developed; these include several that are specific to respiratory disease.

Commonly used asthma-specific QOL questionnaires include the Asthma Quality of Life Questionnaire (Juniper *et al.*, 1992), the Living with Asthma Questionnaire (Hyland *et al.*, 1991), the St George's Respiratory Questionnaire (Jones *et al.*, 1991), and the Asthma Bother Profile (Hyland *et al.*, 1995). There are also some less frequently used questionnaires, such as the Asthma Quality of Life Questionnaire (Marks *et al.*, 1992) and the Respiratory Illness Quality of Life Questionnaire (Maillé *et al.*, 1994). In addition, checklists of activity restriction in asthma also provide a perspective on this aspect of QOL (Creer *et al.*, 1992).

The St George's Respiratory Questionnaire is designed both for asthma and COPD. Disease-specific scales for COPD include the Chronic Respiratory Disease Questionnaire (Guyatt *et al.*, 1987) and the Breathing Problems Questionnaire, which can be used either in the original long form (Hyland *et al.*, 1994) or in a short form (Hyland *et al.*, 1998) that was designed for use as an outcome tool in pulmonary rehabilitation.

Quality of life questionnaires also exist for asthmatic children. For older children these are designed for the child to complete, but for younger children they may be designed for completion with the parent. Child-specific questionnaires include those designed by French & Christie (1995), Juniper *et al.* (1996a), and Usherwood *et al.* (1990).

Each of these questionnaires consists of a series of questions about the impact of asthma on the patient's life and, although they differ in length and layout, there is inevitably a good deal of similarity between questionnaires. Table 9.3 gives details of the different questionnaires in terms of the number of items and the names of the subscales. Subscales can be of two kinds:

- Domain subscales are based on the grouping together of different items by the researchers according to the content of the items.
- Construct subscales are based on the grouping together of items on the basis of the psychometric properties of patients' responses to the items, normally established by factor analysis.

Table 9.3 shows whether the subscales are based on domains or constructs.

A major motivation for developing many of these disease-specific QOL questionnaires was to have a tool which could be used as an outcome measure in clinical trials to evaluate drug treatments. This motivation has an impact on the kinds of deficit of QOL that is assessed. For example, no scale, other than the Asthma Bother Profile, has items about the cost of medicines. Evidently, if an instrument is to be used in a clinical trial, asthma-relevant experiences that occur outside of clinical trials (such as cost) will be irrelevant for the purposes of the trial. The Asthma Bother Profile is the only scale to measure the burden of asthma medication, because the scale was not designed to measure outcome in clinical trials, but as a tool for clinical practice.

Any disease-specific QOL questionnaire consists of a set of items – as does any generic questionnaire. Although there is considerable overlap between the items in different questionnaires, they are not identical, as selection of items for a questionnaire reflects the purpose for which the questionnaire is intended.

Researchers are often asked: 'What is the best respiratory-specific questionnaire?' The answer is that there is no 'best' questionnaire, as the selection between questionnaires depends crucially on the purpose to which a questionnaire is put. In selecting among questionnaires a good course of action is to compare the items in different scales against the kind of purpose for which the questionnaire is to be used. This recommendation stems from the simple observation that any QOL questionnaire is designed, either explicitly or implicitly, for a purpose. Clearly it is desirable to match the purpose of the test constructor with that of the user. Disease-specific scales are implicitly or explicitly purpose-specific.

Table 9.3 Summary of respiratory-specific measures of quality of life

Measure and authors	Mode of administration	Number of items and subscales, target population	Subscales
Asthma Bother Profile (Hyland *et al.*, 1995)	Self-complete	22 items: 2 subscales adult asthma	Domains: (a) bother; (b) management
Asthma Quality of Life Questionnaire (Juniper *et al.*, 1992)	Self-complete or interviewer administered	32 items; 4 subscales: adult asthma	Domains: (a) activity limitations; (b) symptoms; (c) emotional function; (d) exposure to environmental stimuli
Asthma Quality of Life Questionnaire (Marks *et al.*, 1992)	Self-complete	20 items; 4 subscales; adult asthma	Constructs: (a) breathlessness; (b) mood disturbance; (c) social disruption; (d) concerns for health
Breathing Problems Questionnaire – long version (Hyland *et al.*, 1994)	Self-complete	33 items; 13 or 2 subscales; COPD	Domains: (a) walking; (b) bending or reaching; (c) washing and bathing; (d) household chores; (e) social interactions; (f) effects of weather or temperature; (g) effects of smells and fumes; (h) effects of colds; (i) sleeping; (j) medicine; (k) dysphoric states; (l) eating; (m) excretion urgency Constructs: (a) problems; (b) evaluations

Breathing Problems Questionnaire – short version (Hyland *et al.* 1998)	Self-complete	10 items; no subscales; COPD	None
Childhood Asthma Questionnaires (French & Christie, 1995) Form A (4–7 years)	Completed by the child with assistance	14 items (also 10 questions for parents); 2 subscales; child asthma	Constructs: (a) distress; (b) quality of living
Form B (8–11 years)	Completed independently by the child	38 items (also 6 questions to be completed by parents); 3 subscales; child asthma	Constructs: (a) distress; (b) severity; (c) active quality of living
Form C (12–16 years)	Completed independently by the child	46 items; 5 subscales; child asthma	Constructs: (a) distress; (b) severity; (c) reactivity; (d) active quality of living; (e) teenage quality of living
Chronic Respiratory Disease Questionnaire (Guyatt *et al.*, 1987)	Interviewer administered	20 items; 4 subscales; COPD	Domains: (a) dyspnea; (b) fatigue; (c) emotional function; (d) mastery
Index of Perceived Symptoms in Asthmatic Children (Usherwood *et al.*, 1990)	Completed by parent	17 items; 3 subscales; child asthma	Constructs: (a) perceived disability; (b) perceived nocturnal symptoms; (c) perceived daytime symptoms
Life Activities Questionnaire for Adult Asthma (Creer *et al.*, 1992)	Self-complete	70 items; 7 subscales; adult asthma	Domains: (a) physical activities; (b) work activities; (c) outdoor activities; (d) emotions and emotional behaviors; (e) home care; (f) eating and drinking activities; (g) miscellaneous

Table 9.3 *contd.*

Measure and authors	Mode of administration	Number of items and subscales, target population	Subscales
Living with Asthma Questionnaire (Hyland *et al.*, 1997)	Self-complete	68 items; 11 or 4 subscales; adult asthma	Domains: (a) social or leisure; b) sport; (c) holidays; (d) sleep; (e) work and other activities; (f) colds; (g) mobility; (h) effects on others; (i) medication use; (k) sex; (l) dysphoric states and attitudes Constructs: (a) activities; (b) avoidance; (c) preoccupation; (d) distress
Paediatric Quality of Life questionnaire (Juniper *et al.*, 1996a)	Interviewer administered	23 items; 3 subscales; child asthma	Domains: (a) activity limitation; (b) symptoms; (c) emotional function
Paediatric Asthma Caregiver's Quality of Life Questionnaire (Juniper *et al.*, 1996b)	Self-complete	13 items; 2 subscales; asthma caregiver	Domains: (a) activity limitations; (b) emotional function
Respiratory Illness Quality of Life Questionnaire (Maillé *et al.*, 1994)	Self-complete	55 items; 7 subscales; adult asthma	Domains: (a) breathing problems; (b) physical problems; (c) emotions; (d) situations triggering or enhancing breathing problems; (e) daily and domestic activities; (f) social activities, relationships, and sexuality; (g) general activities
St George's Respiratory Questionnaire (Jones *et al.*, 1991)	Self-complete	76 items; 3 subscales; adult asthma or COPD	Constructs: (a) symptoms; (b) activity; (c) impact

An example of the explicit development of a purpose-specific, disease-specific questionnaire is provided by the shortened version of the Breathing Problems Questionnaire. The full (long) version of the Breathing Problems Questionnaire was designed as a general cross-sectional tool, without any particular intention for its use as an outcome tool in pulmonary rehabilitation. However, when the long version was used as an outcome measure in rehabilitation, it became apparent that, although the majority of items showed improvement following rehabilitation, some exhibited deterioration. The deteriorating items included the increased use of oxygen, the increased number of pillows used at night, and the eating of frequent and smaller meals. However, all these changes are actually recommended as part of the educational element of the rehabilitation program. Thus, the apparent deterioration following rehabilitation is in reality compliance with treatment. The shortened version of the Breathing Problems Questionnaire is limited to those items which can and do show some evidence of change following rehabilitation, and therefore comprises a purpose-specific, disease-specific questionnaire, where items have been selected for a particular purpose. Cross-sectional measures that are useful for assessing severity may not function well when used as longitudinal measures for assessing change because of the items used.

Problems with Questionnaire Assessment of Quality of Life

Although questionnaires are the commonly accepted form of QOL assessment, the method can be criticized on several counts.

First, the use of questionnaires has a built-in assumption that patients have reasonably accurate recall about events that happen to them; i.e., there is an implicit assumption that if a problem occurs due to asthma, then the patient will remember that problem. However, human memory is known to be poor, particularly for nonsalient and repeated events (Baddeley, 1996), and so it is quite possible for patients to underestimate the problems they are experiencing simply because they forget them. Indeed, QOL can also be measured by a structured diary, which is like a mini-questionnaire given on a daily basis. Comparisons between QOL diaries and questionnaires show that they are not equivalent – diaries can be more sensitive to change than questionnaires (Hyland & Crocker, 1995). Thus, when patients are asked about activity interference, it is quite possible for some patients to underestimate the effect of their asthma or COPD due to a failure of recall. Quality of life diaries redress this problem to some degree – a minimal form of QOL diary can be a single item added to a symptom diary where the patient indicates whether 'symptoms interrupted or affected any activity today.'

A second problem with QOL questionnaires is that they are highly correlated with personality (Hyland *et al.*, 1994). The reason for this is evident from Fig. 9.1: QOL results from an interaction between physiological and psychological factors, and inevitably personality affects the judgments people make about their lives. Consequently, optimistic, happy individuals are likely to have a more positive impression of the effect of asthma than depressed or unhappy individuals. Standard QOL questionnaires are therefore inevitably related to personality. An alternative approach is not to ask what the patient *cannot* do but what the patient *does*. In effect, the difference in perspective is between asking the patient if the pot is half empty or if it is half full. Activity check lists in which patients indicate what they have done rather than activity restriction are not related to neuroticism, but are related to another personality dimension – openness to experience (Hyland *et al.*, 1998). They are also related to physiological measures of lung function.

A third problem with QOL questionnaires arises from the process of psychological adaptation that occurs with chronic illness. Such psychological adaptation can take several forms, but in particular involves 'disengagement' from previously unattainable goals (Carver & Scheier, 1990), in which patients who are prevented from doing something because of their asthma no longer wish to do that which they are prevented from doing. Patients therefore become unaware of the limitations imposed on them by their asthma. The consequence of psychological adaptation is particularly important in longitudinal studies, as a questionnaire on a second occasion may be interpreted differently from a first. Lack of apparent change between two occasions may actually be the consequence of psychological adaptation.

These three criticisms of questionnaire measures of QOL stem from the psychological processes that affect a patient's responses to questionnaires:

- memory effects
- effects of personality
- effect of adaptation.

The issue is not whether questionnaires are good at measuring retrospective recall of the impact of asthma, but whether, because of psychological processes, the meaning of 'quality of life' is adequately encapsulated by the retrospective recall of negative events, i.e., by questionnaire.

Meaning of Quality of Life in Asthma: Different Perspectives

The objective of assessing the quality of a person's life is predicated on the assumption that life can be *valued*. However, life can only be valued if the purpose of that life is known. In other words, the concept of QOL assessment is based on an implicit assumption that there is something which is 'good' and which life can be measured against. When QOL is measured by any of the disease-specific questionnaires described above, the 'good' which is QOL is absence of complaint. Thus, a person who complains about the burden of asthma on the questionnaire is judged as having a worse QOL than a person who does not complain. The view that good QOL is absence of complaint fits in with a medical model where complaining patients take up scarce health resources whereas a noncomplaining one does not. The purpose of medicine from this perspective could be characterized as keeping patients alive and noncomplaining.

However, the absence of complaint model is not necessarily consistent with lay perceptions of QOL, nor is it the only model of QOL that is possible. Despite the assertion at the beginning of this chapter that the term quality of life is commonly used to refer to the patient's perception of the effect of illness and its treatment on his life, several other perspectives on QOL are also possible.

1. Life may be valued in terms of *either* the type of activity or the *amount* of activity engaged in. For example, work may be valued more than leisure activities and, if that is the case, then treatments which help a patient go back to work are valued more than those which merely facilitate a leisure activity. A logical implication would be that an asthmatic office worker whose only QOL deficit is in terms of leisure pursuits should have lower priority for treatment than an asthmatic manual worker whose work is affected by asthma. Alternatively, the amount or variety of activity can be valued irrespective of the type, in which case the aim of treatment is to restore to patients options of all kinds of activity. This alternative emphasis on activity differs from the absence of complaint model in that some patients adapt to their chronic illness so that they become unaware that they are restricted.

2. Although illness has negative consequences, some patients report that it also has positive consequences; i.e., there is a 'silver lining' to the cloud of disease. The independence of positive and negative affect is well established in psychology (Bradburn, 1969). In a recent study, Sodergren & Hyland (1999) assessed positive consequences of illness in a sample of 40 COPD patients and found substantial levels of positivity. For example, 35 patients felt that their illness had made them 'realize how supportive other people can be,' 40 patients found that their illness had made them 'realize that things can wait until tomorrow,' and 32 that their illness had 'encouraged them to enjoy simple pleasures.' Thus, QOL questionnaires, by focusing on the complaints of patients, fail to capture their positive experiences, which may be important to the patient.

3. Quality of life scales do not take the perspective of the parent, partner, spouse, or friend into account. Partners and health professionals have different perceptions on QOL than patients. The absence of complaint model assumes that it is the patient who is correct and that

everyone else is wrong; i.e., the patient has the best insight into his mind. However, if QOL is defined in terms of objective behaviours, then it is perfectly feasible that others will have a more accurate picture of what a patient can or cannot do. Clinical experience shows that partners will often point out problems not reported by patients, possibly because the patient's dispositional optimism or disengagement has made him unaware of the problem. In addition to the patient and others having differing, and complementary perspectives, the QOL of a partner or parent, or indeed any other family member, may also be affected by asthma. Depending on how the family copes with a chronic illness, family members may be affected in different ways and to a different extent by a chronic illness. The absence of complaint model fails to take into account the complaints of others or other judgments made by people associated with the patient.

Summary

Disease-specific QOL questionnaires form the accepted 'gold standard' for assessing QOL in respiratory disease. Perhaps gold standard is too strong, as there are many different scales, and 'accepted silver standards' would be a more accurate representation of the current state of affairs. These questionnaires, however, reflect a particular perspective on QOL. They are all predicated on an absence of complaint model of QOL as well as, in the main, focusing only on those concerns that are relevant to clinical trials. Thus, disease-specific respiratory questionnaires reflect a particular perspective on QOL, although it would be fair to add that bias of some kind is inevitable whatever kind of scale. However, complementary approaches to QOL assessment also exist. For example, the Paediatric Asthma Caregiver's Quality of Life Questionnaire (Juniper *et al.*, 1996b) reflects another person perspective; scales such as the Satisfaction with Illness (Hyland & Kenyon, 1992) and the Silver Lining Questionnaire (Sodergren & Hyland, 1999) measure the positivity of illness; and activity checklists (Hyland *et al.*, 1999) measure what people do rather than what they complain about being unable to do.

Although this chapter has focused on the more formal kind of QOL assessment provided by questionnaires, it should not be forgotten that interviews also provide a perspective on QOL. Indeed, for many patients in routine clinical care, an interview provides the only opportunity for assessing QOL. However, whatever form of measurement is used, and whatever aspect of quality of life is assessed, consideration of QOL is an important factor in making clinical decisions.

Future Directions

Two topics of research and two literatures have grown independently: the topic of QOL and the topic of compliance. In this final section, I suggest that the future developments in QOL must involve an integration of these two different perspectives.

Quality of Life and Drug Research

Research into QOL has been influenced to a very great degree by the need for pharmaceutical companies to demonstrate the superiority of their product (i.e., chemical entity) in comparison with some other product. Many of the QOL scales were developed as outcome measures for pharmaceutical studies. The result has been an emphasis, perhaps an overemphasis, on the contribution of pharmaceutical products to QOL. In retrospect, the value of showing that a pharmaceutical product improves QOL can be questioned. A drug improves QOL only because it achieves better asthma control; hence, the more direct variable is that of asthma control. Experience with clinical trials shows that QOL does not improve if PEF does not improve. QOL is important is not so much for the efficacy of a drug, but for the effectiveness for the total treatment package as a whole, where the package includes the drug, inhaler device, instructions, and ancillary support.

The difference between efficacy and effectiveness is crucial. Efficacy studies are carried out under controlled, double-blind conditions so that only the effect of the drug is evaluated. Efficacy studies create an environment for care that is not realized in clinical practice. By contrast, effectiveness studies are designed to match as far as possible real-life situations, where the effectiveness of treatment depends not only on the treatment provided to the patient but also on how the patient uses that treatment. Effectiveness studies are designed to be sensitive to patient compliance. In an efficacy study, it is simply assumed that patients are compliant.

Compliance

It is common to distinguish between intentional and unintentional noncompliance. Unintentional noncompliance includes forgetting to use an inhaler and errors with inhaler device technique. By contrast, intentional noncompliance occurs where the patient intentionally fails to comply with the instruction given. Intentional noncompliance is common. In a study where patients were asked about how they used their inhalers (Kleiger & Dirks, 1979), 46% of patients indicated that they complied, 11% that they overused their prophylactic medicine, 28% reported underuse, and 15% cyclical use, i.e., variable over- and underuse. In particular, patients dislike taking medicine regularly (Osman *et al.*, 1993). In an evaluation of parent's views on medicines (Donelly *et al.*, 1987), 86% of the parents of asthmatic children said that medicine should not be used for long periods, 43% said that the medicine was unnatural and harmful to children, and 31% said children's bodies were too small to cope.

One interpretation of intentional noncompliance is that patients are trying to improve their QOL, but not the kind of QOL advocated by health professionals. The way patients treat themselves with asthma medicines is part of their life, and contributes to QOL. Some patients believe that they obtain a better QOL if they behave in a way different from that of the health professional. This decision to behave in a noncompliant fashion may be motivated by a number of factors, but an important one is the dislike of long-term, regular use of inhalers.

Compliance and QOL

Traditionally, the aim of asthma care has been good asthma control. However, an alternative aim is good asthma control using the technique preferred by the patient, which may also be the technique which the patient will comply with. The important aspects of life that contribute to its quality differ between people, and in the same way, patients want to treat themselves in different ways. They do not all want to manage their illness in the same way.

Therefore, the future of QOL research should involve an integration between compliance and QOL. That integration should be based on individualization of treatment. There is no one treatment, or set of instructions, that works for all patients. Just as patients have different physiologies, they also have different psychologies, and these different psychologies need to be managed in different ways.

Good clinical care involves finding out (a) what the patient wants to achieve in life and (b) how the patient wants to achieve it. Ten years ago there were relatively few treatment options open to the clinician. Now there are a range of steroids with differing properties (one with a once per day option), a range of inhaler devices, as well as oral medications (anti-leukotrienes) that have some degree of anti-inflammatory properties. There are now long-acting β_2-agonists as well as cromolyns, and new drugs are being developed. In addition to the choice of drug and device, the clinician also has a range of options for advice and self-management, e.g., in terms of complexity of regimen. The secret to achieving good QOL is not just getting the drugs right, it is getting the total package right for the individual patient.

References

Andrews, F.M. & Withey, S.B. (1976). *Social indicators of well-being: America's perception of life quality.* New York: Plenum Press.

Baddeley, A. (1996). *Human memory: theory and practice.* London: Earlbaum.

Bandura, A. (1997). *Self-efficacy. The exercise of control.* New York: W.H. Freeman and Company.

Bradburn, N.M. (1969). *The structure of psychological well-being.* Chicago: Aldine.

Carver, C.S. & Scheier, M.F. (1990). Origins and functions of positive and negative affect: a control process view. *Psychological Review*, 97, 19–35.

Carver, C.S., Scheier, M.F., & Weintraub, J.K. (1989). Assessing coping strategies: a theoretically based approach. *Journal of Personality and Social Psychology*, 56, 267–283.

Costa, P.T. & McCrae, R.R. (1980). Influence of extraversion and neuroticism on subjective well-being: happy and unhappy people. *Journal of Personality and Social Psychology*, 38, 668–678.

Creer, T.L., Wigal, J.K., Kotses, H., McConnaughy, K., & Winder, J.A. (1992). A life activities questionnaire for adult asthma. *Journal of Asthma*, 29, 393–399.

Donelly, J.E., Donelly, W.J., Thong, Y.H. (1987). Parental perceptions and attitudes towards asthma and its treatment: a controlled study. *Social Science and Medicine*, 24, 431–437.

French, D.J. & Christie, M.J. (1995). Developing outcome measures for children: the example of "Quality of Life" assessment for paediatric asthma. In: A. Hutchinson, E. McColl, M.J. Christie, & C.L. Riccalton (Eds), *Health outcomes in primary and outpatient care* (pp. 157–180). Chur: Harwood Academic.

Guyatt, G.H., Berman, L.B., Townsend, M., Pugsley, S.O., & Chambers, L.W. (1987). A measure of quality of life for clinical trials in chronic lung disease. *Thorax*, 42, 773–778.

Hyland, M.E. (1992). A reformulation of quality of life for medical science. *Quality of Life Research*, 1, 267–272.

Hyland, M.E. (1994). Antiasthma drugs. Quality of life rating scales and sensitivity to longitudinal change. *PharmacoEconomics*, 6, 324–329.

Hyland, M.E. & Crocker, G.R. (1995). Validation of an asthma quality of life diary in a clinical trial. *Thorax*, 50, 724–730.

Hyland, M.E. & Kenyon, C.A.P. (1992). A measure of positive health-related quality of life: the satisfaction with illness scale. *Psychological Reports*, 71, 1137–1138.

Hyland, M.E., Sodersgren, S.C., & Singh, S.J., (1999). Variety of activity: relationship with health status, demographic variables and global quality of life. *Psychology, Health & Medicine*, 3, 241–254.

Hyland, M.E., Finnis, S., & Irvine, S.H. (1991). A scale for assessing quality of life in adult asthma sufferers. *Journal of Psychosomatic Research*, 35, 99–110.

Hyland, M.E., Bott, J., Singh, S., & Kenyon, C.A.P. (1994). Domains, constructs and the development of the breathing problems questionnaire. *Quality of Life Research*, 3, 245–256.

Hyland, M.E., Ley, A., Fisher, D.W., & Woodward, V. (1995). Measurement of psychological distress in asthma and asthma management programmes. *British Journal of Clinical Psychology*, 34, 601–611.

Hyland, M.E., Bellesis, M., Thompson, P.J., & Kenyon C.A.P. (1996). The constructs of asthma quality of life: psychometric, experimental and correlation evidence. *Psychology and Health*, 12, 101–121.

Hyland, M.E., Singh, S.J., Sodergren, S.C., & Morgan, M.D.L. (1998). Development of a shortened version of the Breathing Problems Questionnaire suitable for use in a pulmonary rehabilitation clinic: a purpose-specific, disease-specific questionnaire. *Quality of Life Research*, 7, 227–233.

Jones, P.W., Quirk, F.H., & Baveystock, C.M. (1991). The St. George's Respiratory Questionnaire. *Respiratory Medicine*, 85, 25–31 (supplement B).

Juniper, E.F., Guyatt, G.H., Epstein, R.S., Ferrie, P.J., Jaeschke, R., & Hiller, T.K. (1992). Evaluation of impairment of health related quality of life in asthma: development of a questionnaire for use in clinical trials. *Thorax*, 47, 76–83.

Juniper, E.F., Guyatt, G.H., Feeny, D.H., Ferrie, P.J., Griffith, L.E., & Townsend, M. (1996a). Measuring quality of life in children with asthma. *Quality of Life Research*, 5, 35–46.

Juniper, E.F., Guyatt, G.H., Feeny, D.H., Ferrie, P.J., Griffith, L.E., & Townsend, M. (1996b). Measuring quality of life in the parents of children with asthma. *Quality of Life Research*, 5, 27–34.

Kendrick, A.H., Higgs, C.M.B., Whitfield, M.J., & Laszlo, G. (1993). Accuracy of perception of severity of asthma: patients treated in general practice. *British Medical Journal*, 307, 422–424.

Kleiger, J.H. & Dirks, J.F. (1979). Medication compliance in chronic asthmatic patients. *The Journal of Asthma Research*, 16, 93–96.

Maillé, A.R., Kaptein, A.A., Koning, C.J.M., & Zwinderman, A.H. (1994). Developing a quality of life questionnaire for patients with respiratory illness. *Monaldi Archives of Chest Disease*, 49, 76–78.

Marks, G.B., Dunn, S.M., & Woolcock, A.J. (1992). A scale for the measurement of quality of life in adults with asthma. *Journal of Clinical Epidemiology*, 45, 461–472.

McSweeny, A.J. & Creer, T.L. (1995). Health-related quality of life assessment in medical care. *Disease-a-Month*, 41, 1–72.

O'Boyle, C.A., McGee, H., Hickey, A., O'Malley, K., Joyce, C.R.B. (1992). Individual quality of life in patients undergoing hip replacement. *Lancet*, 339, 1088–1091.

Osman, L.M., Russell, I.T., Friend, J.A., Legge, J.S., & Douglas, J.G. (1993). Predicting patient attitudes to asthma medication. *Thorax*, 48, 827–830.

Pennebaker, J.W. (1982). *The psychology of physical symptoms*. New York: Springer.

Rijken, M., Komproe, I.H., Ros, W.J.G., Winnubst, J.A.M., & van Heesch, N.C.A. (1995). Subjective well-being of elderly women: conceptual differences between cancer patients, women suffering from chronic ailments and healthy women. *British Journal of Clinical Psychology*, 34, 289–300.

Sodergren, S.C. & Hyland, M.E. (2000). What are the positive consequences of illness? *Psychology and Health*, 15, 85–97.

Suh, E., Diener, E., & Fujita, F. (1996). Events and subjective well-being: only recent events matter. *Journal of Personality and Social Psychology*, 70, 1091–1102

Usherwood, T.P., Scrimgeour, A., & Barber, J.H. (1990). Questionnaire to measure perceived symptoms and disability in asthma. *Archives of Disease in Childhood*, 65, 779–781.

Ware, J.E. & Sherbourne, C.D. (1992). The MOS 36 item Short-form Health Survey. *Medical Care*, 30, 473–483.

Watson, D. & Pennebaker, J.W. (1989). Health complaints, stress and distress: exploring the central role of negative affectivity. *Psychological Review*, 96, 234–254.

10
Cystic fibrosis: A biopsychosocial perspective

Kathryn E. Gustafson and Melanie J. Bonner

Editors' note—*In this chapter, Gustafson and Bonner describe cystic fibrosis (CF) and its impact on patients and families. As they note, CF is the most common life-shortening genetic disorder in the white population throughout the world. Gustafson and Bonner describe recent medical approaches, particularly the introduction of inhaled antibiotics and inhaled enzyme therapy, to the management of CF. It is hoped that these medical innovations, when included in an interdisciplinarian approach to treatment, will lead to breakthroughs in the control of CF.*

The goal of controlling cystic fibrosis cannot occur soon enough. As Gustafson and Bonner note, CF represents an overwhelming presence in the lives of those with the condition and their families. In addition, it continues to limit the duration of life of those afflicted with the condition, as well as drain away finite moneys needed for its care. Survival estimates for adults with CF in the United Kingdom were recently described by Lewis et al. (1999). Based upon observed cohort survival data for patients with CF born since 1968 in the UK, two prominent trends were noted:

- *it was found that the number of patients surviving into later adulthood is increasing – this is encouraging news*
- *on the down side, however, Lewis and his colleagues found that the mortality rate in adults shows no evidence of improvement.*

Based upon the data, the authors concluded that it was impossible to determine whether the high mortality rates in adulthood will be improved with enhanced adult clinics or improved treatment for CF patients in childhood.

Cystic fibrosis is also an expensive disorder. Lieu et al. (1999) analyzed average annual costs for 136 CF patients served by a health maintenance organization with a CF center. The average cost of medical care for CF in 1996 was US$13,300 for patients. However, costs varied by severity, in that they ranged from US$6,200 among patients with mild CF to US$43,300 among patients with severe CF. These findings led Lieu and his colleagues to conclude that the cost of CF is substantial, even among those with mild forms of the disorder. The two factors alone – limits in life expectancy and financial costs – emphasize the significance of the research and services provided by professionals such as Gustafson and Bonner.

> *Growing up with cystic fibrosis is really hard. I feel, think, and desire all the same things other healthy kids do only in the back of my mind, I am never really sure if things will work out. I try not to think*

about it, but it is always there. And, I try to do everything the doctors tell me to do, like my therapy, take my pills and keep a positive attitude. But, still over time, I feel my illness getting worse, and I wonder . . .

(Allison, aged 16)

Introduction

Among respiratory disorders, cystic fibrosis (CF) is a disease with far-reaching emotional and psychological consequences for children and parents who confront the disease. The birth of a child with cystic fibrosis genetically links both parents to this lethal disorder, in many cases when the parents were not even aware that they were carriers of the disorder. Parents often experience feelings of grief, guilt, and fear for the future. The children experience a time-consuming, rigorous daily treatment regimen, swallow handfuls of pills per day, and demonstrate symptoms such as coughing up sputum or emitting foul-smelling flatulence or stools that are embarrassing to them. Physically, they may demonstrate poor growth or delayed development, clubbing of the fingers or toes, and a barrel-chested appearance. Many of these children miss extended periods of school and social activities because periodic hospitalizations for pulmonary 'tune-up' are necessary. And, as they grow up, they face declining health and an inevitably foreshortened future, while simultaneously confronting the normal developmental tasks of establishing autonomy, achieving an identity, and forming relationships. Yet, in the face of this devastating illness, most children and parents demonstrate a remarkable resilience that motivates and inspires health care professionals who work with individuals with cystic fibrosis.

Medical Overview

Cystic fibrosis is the most common lethal genetic disease in the Caucasian population, with an incidence of 1 in 2500 births and a carrier frequency of approximately 5% (Boat *et al.*, 1989). There are approximately 21,000 patients currently under care at CF Care Centers in the US (Cystic Fibrosis Foundation, 2000). Patients are typically diagnosed in infancy after referral, secondary to persistent respiratory symptoms, failure to thrive despite adequate food intake, steatorrhea, meconium ileus, or intestinal obstruction. Diagnosis is typically made by elevated levels of sodium chloride in sweat collected during a sweat test. Although there is no cure for the disease, the prognosis for CF has improved drastically in recent years. The median survival from birth was only 10.4 years in 1966

(Orenstein & Wachnowsky, 1985), but 33 years later in 1999 the median survival from birth was 29.1 years (Cystic Fibrosis Foundation, 2000). Therefore, it is now likely that an individual born with CF will reach adulthood and enjoy a productive life. Indeed, 38% of all patients with CF followed by the CF Centers in the US are 18 years of age or older, and of these 37% are employed full time, 11% are employed part time, and 25% are students (Cystic Fibrosis Foundation, 2000).

Cystic fibrosis is an autosomal recessive disorder that affects the exocrine glands in several major organ systems, including the respiratory, digestive, pancreas, liver, and reproductive systems. Mucus secretions in the ducts of the exocrine glands are abnormally viscous, due to the faulty transport of sodium and chloride within the cells. In the respiratory system, the thick mucus leads to both obstruction and infection, which over time results in damage to the lungs and gradual deterioration of pulmonary functioning. Cardiorespiratory factors are the primary causes of death in patients with CF (Cystic Fibrosis Foundation, 2000). As a result, the primary treatment objective is to prevent and treat the pulmonary disease in order to delay the progression of deterioration of the lungs. Keeping the airways clear of obstruction is believed to be important to delaying lung deterioration, so chest physical therapy, involving postural drainage and clap percussion to loosen sputum and facilitate expectoration of the mucus through coughing, is recommended from one to four times daily. Patients may also use new mucus-thinning medications such as Pulmozyme. Exercise is also sometimes used as an adjunct or supplement to chest physical therapy to loosen mucus secretions.

Because patients with CF are also susceptible to bacterial infections in the lungs, prevention and treatment of infection with antibiotic therapy is recommended. Oral antibiotics are used prophylactically as well as to treat acute infections, and intravenous antibiotic therapy may also be necessary for more serious infections or in situations when there is no response to the oral antibiotics. In recent years, aerosolized antibiotics have been developed that allow for the delivery of more concentrated doses of antibiotics directly to the site of lung infections. Moreover, clinical trials are currently underway to develop new forms of antibiotics as well as drugs to correct the protein product of the gene. There is increasing concern about antibiotic-resistant organisms, as infection with such organisms can be associated with rapid clinical deterioration.

More recently it has been recognized that airway inflammation is also a problem in individuals with CF as it is associated with lung deterioration. Thus, prevention of deleterious inflammatory response using oral or inhaled steroids and nonsteroidal anti-inflammatory drugs (NSAIDs) is being investigated (Wallis, 1996).

Heart–lung and bilateral lung transplantation are increasingly being used to treat end-stage pulmonary disease in some children and adults with CF, with almost 1000 such operations having occurred by 2000 (Cystic Fibrosis Foundation, 2000). Survival at 1 year is 80% and at 4 years is 60%, with the major postoperative complications being rejection and infection (Conway, 1996). Lobar transplants using cadaver donors or living-related donors have recently been used and are on the increase.

Another major problem in CF is related to nutrition and growth. Most patients with CF exhibit pancreatic insufficiency due to blockage of the ducts of the pancreas by the viscous secretions. Inadequate secretion of pancreatic enzymes means that patients with CF have inadequate digestion and malabsorption of fat, protein, and fat-soluble vitamins. Thus, enzyme-replacement supplements are required with every meal. Moreover, both CF metabolism and lung disease seem to dictate the need for increased calories, so individuals with CF should consume 125–150% of expected caloric requirements. Patients are also typically prescribed fat-soluble vitamin supplements, including vitamins A, D, and E. Because good nutritional management is associated with improved survival and better lung function, regular monitoring of nutritional status with appropriate modification of treatment protocols is strongly recommended (Wallis, 1996).

Additional complications in individuals with CF emerge as life expectancy increases (Conway, 1996). Such difficulties include abnormal glucose tolerance, and diagnosis with diabetes mellitus. Liver disease may also occur. Moreover, male patients are usually infertile. Although female patients can have healthy babies without compromising their own health in certain situations, it is important that the woman has reasonable lung function, good nutritional status, and collaborative care between the CF Center and her obstetrician.

In recent years, there has been much progress towards a cure for this debilitating disease. A major medical advance was the identification of the CF gene (Kerem *et al.*, 1989). Then, in 1990, scientists successfully made copies of the normal gene and corrected defective cells in laboratory dishes. In 1993, the first experimental gene therapy treatment was given to a patient with CF, and gene therapy clinical trials are ongoing to date.

As we have now reviewed the medical aspects of CF, in the remainder of this chapter we will discuss the existing literature that examines:

- the psychological adjustment of children with CF,
- the psychological adjustment of parents of children with CF, and
- adherence to medical treatment in patients with CF.

Future research directions and suggestions for biopsychosocial interventions are identified.

Psychological Adjustment in Children with Cystic Fibrosis

Chronic childhood illness is recognized as a significant stressor both for children with the illnesses and for their families (Perrin & MacLean, 1988). Although the rates of difficulties in adjustment to chronic illness vary across illnesses and across different types of studies (Thompson & Gustafson, 1996), it is estimated that children with chronic illness have a risk for adjustment difficulties that is 1.5–3 times as high as children without chronic illness (Pless, 1984). Despite the risk for adjustment problems, good adjustment to chronic illness is also possible, and indeed, good adjustment in the face of chronic illness is the most likely outcome (Thompson & Gustafson, 1996).

There have been numerous studies of psychological adjustment in children with CF. Although some of the early clinical research suggested a high incidence of emotional problems in children with CF, most of these studies were characterized by significant methodological problems such as small sample sizes, a lack of comparison groups, or dependent variables that were subjective, or lacked reliability and validity (Drotar *et al.*, 1981). Moreover, the substantial advances in the medical treatment for children with CF have improved the quality of life for children with CF such that these early studies, even if methodologically adequate, may be irrelevant to the challenges confronting children with CF today.

Most studies of adjustment in children with CF have been cross-sectional studies. For example, representative studies include those by Simmons and colleagues, who examined adjustment in children with CF at four different ages: preschool age (Cowen *et al.*, 1985), latency age (Simmons *et al.*, 1987), early adolescence (Simmons *et al.*, 1985), and late adolescence and adulthood (Cowen *et al.*, 1984).

In the preschool-age study, psychosocial adjustment in 41 children aged 2–5 with CF was rated by parents as better than that of a control group of 31 healthy children (Cowen *et al.*, 1985). In the latency-age study, psychosocial adjustment in 108 children with CF, ages 6–11, was evaluated in comparison to a healthy sibling control group and relative to normative data on several self- and parent-report measures (Simmons *et al.*, 1987). Male patients with CF had statistically significant higher scores on the total, internalizing, and externalizing behavior problems scales of the Child Behavior Checklist (CBCL: Achenbach, 1991), whereas female patients with CF had higher scores on the total and internalizing scales. Moreover, male patients had higher scores on the total behavior problem scale than did healthy sibling controls. Twenty-three percent of the patients with CF (19% of the girls and 26% of the boys) obtained total behavior problem scores greater than the 90th percentile, which was deemed to be clinically significant.

Similar findings were reported for the sample of 62 early adolescent patients (ages 12–15) with CF (Simmons *et al.*, 1985). Compared with the normative data for the CBCL, male patients exhibited elevations on the total, internalizing, and externalizing scales, whereas female patients exhibited elevations on the total behavior problem scale. For this study, the authors used a T score of 70 or over (2 SD from the mean) as reflecting clinical significance, and found that 6.5% of the patients (4% of the girls and 9% of the boys) showed such marked elevations on the total behavior problem scale.

In the study of late adolescents and adults (Cowen *et al.*, 1984), 59% of women and 20% of men, aged 20 or over, showed moderate to severe disturbance on a measure of general emotional disturbance, whereas only 30% of women and 12% of men aged 16–19 demonstrated comparable levels of emotional distress. Similar findings were obtained on a measure of self-esteem.

Although most studies have assessed psychological distress through symptom checklists, the nature of psychological adjustment difficulties in patients with CF has been further clarified in studies that have utilized structured diagnostic interviews. Kashani *et al.* (1988) examined psychological adjustment in 30 children and adolescents (ages 7–17) with CF in comparison with that of a matched control group of healthy peers. These researchers used the parent report on the CBCL, as well as both the child and parent versions of a structured diagnostic interview that generates psychiatric diagnoses. Child self-reports of hopelessness and self-concept were also obtained. Based on child and parent reports on the diagnostic interview, no differences emerged between the children with CF and the control children with regard to the number and types of psychiatric diagnoses. However, children with CF were rated by their parents as having more psychiatric symptoms than were the control children, primarily in terms of a larger number of somatic symptoms. The children with CF were rated as higher on the internalizing and externalizing scales of the CBCL than were the control children, although all scores were within one-half of a standard deviation of the norms for the CBCL nonclinical sample. The CF children did not differ significantly from controls in self-reported hopelessness or self-concept.

A structured diagnostic interview was also used by Thompson *et al.* (1990), who compared psychological adjustment in children with CF with that of psychiatrically referred children and nonreferred children. The criteria for a Diagnostic and Statistical Manual of Mental Disorders, 3rd Edition DSM-III (American Psychiatric Association, 1980) diagnosis were met for 58% of the children with CF, 23% of the nonreferred children, and 77% of the psychiatrically referred children. In terms of symptoms, the children with CF did not report higher numbers of symptoms than nonreferred children. It was only in terms of the internalizing symptoms of worries, self-image, and anxiety, particularly separation anxiety, that the children with CF were similar to the psychiatrically referred children.

All of these studies reflected advancements in our understanding of psychological functioning in children with CF over earlier research. In particular, these studies reflected improvements in methodology, as these were among the first studies of adjustment in children with CF that used multiple methods of assessment using standardized, psychometrically sound instruments. These studies demonstrated that although a subset of children and adolescents with CF demonstrated adjustment problems, there were also many children in these studies who did not. Thus, it became necessary to understand what factors differentiate those with good psychological adjustment from those with poor psychological adjustment. Moreover, these studies were cross-sectional in nature and therefore failed to provide us with an understanding of the stability of adjustment patterns over time and how patterns of adjustment change across different phases of the illness or across children's development. To answer these important questions about adjustment to CF, within-group research using longitudinal designs was necessary (Thompson et al., 1994b).

A series of studies of children with CF by Thompson and colleagues at Duke University Medical Center were guided by the transactional stress and coping model of adjustment to chronic illness (Thompson & Gustafson, 1996). The studies sought to

1 identify the types and frequencies of psychological adjustment problems in children with CF and their mothers;
2 delineate the role of hypothesized mediational processes in psychological adjustment; and
3 determine how psychological adjustment, mediational processes, and their interrelationship change over time.

The protocol assessed psychological adjustment of children with CF and their mothers and the hypothesized mediational processes at three points in time, approximately 1 year apart. The focus of the transactional stress and coping model (Fig. 10.1) is on the contribution of mediational processes hypothesized to influence psychological adjustment of children and their mothers over and above the contributions of illness parameters (e.g., severity) and demographic parameters (e.g., socioeconomic status [SES], patient age, and gender). Child adjustment is hypothesized to be mediated by the child's self-esteem and health locus of control and by maternal adjustment. The mother's adjustment is hypothesized to be mediated by:

- cognitive processes of appraisal of stress, expectations of efficacy, and health locus of control;
- coping methods;
- social support in terms of family functioning; and
- child psychological adjustment.

In these studies, child adjustment is assessed in terms of child report on a standardized diagnostic interview, the Child Assessment Schedule

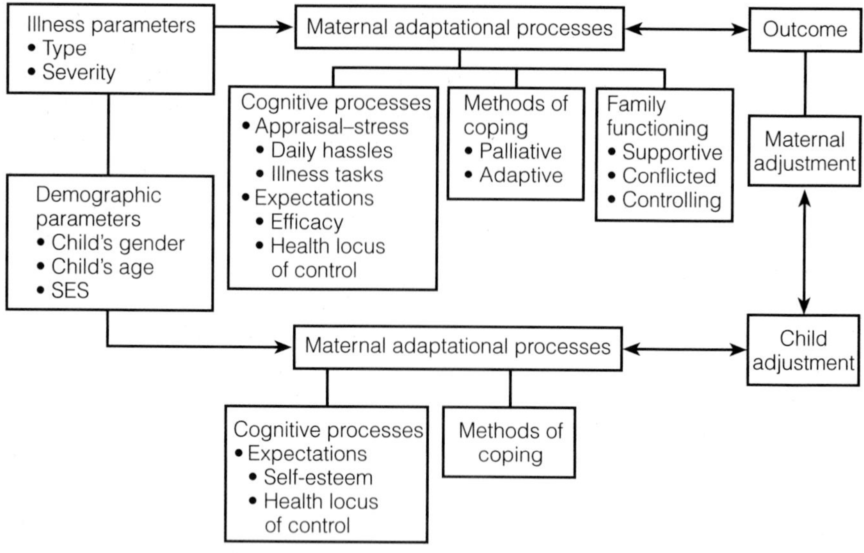

Figure 10.1

The Transactional Stress and Coping Model. Reproduced with permission from Thompson *et al.* (1994b).

(CAS: Hodges *et al.*, 1982) which generates DSM-III diagnoses and a total symptom score, as well as in terms of parent report on the Missouri Children's Behavior Checklist (MCBC: Sines *et al.*, 1969). The MCBC yields internalizing and externalizing behavior problem factor scores and seven behavior patterns, including four problem patterns and three problem-free patterns (Thompson *et al.*, 1989). Maternal adjustment was assessed using the Symptom Checklist-90-Revised (SCL-90-R; Derogatis, 1983). Illness severity was assessed using the Shwachman Clinical Evaluation System (Shwachman & Kulczycki, 1958).

The initial (Time 1) study of adjustment in children aged 7–12 with CF ($n = 45$) found that 60% of the children with CF had a mother-reported behavior problem, with the mixed internal and external behavior problem pattern the most frequent, followed by an undifferentiated behavior problem pattern (Thompson *et al.*, 1992a). On the child-reported CAS, 62% of children with CF met criteria for a DSM-III diagnosis, with anxiety disorders and oppositional disorders the most frequent. Forty-four percent of the children demonstrated poor adjustment on both the parent- and self-report instruments, with three-quarters of these children having a mixture of internalizing and externalizing problems. Children with poor adjustment on both measures had lower SES and lower levels of self-esteem than those with good adjustment. Multiple regression analyses were utilized to evaluate the unique and combined contributions of the variables of the transactional stress and coping model. In terms of mother-reported internalizing and externalizing behavior problems, maternal anxiety and child's self-worth accounted for additional significant increments in variance above and beyond the variance accounted for by illness and demographic variables. The variables of the transactional stress and coping model accounted for 39% of the variance in internalizing behavior problems and 43% of the variance in externalizing behavior problems. In terms of child-reported symptoms on the CAS, child's self-worth, chance health locus of control beliefs, and maternal anxiety accounted for additional significant increments in variance above that accounted for by the illness and demographic variables. The variables of the stress and coping model accounted for 68% of the variance in child's total symptom score.

A similar study of adjustment in adolescents (age 13–17) with CF ($n = 37$) was conducted (Thompson *et al.*, 1995). Criteria for DSM-III diagnoses were met by 51% of the adolescent sample, with oppositional disorder and the anxiety disorders the most frequent diagnoses. When good and poor adjustment subgroups were formed based on the presence or absence of a DSM-III diagnosis, adolescents with poor adjustment had lower SES relative to those with good adjustment. In addition to lower SES, adolescents with poor adjustment were more likely to believe that chance and powerful others (e.g., physicians) influence their health (i.e., external health locus of control beliefs). There were no significant subgroup differences in terms of illness severity, age, gender, or maternal adjustment. Multiple regression analyses revealed that maternal coping, illness severity and powerful other health locus of control beliefs accounted for 52% of the variance in total symptom score.

A follow-up study (Time 2) of change and stability in psychological adjustment was conducted with 41 of the children with CF approximately 1 year later (Thompson *et al.*, 1994). In terms of child report of adjustment as assessed with the CAS, the rate of adjustment problems was nearly identical from Time 1 (63%) to Time 2 (61%). However, there was considerable change at the level of the individual. Forty-nine percent of the children demonstrated poor adjustment at both time points, 24% had good adjustment at both time points, and 27% changed classification. Although anxiety diagnoses and oppositional disorders were most frequent at both time points, only 37% of children had the same diagnosis at both points. In terms of mother-reported adjustment as assessed by the MCBC, the rate of behavior problem patterns was comparable at Time 1 (63%) and Time 2 (58%), and classification of individual children was relatively stable. Fifty-four percent had poor adjustment at both time points, 32% had good adjustment at both time points, and only 15% changed classification over time. Although the mixed internal and external behavior problem profile was the most frequent at Time 1, the internal profile was most frequent 1 year later at Time 2. Fifty-four percent of the subjects had the same behavior pattern at both time points.

Stable good and stable poor adjustment subgroups were formed based on having good or poor adjustment at both time points. Based on child report on the CAS, children with stable poor adjustment demonstrated a significantly lower level of self-worth at Time 2, and a trend toward lower self-worth and higher maternal distress at Time 1. Based on parent report on the MCBC, the stable poor adjustment subgroup exhibited a trend for lower self-worth at Time 2.

Hierarchical multiple regression analyses were completed to determine whether the variables of the transactional stress and coping model would account for the variance in adjustment at Time 2, with initial (Time 1) levels of adjustment controlled. For mother-reported internalizing behavior problems at Time 2, self-worth at Time 2 accounted for a significant amount of the variance. For externalizing behavior problems at follow-up, none of the variables of the transactional stress and coping model contributed additional variance. For child report of total symptoms on the CAS, significant increments in variance were accounted for by lower self-worth at Time 2, younger age at Time 1, and maternal distress at Time 2.

A second follow-up assessment (Time 3) was conducted approximately 12 months later to further examine changes and stability in adjustment, hypothesized mediational processes, and patterns of interrelationships (Thompson *et al.*, 1999). Fifty-nine children with CF and their mothers participated in the Time 3 assessment. As with the earlier assessment point, the rate of adjustment problems was relatively high; 44% of the children with CF met criteria for a DSM-III diagnosis at Time 3. However, there was relatively little stability in classification of individual adjustment as good or poor. Across the three assessment points, stable good adjustment was demonstrated by 19% of the subjects and stable poor adjustment was demonstrated by 12% of the subjects. Internalizing disorders were the most frequent at each time point, although there was a low correspondence of specific diagnoses across individuals from Time 1 to Time 3.

In terms of mother report of psychological adjustment on the MCBC, there was a significant decrease in externalizing scores over time. The rate of mother-reported adjustment problems remained high at Time 3, with 69% of the subjects receiving a behavior problem pattern. Across the three time points, stable good adjustment was demonstrated by 19% and stable poor adjustment was demonstrated by 47%. Overall, there was a moderate level of consistency in classification of adjustment as good or poor based on the presence of a behavior problem profile. Internalizing behavior problems were most frequent and externalizing problems were relatively infrequent, and there was a moderate level of consistency in specific behavior profiles across individuals.

In summary, the research on the adjustment of children with CF has been consistent with the research on adjustment to chronic illness in general; i.e., children with CF are at increased risk for psychological adjustment problems. Children with CF appear to be primarily at risk for internalizing difficulties, or internalizing difficulties mixed with milder forms of externalizing problems such as oppositional disorder, perhaps related to medical compliance. More serious externalizing disorders, such as conduct disorder, are rare. Longitudinal studies are relatively scarce, but those such as the series of studies by Thompson and colleagues demonstrate that although the overall rates of adjustment problems remain relatively stable, there is considerably less stability at the level of the individual in terms of good versus poor adjustment and in terms of specific diagnoses or behavior problem profiles. However, there is somewhat more stability in mother-reported than in child-reported adjustment. Given these cumulative findings, it is necessary to engage in research that will not only identify markers of risk and resilience but will also identify variables and processes that are associated with transition into or out of good adjustment categories. Moreover, intervention efforts may be best applied to those children who demonstrate stable poor adjustment over time (Thompson *et al.*, 1999).

There has been almost no research on interventions that target the psychological adjustment and coping difficulties in patients with CF. One notable exception is a cognitive–behavioral intervention using a multiple baseline design across five adolescents with CF who were referred for treatment by medical staff (Hains *et al.*, 1997). The patients participated in a nine-session weekly intervention, targeting cognitive restructuring and problem-solving skills. With treatment, the adolescents demonstrated decreased anxiety, an increase in the use of positive coping techniques and a decrease in the use of negative coping techniques on problems related to CF, and a decrease in perceived functional disability. At 3-month follow-up, most youths maintained their improvement in anxiety and perceived functional disability. Although this study included only a small number of patients, it does support the potential role of cognitive–behavioral interventions for individuals with a chronic illness such as CF (Thompson & Gustafson, 1996).

Psychological Adjustment of Parents of Children with Cystic Fibrosis

The chronic nature and severity of CF have a potentially significant impact on the parents and family of the child or adolescent with CF. In addition to the burdens associated with the complex daily treatment regimen, parents must confront the challenges associated with the potential emotional impact of the disease on the child, the siblings, and on the parents themselves. Moreover, the psychological adjustment of parents of children with CF is also important because of the potential impact of parental adjustment on the adjustment of the children with CF. Research on parental adjustment has examined several areas:

- What are the rates and patterns of adjustment problems in mothers and fathers of children with CF?
- How does parental adjustment change over time?
- What illness, demographic or psychosocial factors are correlates of adjustment in parents of children with CF?

Parents of children with CF are at increased risk for psychological adjustment problems, although resilience in the face of this stressor is possible, and, in fact, good adjustment is the most likely outcome (Thompson & Gustafson, 1996). However, rates of adjustment problems have varied somewhat across studies, perhaps associated with how adjustment was measured or due to study characteristics such as age of child, illness severity, or phase of illness. Studies by Thompson and colleagues found that 34% of mothers of children with CF (Thompson *et al.*, 1992b) and 24% of mothers of adolescents with CF (Thompson *et al.*, 1995) reported poor psychological adjustment on a self-report measure of psychological symptoms.

Elevations into the clinical range of distress occurred for 21% of the mothers on a scale of depressive symptoms and for 18% of the mothers on a scale of anxiety symptoms (Thompson *et al.*, 1992b). Similarly, Walker *et al.* (1987) found that mothers of children with CF scored higher on a measure of depressive symptoms than a control group of mothers with healthy children, but that this finding was significant only for mothers of preschool or early adolescent children and not for mothers with school-age or late-adolescent children. Moreover, Mullins *et al.* (1991) found that although mothers of children with CF had higher scores than the published nonpsychiatric norms on subscales assessing symptoms of depression, anxiety, and hostility, as well as on the overall distress scale, the mean scores for each of these scales were within one standard deviation of the general population norms. This suggests that elevations in the CF sample may not be clinically significant.

Most studies of adjustment in parents of children with CF have focused on mothers. Relatively few studies have included fathers or compared adjustment patterns in mothers and fathers of children with CF. An early study assessed personality functioning in mothers and fathers of children with CF using the Minnesota Multiphasic Personality Inventory (MMPI) (Gayton *et al.*, 1977) and found that 32% of the fathers and 22% of the mothers had one or more MMPI scales in the clinical range and that mothers and fathers differed in terms of which scales were elevated. In another study of adjustment of mothers and fathers of children with CF (Nagy & Ungerer, 1990), mothers reported lower levels of emotional and behavioral control on a mental health inventory than did fathers. There were no differences between mothers and fathers on state and trait anxiety, however, although mothers reported greater trait anxiety and fathers reported lower state anxiety than the normative population.

Mothers and fathers did not differ significantly in their perceptions of the stresses associated with rearing a child with CF. In contrast, a study by Goldberg *et al.* (1990) did find some differences in parenting stress as reported by mothers and fathers of infants with CF, congenital heart disease, or no chronic illness. Fathers reported more stress than mothers in the Child domain of the Parenting Stress Index (Abidin, 1986), whereas mothers reported more stress than fathers in the Parent domain. The authors concluded that mothers reported more stress in areas that often affect mothers of young children, including depression, role restrictions, personal health, and marital problems, whereas fathers reported more stress in areas related to forming a relationship with the child, including attachment to child, child reinforcement of parent, and child distractibility/hyperactivity. Similarly, a study of parents' functioning during the first 2 years after a child's CF diagnosis found that mothers reported more role strain related to functioning as caregivers and greater levels of depressive symptoms than did fathers (Quittner *et al.*, 1992a).

Although most studies of adjustment in parents of children with CF have been cross-sectional in nature, Thompson and colleagues have examined patterns of adjustment and change over time (Thompson *et al.*, 1994a, 1999). In a follow-up sample of 57 mothers of children and adolescents with CF (Thompson *et al.*, 1994a), 30% of mothers demonstrated poor adjustment on a self-report measure of psychological distress at Time 1 and 19% demonstrated poor adjustment at Time 2. Fourteen percent of mothers demonstrated stable poor adjustment across both points in time, whereas 65% demonstrated stable good adjustment over time. Mothers demonstrating stable poor adjustment had higher levels of daily stress, more use of palliative coping, and higher levels of family conflict than mothers demonstrating stable good adjustment. When controlling for initial levels of maternal adjustment, demographic variables, and follow-up interval, significant increments in variance in maternal adjustment at follow-up were accounted for by illness severity, child adjustment, daily stress, and family conflict.

Fifty-nine mothers completed a third assessment point (Thompson *et al.*, 1999). There was a significant decrease in rate of poor adjustment over time, with 31% reporting poor adjustment at Time 1, 18% reporting poor adjustment at Time 2, and 16% reporting poor adjustment at Time 3. Across the three time points, consistently good adjustment was demonstrated by 67% of the mothers and consistently poor adjustment was demonstrated by 11% of the mothers, resulting in moderate stability in classification. The mothers with stable poor adjustment over time exhibited higher levels of daily stress, greater use of palliative coping in general, and relative to adaptive coping, and higher levels of family conflict than mothers with stable good adjustment over time. Higher levels of daily stress at Time 1 accounted for a 25% increment in mother's distress at Time 3 over and above that accounted for by the demographic variables. This line of research indicates that although mothers of children with CF are at risk for adjustment difficulties, some of these difficulties may resolve over time. However, there is a subset of individuals who demonstrate stable adjustment difficulties over time, and these adjustment difficulties are associated with mediational variables that could serve as salient intervention targets, such as enhancing management of daily stressors, decreasing family conflict and increasing family support, and decreasing reliance on palliative coping methods.

Although research has identified potentially salient targets for intervention, interventions specifically targeting adjustment or coping difficulties in parents of children with CF are virtually nonexistent. Schroeder and colleagues described a pilot study of a 2-day educational workshop to improve communication and problem-solving skills for parents of children with CF (Schroeder *et al.*, 1988). Significant improvements in self-esteem, marital adjustment, and family functioning were noted at the 2-month follow-up in those families initially acknowledging problems. Some benefit to parents' adjustment may also be obtained from interventions specifically targeting self-management (Bartholomew *et al.*, 1997), feeding problems in children (Stark *et al.*, 1994), and adherence to medical treatments (Quittner *et al.*, 2000).

Treatment Adherence

Adherence to treatment recommendations is problematic across illness types, particularly chronic illnesses with complex treatment regimens (Rapoff & Christophersen, 1982). Indeed, findings within and across illnesses, both acute and chronic, reveal a great deal of variability in adherence estimates, with many studies revealing rates around 50% adherence (see Epstein & Cluss, 1982; Dunbar-Jacob *et al.*, 1993). This variability is accounted for in part by the use of different adherence definitions, measures, target behaviors, and informants. Several models of adherence have been developed to help explain some of the variance in treatment outcome, although most of these models lack a theoretical and/or developmental framework (Thompson & Gustafson, 1996). Collectively, however, the research findings highlight the importance of assessing multiple parameters, including biomedical (e.g., complexity of the regimen, chronicity of the disease), child, and socio-ecological (e.g., family functioning, patient–physician relationship) when examining treatment adherence in a chronic illness population.

When considering that CF is a terminal illness with a complex treatment regimen (Matthews & Drotar, 1984), it is not surprising that adherence in the CF population is considered a significant problem (Czajkowski & Koocher, 1986; Koocher *et al.*, 1990; Lask, 1994; Stark *et al.*, 1995a). Moreover, much like other chronic illnesses, there is variability in adherence within the treatment regimen; i.e., most studies have documented good adherence overall in patients with CF, but have found that adherence to medication regimens is better than adherence to dieting needs and chest physiotherapy (Stark *et al.*, 1995a). Thus, interventions that target both the challenges of adherence that are shared with other chronic illnesses and the unique aspects of the CF treatment regimen are needed.

Koocher *et al.* (1990) have identified typologies of nonadherence in the CF population based on reviews of more than 1200 anecdotal reports of 223 patients with CF and their family members. The framework that emerged conceptualizes nonadherence as reflecting three general categories: inadequate knowledge or developmentally sensitive understanding of CF, psychosocial resistance factors, and educated nonadherence (quality of life). Studies that highlight some of these aspects are summarized below and interpreted more broadly within a biopsychosocial framework.

Medication Adherence

As noted earlier, compliance with medication (e.g., antibiotics) is important given that pulmonary infections pose life-threatening problems in patients with CF. Gudas *et al.* (1991) conducted a study that highlights the importance of sociobehavioral factors and a developmental perspective when evaluating adherence in a CF population. Their sample included 100 patients with CF, ranging in age from 5 to 20 years, who were divided into four age groups (5–7; 8–11; 12–15; 16–20). Compliance with medication, chest physiotherapy, and dietary recommendations was assessed with self-report, parent report, and physician report. Direct measures of compliance (e.g., blood, urine samples) were not taken; however, acceptable levels of reliability were achieved across informants. Compliance attitudes were assessed by the Medical Compliance Incomplete Stories Test (MCIST: Koocher *et al.*, 1987), an instrument found to discriminate between compliant and noncompliant patients in a previous study (Czajkowski & Koocher, 1986). The MCIST is a series of incomplete stories about children who are confronted with different medical treatments. The patients with CF were asked to complete these stories, which were transcribed and scored according to three dimensions:

- compliance/coping;
- optimism; and
- self-efficacy.

Ratings of sociobehavioral variables were also obtained across informants, including perceived severity of the disease, level of independence for care, and optimism of the patient. Additionally, data on knowledge of CF treatment were obtained from the child. The knowledge measure included an assessment of the child's understanding of facts (e.g., types of medications taken) and his/her knowledge of the impact of these medications. The latter is thought to require more sophisticated cognitive conceptualizations and, thus, has developmental implications. The results demonstrated that, overall, patients with CF are generally compliant, although the rate of compliance varied with regimen components. Patients with CF were most compliant with their medications, less compliant with chest physiotherapy, and least compliant with dietary recommendations. Additionally, although the relationship between age and compliance indices was not significant overall, it was found that the older the child, the less compliant he/she was with medication.

The latter finding lends further support for the general finding that compliance with chronic illness regimens decreases with time (Haynes, 1979; La Greca, 1988). More specific to CF is that the complexity of the treatment regimen increases with length of disease given the progression of symptoms. Additionally, regarding child/developmental parameters, lower compliance with age may parallel noncompliance outside of the medical context (e.g., during adolescence). Finally, from both a developmental and a socio-ecological perspective, lower compliance with age may reflect decreased parental involvement in the medical regimen. Although older children were less compliant overall, there was a positive relationship between age and optimism in predicting medication compliance in older children.

Related to medication adherence is the use of vitamin supplementation. It is expected that all patients with CF will require vitamin supplementation at some point in the disease process. Using questionnaire responses from 80 pancreatic-insufficient adult and child patients, Borowitz *et al.* (1994) found that less than half of the respondents reported adherence to their prescribed daily regimen. Variability in adherence was not related to demographic variables (age, gender, or education). Rather, the authors explained the variability using the typologies of nonadherence described above (Koocher *et al.*, 1990), including forgetting, cost, inconvenience, and judgment about the importance of vitamins in the overall treatment process.

Dietary Adherence/Feeding Interventions

Another important aspect of the CF treatment regimen is management of dietary intake, given its relation to lung disease and recovery from illness (Stark *et al.*, 1995a, Stark, 2000). Although adequate nutrition is regarded as important to the long-term survival of patients with CF, it is considered one of the more difficult aspects of the treatment regimen. Indeed, a survey completed by Sanders *et al.* (1991) revealed that dietary compliance and mealtime behaviors were considered problematic by 70% of a CF sample. Moreover, Quittner *et al.* (1991) reported that mealtime was the most common problem identified by parents of children with CF between the ages of 2 to 5. Given the difficulties with absorption of calories and high risk for malnutrition, patients with CF generally have a need for increased consumption of calories. However, Stark *et al.* (1995b) found that patients with CF only consumed 100% of the RDA for calories instead of the recommended 125–150%. Additionally, some patients will require enteral feeds or even total parenteral nutrition to address severe malabsorption and anorexia. More specific recommendations for assessing the nutritional needs of patients with CF are outlined in a consensus report (Ramsey *et al.*, 1992) to help guide clinicians and caregivers in achieving optimal nutritional status.

Factors that may impact adherence to caloric recommendations include direct effects of the disease on the patient's appetite (e.g., recurrent vomiting, reflux, respiratory infections) or indirect effects of psychosocial processes. Regarding the latter, Stark *et al.* (1995b) raised concern about the impact of societal values on the fat intake of patients with CF given the increasingly fat-conscious behaviors of our nation. Moreover, Gudas *et al.* (1991) found a lack of consensus between the parents of patients with CF and their physicians regarding expectations for dietary adherence. This finding lends support to the importance of cooperative treatment planning and clear communication described by La Greca (1988). Adherence to dietary guidelines is also thought to vary as a function of age. For example, adolescent patients may have the highest nutritional needs due to puberty development and accelerated growth, while also experiencing social pressures that may negatively impact their food intake (Ramsey *et al.*, 1992).

Psychosocial factors have also been investigated by Stark and her colleagues who have found that negative parent–child interactions at mealtime are reported in both underweight and weight-appropriate children (Bowen & Stark, 1991). This finding led to the identification of 'critical family behaviors' during mealtime – including parental coaxing, ineffective parental commands, and a slower rate of food intake by children with CF – that contribute to poorer adherence to dietary recommendations (Stark *et al.*, 1993). They further demonstrated the efficacy of behavioral parent management training in ameliorating these maladaptive mealtime behaviors, with treatment results generalizing to improved caloric intake and weight gain (Stark *et al.*, 1993, 1994). Similar results using a behavioral intervention were demonstrated in young patients with CF (ages 10–42 months) who were malnourished (Singer *et al.*, 1991). Such interventions highlight the importance of socio-ecological factors, especially parental coping strategies, in improving adherence.

The importance of psychosocial factors was further supported in a recent study by Sanders *et al.* (1997) who outlined a 'descriptive profile' of the adjustment problems and mealtime interactions of children with CF ages 1–7 years and their parents. They utilized comparison groups of 25 non-CF children with feeding problems and 20 nonclinic children matched for age, gender, and SES in order to estimate the relative contribution of disease status to the problematic mealtime interactions. Assessment of parental perceptions of feeding, as well as observational methods of mealtime interactions, revealed that children with CF did not differ significantly from either comparison group in terms of disruptive behaviors. However, the parents of the CF and feeding problem groups perceived these behaviors to be more troublesome. Observations of the CF group revealed that mothers exhibited higher levels of aversive behavior when compared with nonclinic controls and lower levels of positive attention when compared with mothers of the feeding problem group. Mothers of children with CF also gave more instructions that did not result in compliance when compared with nonclinic controls.

Measures of general child adjustment (CBCL: Achenbach, 1991, 1992) completed by mothers revealed lower levels of externalizing and total behavior problems reported in the CF and nonclinic control groups relative to the feeding problem group, although all groups exhibited profiles in the normal range for this measure. Measures of parental adjustment revealed that mothers of children with CF report significantly lower levels of parenting efficacy than both comparison groups; however, no group differences emerged for measures of mother's depression, social support, marital satisfaction, or parent-role satisfaction. Assessment of fathers' adjustment revealed similarly low levels of parenting efficacy in the CF sample and lower marital satisfaction when compared with nonclinic controls.

Combined, these findings of low parent self-efficacy and greater perception of disruptive behaviors by parents – despite contrary observational data – lend further support to the need for interventions that address psychosocial stressors faced by families of the chronically ill patient (Quittner *et al.*, 1992b).

CPT Adherence

Chest physiotherapy (CPT) is an important aspect of the CF treatment regimen that may be particularly sensitive to nonadherence, given that it is demanding and disruptive to daily routines (Lask, 1994). This finding has been cited in early studies (Passero *et al.*, 1981); however, in a more recent survey of parents of patients with CF, 89% reported CPT compliance to be problematic (Sanders *et al.*, 1991). Although clinician ratings explained very little of the variance in an adherence problem measure, in this study a relationship was found between clinician's ratings and parent-reported problems with CPT in their children. One explanation for poor adherence to CPT is that, although it provides relief in some situations (e.g. acute pulmonary infection), long-term benefits are less clear, a situation associated with nonadherence in other illnesses (La Greca, 1988; Stark *et al.*, 1995a). This may also explain why CPT was negatively associated with perceived severity in one study of children with CF (Gudas *et al.*, 1991). Specifically, CPT may not produce immediate relief, but serves the negative, although important function, of prophylactic cough production.

The importance of parental efficacy was also demonstrated in relation to CPT. Using linear structural modeling with data from a sample of 199 patients with CF and their primary caregivers, Parcel *et al.* (1994) found that perceived self-efficacy regarding one's performance of treatment-related behaviors was a significant factor in predicting self-management behavior associated with respiratory problems in patients with CF. Moreover, although knowledge predicted coping behaviors, it was not directly related to treatment-adherence behaviors. Thus, it appears that patients with CF and their primary caregivers not only need to have some level of knowledge to cope with the CF demands but also must feel confident that they can apply that knowledge. This expands the concept of adherence to include other important cognitive variables in conjunction with behavioral skills to manage CF.

As with the feeding interventions described above, behavioral modification strategies have been successfully applied to CPT. Stark *et al.* (1987) used behavioral contracting between an 11-year-old patient with CF and her parents; this included specification for rewards contingent upon meeting daily CPT goals. This intervention was effective in increasing CPT adherence and in decreasing parent–child conflict surrounding the procedure. Replication of this methodology and development of other CPT intervention studies are needed to better determine the effects of CPT on health outcome variables.

Additional Psychosocial Factors and Adherence

Findings from the aforementioned studies highlight the complexity of the CF regimen as a primary explanation for variance in adherence rates. Additionally, variability also seems to be strongly related to parent/family perceptions, behaviors, and adjustment. Indeed, several studies described the incongruence between parents' and physicians' opinions about adherence, a finding that is not specific to CF regimens (Lask, 1994).

An earlier study (Patterson, 1985) described 'critical factors' that impact family adherence to prescribed CF regimens in a sample of 72 families with a child with CF. Using the conceptual framework of the Family Adjustment and Adaptation Response Model (FAAR: McCubbin & Patterson, 1982), 51% of the variance in family compliance was predicted. The FAAR model emphasizes the family variables such as demands, resources, perception, and coping that are thought to interact over time to produce a certain level of adjustment. Several instruments were employed to assess the parameters of the FAAR model. Results revealed that the family resource of expressiveness was positively associated with adherence whereas active orientation was negatively related. Personal resources including paternal education and maternal unemployment were also positively associated with treatment adherence. Family coping methods of integration, cooperation, and optimism were positively associated with adherence. Additionally, several demographic variables were associated with lower levels of adherence, including longer marriages, male gender, older age of the patient, and greater number of children in the family. Although positively related, the correlation between family compliance and pulmonary functions was not significant. More recently, however, Patterson *et al.* (1993) predicted 33% of the variance in a 10-year pulmonary health trend (i.e., forced expiratory volume; FEV1) in a sample of 91 children with CF. The importance of family factors such as integration and support was upheld as important predictors of outcome.

Findings from a recent study of mothers of 24 patients with CF, ranging from 6 months to 17 years of age, also revealed the potential relation between adherence and family dynamics (Geiss *et al.*, 1992). Adherence in this study was measured by combined physician, patient, and family reports, as well as physical findings, to produce a composite adherence rating. Results revealed that higher levels of perceived adherence were related to less satisfactory marital relations and greater social isolation in the parents of the patients with CF. The authors explained this unexpected finding by noting that mothers with few positive marital and social interactions may become more involved with the treatment regimen as a substitute, thereby leading to higher levels of perceived compliance. Alternatively, the authors suggest a more direct impact of a mother's inability to maintain satisfactory marital and social relations as a result of the demanding nature of the treatment regimen.

A related issue concerns the transfer of regimen responsibilities from parents to the patients as part of the normal transition from dependency to autonomy. Given the necessary involvement of parents in the daily lives of children with CF, this transition may be experienced as particularly unsettling. The feeding studies reviewed earlier, which revealed greater parental involvement and instruction during mealtime when compared with control groups, highlight concerns about dependency patterns being established early in a chronic illness sample. Indeed, because patients with CF are living to adulthood, the need for interventions geared at self-management has become increasingly important.

Cappelli *et al.* (1989) developed a caregiver questionnaire to assess caregiver 'readiness' to transfer responsibilities that may help medical staff identify areas of relative weakness for families. A careful approach to this transfer is underscored by findings that age and length of disease are positively related to symptom exacerbation.

Using CF and diabetes samples, Drotar & Levers (1994) considered the impact of multiple parental role demands and the transference of treatment responsibilities to older patients. This study was designed, in part, to address the significant disparities found among professionals regarding the age at which increased independence in regimen responsibilities was expected in a diabetes sample (Wysocki *et al.*, 1990). Mothers of patients (ages 4–14) with IDDM (insulin-dependent diabetes mellitus) ($n = 26$) and CF ($n = 26$) were interviewed and completed several questionnaires regarding regimen responsibilities and their child's level of independence outside of regimen behaviors. Results revealed comparable levels of independence in patients across illness groups. As expected, independence varied with age, with older children assuming greater responsibility for regimen behaviors. Although this increase in independence was evident, there was still substantial sharing of responsibilities with the patients' mothers. Additionally, the level of independence varied as a function of specific regimen behaviors, with parents maintaining the majority of the responsibility for making and remembering clinic appointments and interacting with clinic staff. Independence with treatment regimen behaviors was significantly related to independence regarding nonillness responsibilities, which suggests that general adaptive behavioral functioning is important to CF management.

The authors note, however, that greater independence does not necessarily translate into improved adherence. This may explain, in part, why mothers continue to stay highly involved with the treatment regimen, despite age-related increases in independence in their children. The authors noted, however, that the strain and ambivalence experienced by caregivers and the quest for normal developmental levels of independence by the patients can lead to family conflict. Thus, interventions to enhance independence in the context of well-defined parent–child responsibilities for regimen behaviors are needed. Given the above findings, such interventions should include some method of providing emotional support for the primary caregivers.

Several studies have assessed treatment compliance in an adult CF population. In general, the findings are similar to the child population, with better adherence reported for medication versus CPT (Abbott *et al.*, 1994). Additionally, a recent study of adult compliance found that patients who perceived their disease to be controlled by others (i.e., family members and health care providers) reported better adherence to their regimen (Abbott *et al.*, 1996). Another recent assessment of adult patients with CF found that while most had attained adult developmental tasks (e.g., living independently, marriage), many continued to share treatment responsibilities with parents, such as management of medical insurance and monitoring nutritional status (Hamlett *et al.*, 1996). These findings suggest that concerns with adherence and underlying psychosocial factors do not end with adulthood. Given the improved survival rate of patients with CF, assessing the special needs of this age group will become increasingly important.

Self-Management

Given the complexity of the CF regimen, variable adherence rates, and multiple parameters of adherence, self-management programs may offer promise for enhancing disease management and improving quality of life.

Bartholomew and colleagues developed the Cystic Fibrosis Family Education Program, a comprehensive health education program that targets knowledge, self-efficacy, and self-management behaviors to improve health and quality of life (Bartholomew *et al.*, 1991). Recently, the efficacy of this program was demonstrated in a short-term outcome study (Bartholomew *et al.*, 1997). A sample of 195 patients between the ages of 1 and 18 years (mean = 8.6) and their primary caregivers were enrolled in the study. One-hundred and four of the patient–caregiver dyads made up the intervention group and 95 dyads comprised a 'usual care' comparison group. The intervention included a self-paced print curriculum developed within a social cognitive framework. The curriculum included instruction on medical care (respiratory care, nutrition) as well as communication and coping. Additionally, developmentally sensitive intervention methods – including goal setting, reinforcement, modeling, skills training, and self-monitoring – were provided, with specific strategies and learning activities for parents and children.

Measures included cognitive variables of knowledge of CF, self-efficacy, and outcome expectations; behavioral variables of self-management activities, problem solving/coping strategies; quality of life variables, including adaptive behavioral development, behavioral–emotional functioning (CBCL), quality of well-being, family impact, and parenting stress; and health status variables, including NIH (National Institutes of Health) index of physical health status (pulmonary functions, chest X-ray, and height/weight). Analysis of covariance for each dependent measure was used to determine intervention effects. Age, SES, and pretest results were used as covariates for each measure. Results revealed significant differences between the intervention and control groups for caregiver and child knowledge, caregiver and child self-efficacy, adolescent and parent self-management, three aspects of parental problem solving, CBCL scores, NIH total and pulmonary function scores, and chest X-ray. Self-efficacy findings for caregivers and patients were moderated by a significant interaction between treatment group and pretest scores, suggesting that increases in self-efficacy were found only for subjects with low pretest self-efficacy. A similar interaction was found for caregivers and problem solving. Although this study focused on outcome variables at one point in time and did not use random assignment to groups, the results are compelling and provide further evidence that a multifaceted approach to CF treatment is indicated.

In a similar, smaller study of self-management of patients with CF (Cottrell *et al.*, 1996) children in the self-management group demonstrated a significant weight gain relative to the children in the control group. Moreover, more children in the self-management group demonstrated improved compliance with aerosol treatments and with CPT. These findings are especially compelling, in light of the fact that the low number of subjects ($n = 20$) reduced the power of the statistical procedures and the sample was a highly motivated group who already practiced self-management, resulting in a limited range for improvement.

Summary and Future Directions

With the dramatic advances in medical care and life expectancies in individuals with CF, an understanding of the biopsychosocial processes that are associated with stable psychological functioning and treatment adherence are crucial. Although there is evidence of increased risk for psychological adjustment problems in the face of this significant medical illness in both patients and family members, good adjustment is the most likely outcome. Indeed the resilience evident in most patients is remarkable. Only a subset of patients and parents demonstrate persistent difficulties in adjustment, and these difficulties in adjustment are associated with particular psychosocial processes that could serve as salient intervention targets. Although additional research is warranted to more fully identify those psychosocial parameters most relevant to adjustment in patients with CF, there is accumulated evidence that stress management, family functioning, and coping skills enhancement would serve as salient targets for intervention for mothers of CF patients. However, to date, there has been little empirical investigation of such interventions. What is required now are clinical investigations of the impact of these interventions on the psychosocial outcomes for patients with CF and their families.

There have been more intervention studies with treatment adherence. The relationship between adherence and outcome in the CF population is not direct, but rather is subject to multiple influences, including psychosocial and developmental factors. Furthermore, adherence to one aspect of the treatment regimen is not predictive of adherence to others, which suggests the need for target-specific interventions. Given the significant role of caregivers, particularly mothers, interventions that also address their roles are indicated. To date, behavioral interventions designed to address both parent and child behaviors have been successfully employed in the CF population, although these are generally limited to nutrition and feeding.

Moreover, findings from the above-reviewed studies suggest that management of CF complications requires more than just adherence to the prescribed medical regimen. Rather, concerns about the quality of life of patients with chronic illnesses such as CF call into question what level of adherence is necessary to directly affect clinical status while not severely compromising the daily life of the patient (Sanders *et al.*, 1991). Interventions that strive to achieve a balance between adherence and quality of life are necessary. Self-management programs have begun to and will likely continue to play a significant role in the treatment and management of CF. Finally, an integration of intervention targets such as stress management, family therapy, and coping skills enhancement – as identified in the stress and coping literature – with the techniques and principles of self-management, would provide the most comprehensive approach to maximizing the biopsychosocial outcomes of individuals with CF.

References

Abbott, J., Dodd, M., Bilton, D., & Webb, A.K. (1994). Treatment compliance in adults with cystic fibrosis. *Thorax*, 49, 115–120.

Abbott, J., Dodd, M., & Webb, A.K. (1996). Health perceptions and treatment adherence in adults with cystic fibrosis. *Thorax*, 51, 1233–1238.

Abidin, R.R. (1986). *Parenting stress index*, 2nd edn. Charlottesville, VA: Pediatric Psychology Press.

Achenbach, T.M. (1991). *Manual for the child behavior checklist/4–18 and 1991 profile.* Burlington: University of Vermont Department of Psychiatry.

Achenbach, T.M. (1992). *Manual for the child behavior checklist/2–3 and 1992 profile.* Burlington: University of Vermont Department of Psychiatry.

American Psychiatric Association (1980). *Diagnostic and statistical manual of mental disorders*, 3rd edn. Washington, DC: American Psychiatric Association.

Bartholomew, L.K., Parcel, G.S., Seilheimer, D.K., Czyzewski, D., Spinelli, S.H., & Congdon, B. (1991). Development of a health education program to promote the self-management of cystic fibrosis. *Health Education Quarterly*, 18, 429–443.

Bartholomew, L.K., Czyzewski, D.I., Parcel, G.S., *et al.* (1997). Self-management of cystic fibrosis: short-term outcomes of the Cystic Fibrosis Family Education Program. *Health Education and Behavior*, 24, 652–666.

Boat, T.F., Welsh, M.J. & Beaudet, A.L. (1989). Cystic fibrosis. In: C.L. Scriver, A.L. Beaudet, S. Sly, & D. Valle (Eds), *The metabolic bases of inherited disease* (pp. 2469–2680). New York: McGraw-Hill.

Borowitz, D., Wegman, T., & Harris, M. (1994). Preventive care for patients with chronic illness: multivitamin use in patients with cystic fibrosis. *Clinical Pediatrics*, 12, 720–725.

Bowen, A.M. & Stark, L.J. (1991). Malnutrition in cystic fibrosis: a behavioral conceptualization of cause and treatment. *Clinical Psychology Review*, 11, 315–331.

Cappelli, M., MacDonald, N.E., & McGrath, P.J. (1989). Assessment of readiness to transfer to adult care for adolescents with cystic fibrosis. *Children's Health Care*, 18, 218–224.

Conway, S.P. (1996). Cystic fibrosis: adult clinical aspects. *British Journal of Hospital Medicine*, 55, 248–252.

Cottrell, C.K., Young, G.A., Creer, T.L., Holroyd, K.A., & Kotses, H. (1996). The development and evaluation of a self-management program for cystic fibrosis. *Pediatric Asthma Allergy & Immunology*, 10, 109–118.

Cowen, L., Corey, M., Simmons, R., Kennan, N., Robertson, J., & Levison, H. (1984). Growing older with cystic fibrosis: psychological adjustment of patients more than 16 years old. *Psychosomatic Medicine*, 46, 363–375.

Cowen, L., Corey, M., Keenan, N., Simmons, R., Arndt, E., & Levison, H. (1985). Family adaptation and psychosocial adjustment to cystic fibrosis in the preschool child. *Social Science and Medicine*, 20, 553–560.

Cystic Fibrosis Foundation (2000). *Patient Registry 1999 Annual Report.* Bethesda, Maryland: Cystic Fibrosis Foundation.

Czajkowski, D.R. & Koocher, G.P. (1986). Predicting medical compliance among adolescents with cystic fibrosis. *Health Psychology*, 5, 297–305.

Derogatis, L.R. (1983). *SCL-90-R: administration, scoring, and procedures manual II.* Baltimore: Johns Hopkins University, Clinical Psychometric Research Unit.

Drotar, D. & Levers, C. (1994). Age differences in parent and child responsibilities for management of cystic fibrosis and insulin-dependent diabetes mellitus. *Journal of Developmental and Behavioral Pediatrics*, 15, 265–272.

Drotar, D., Doershuk, C.F., Stern, R.C., Boat, T.F., Boyer, W., & Matthews, L. (1981). Psychological functioning of children with cystic fibrosis. *Pediatrics*, 67, 338–343.

Dunbar-Jacob, J., Dunning, E.J., & Dwyer, K. (1993). Compliance research in pediatric and adolescent populations. Two decades of research. In: N.P. Krasnegor, L. Epstein, S.B. Johnson, & S.J. Yaffee (Eds), *Developmental aspects of health compliance behavior* (pp. 29–51). Hillsday, NJ: Erlbaum.

Epstein, L.H. & Cluss, P.A. (1982). A behavioral medicine perspective on adherence to long-term medical regimens. *Journal of Consulting and Clinical Psychology*, 50, 950–971.

Gayton, W.F., Friedman, S.B., Tavormina, J.B., & Tucker, F. (1977). Children with cystic fibrosis: I. psychological test findings of patients, siblings, and parents. *Pediatrics*, 59, 888–894.

Geiss, S.K., Hobbs, S.A., Hammersley-Maercklein, G., Kramer, J.C., & Henley, M. (1992). Psychosocial factors related to perceived compliance with cystic fibrosis. *Journal of Clinical Psychology*, 48, 99–103.

Goldberg, S., Morris, P., Simmons, R.J., Fowler, R.S., Levison, H. (1990). Chronic illness in infancy and parenting stress: a comparison of three groups of parents. *Journal of Pediatric Psychology*, 15, 347–358.

Gudas, L.J., Koocher, G.P., & Wypij, D. (1991). Perceptions of medical compliance in children and adolescents with cystic fibrosis. *Journal of Developmental and Behavioral Pediatrics*, 12, 236–242.

Hains, A.A., Davies, W.H., Behrens, D., & Biller, J.A. (1997). Cognitive-behavioral interventions for adolescents with cystic fibrosis. *Journal of Pediatric Psychology*, 22, 669–687.

Hamlett, K.W., Murphy, M., Hayes, R., & Doershuk, C.F. (1996). Health independence and developmental tasks of adulthood in cystic fibrosis. *Rehabilitation Psychology*, 41, 149–160.

Haynes, R.B. (1979). Strategies to improve compliance with referrals, appointments, and prescribed medical regimens. In: R.B. Haynes, D.W. Taylor, & D.L. Sackett (Eds), *Compliance in health care* (pp. 121–143). Baltimore: Johns Hopkins University Press.

Hodges, K., Kline, J., Stern, L., Cytryn, L., & McKnew, D. (1982). The development of a child assessment interview for research and clinical use. *Journal of Abnormal Child Psychology*, 10, 173–189.

Kashani, J.H., Barbero, G.J., Wilfley, D.E., Morris, D.A., & Sheppard, J.A. (1988). Psychological concomitants of cystic fibrosis in children and adolescents. *Adolescence*, 23, 873–880.

Kerem, B., Rommens, J.M., Buchanan, J.A. *et al.* (1989). Identification of the cystic fibrosis gene: genetic analysis. *Science*, 245, 1073–1080.

Koocher, G.P., Czajkowski, D., & Fitzpatrick, J. (1987). Manual for the medical incomplete stories test (MCIST), unpublished research instrument. Children's Hospital, Boston, MA.

Koocher, G.P., McGrath, M.L., & Gudas, L.J. (1990). Typologies of nonadherence in cystic fibrosis. *Journal of Developmental and Behavioral Pediatrics*, 11, 353–358.

La Greca, A.M. (1988). Adherence to prescribed medical regimens. In: D.K. Routh (Ed.), *Handbook of pediatric psychology* (pp. 299–320). New York: Guilford Press.

La Greca, A.M. (1990). Issues in adherence with pediatric regimens. *Journal of Pediatric Psychology*, 15, 423–436.

Lask, B. (1994). Non-adherence to treatment in cystic fibrosis. *Journal of the Royal Society of Medicine*, 87 (suppl. 21), 25–27.

Lewis, P.A., Morison, S., Dodge, J.A., *et al.* (1999). Survival estimates for adults with cystic fibrosis born in the United Kingdom between 1947 and 1967. *Thorax*, 54, 420–422.

Lieu, T.A., Ray, C.T., Farmer, G., & Shay, G.F. (1999). The cost of medical care for patients with cystic fibrosis in a health maintenance organization. *Pediatrics*, 103(6), e72.

McCubbin, H. & Patterson, J. (1982). Family adaptation to crisis. In: H. McCubbin, A. Cauble, & J. Patterson (Eds), *Family stress, coping and social support* (pp. 26–47). Springfield, IL, C.C. Thomas.

Matthews, L.W., & Drotar, D. (1984). Cystic fibrosis: a challenging long-term chronic disease. *Pediatric Clinics of North America*, 31, 133–152.

Mullins, L.L., Olson, R.A., Reyes, S., Bernardy, N., Huszti, H.C., & Volk, R.T. (1991). Risk and resistance factors in the adaptation of mothers of children with cystic fibrosis. *Journal of Pediatric Psychology*, 16, 701–715.

Nagy, S. & Ungerer, J.A. (1990). The adaptation of mothers and fathers to children with cystic fibrosis: a comparison. *Children's Health Care*, 19, 147–154.

Orenstein, D.M. & Wachnowsky, D.M. (1985). Behavioral aspects of cystic fibrosis. *Annals of Behavioral Medicine*, 7, 17–20.

Parcel, G.S., Swank, P.R., Mariotto, M.J. *et al.* (1994). Self-management of cystic fibrosis: a structural model for educational and behavioral variables. *Social Science and Medicine*, 38, 1307–1315.

Passero, M.A., Remor, B., & Solomon, J. (1981). Patient-reported compliance with cystic fibrosis therapy. *Clinical Pediatrics*, 20, 264–268.

Patterson, J.M. (1985). Critical factors affecting family compliance with home treatment for children with cystic fibrosis. *Family Relations*, 34, 78–89.

Patterson, J.M., Budd, J., Goetz, D., & Warwick, W.J. (1993). Family correlates of a 10-year pulmonary health trend in cystic fibrosis. *Pediatrics*, 91, 383–389.

Perrin, J.M., & MacLean, W.E., Jr. (1988). Children with chronic illness: the prevention of dysfunction. *Pediatric Clinics of North America*, 35, 1325–1337.

Pless, I.B. (1984). Clinical assessment: physical and psychological functioning. *Pediatric Clinics of North America*, 31, 33–45.

Quittner, A.L., DiGirolamo, A.M., & Winslow, E.B. (1991). *Problems in parenting a child with cystic fibrosis. A contextual analysis.* Paper presented at the meeting of the Florida Conference on Child Health Care Psychology, April 1991, Gainesville, FL.

Quittner, A.L., DiGirolamo, A.M., Michel, M., & Eigen, H. (1992a). Parental response to CF: a contextual analysis of the diagnostic phase. *Journal of Pediatric Psychology*, 17, 683–704.

Quittner, A.L., Drotar, D., Iveres-Landis, C., Slocum, N., Seidner, D., & Jacobsen, J. (2000). Adherence to medical treatments in adolescents with cystic fibrosis: The development and evaluation of family based interventions. In D. Drotar (Ed). *Promoting Adherence to Medical Treatment in Chronic Childhood Illness: Concepts, Methods and Interventions.* (pp. 383–487). New Jersey: Lawrence Elbaum Associates Inc.

Quittner, A.L., Opipari, L.C., Regoli, M.J., Jacobson, J., & Eigen, H. (1992b). The impact of caregiving and role strain on family life: comparisons between mothers of children with cystic fibrosis and matched controls. *Rehabilitation Psychology*, 37, 275–290.

Ramsey, B.W., Farrell, P.M., Pencharz, P., & the Consensus Committee (1992). Nutritional assessment and management in cystic fibrosis: a consensus report. *American Journal of Clinical Nutrition*, 55, 108–116.

Rapoff, M.A. & Christophersen, E.R. (1982). Compliance of pediatric patients with medical regimens: a review and evaluation. In: R.B. Stuart (Ed.), *Adherence, compliance and generalization in behavioral medicine* (pp. 79–124). New York: Brunner/Mazel.

Sanders, M.R., Gravestock, F., Wanstall, K., & Dunne, M. (1991). The relationship between children's treatment-related behavior problems, age and clinical status in cystic fibrosis. *Journal of Paediatric Child Health*, 27, 290–294.

Sanders, M.R., Turner, K.M., Wall, C.R., Waugh, L.M., & Tully, L.A. (1997). Mealtime behavior and parent–child interaction: a comparison of children with cystic fibrosis, children with feeding problems, and nonclinic controls. *Journal of Pediatric Psychology*, 22, 881–900.

Schroeder, K.H., Casadaban, A.B., & Davis, B. (1988). Interpersonal skills training for parents of children with cystic fibrosis. *Family Systems Medicine*, 6, 51–68.

Shwachman, H. & Kulczycki, L.L. (1958). Long-term study of one hundred and five patients with cystic fibrosis: studies made over a 5 to 14 year period. *American Journal of Diseases in Children*, 96, 6–15.

Simmons, R.J., Corey, M., Cowen, L., Keenan, N., Robertson, J., & Levison, H. (1985). Emotional adjustment of early adolescents with cystic fibrosis. *Psychosomatic Medicine*, 47, 111–122.

Simmons, R.J., Corey, M., Cowen, L., Keenan, N., Robertson, J., & Levison, H. (1987). Behavioral adjustment of latency age children with cystic fibrosis. *Psychosomatic Medicine*, 49, 291–301.

Sines, J.O., Pauker, J.D., Sines, L.K., & Owen, D.R. (1969). Identification of clinically relevant dimensions of children's behavior. *Journal of Consulting and Clinical Psychology*, 33, 728–734.

Singer, L.T., Nofer, J.A., Benson-Szekely, L.J., & Brooks, L.J. (1991). Behavioral assessment and management of food refusal in children with cystic fibrosis. *Journal of Developmental and Behavioral Pediatrics*, 12, 115–120.

Stark, L.J. (2000). Adherence to diet in chronic conditions: The example of cystic fibrosis. In D. Drotar (Ed). *Promoting Adherence to Medical Treatment in Chronic Childhood Illness: Concepts, Methods, and Interventions.* (pp. 409–427). New Jersey: Lawrence Erlbaum Associates, Inc.

Stark, L.J., Miller, S.T., Plienis, A.J., & Drabman, R.S. (1987). Behavioral contracting to increase chest physiotherapy. A study of a young cystic fibrosis patient. *Behavior Modification*, 11, 75–86.

Stark, L.J., Knapp, L., Bowen, A.M., *et al.* (1993). Behavioral treatment of calorie consumption in children with cystic fibrosis: replication with two year follow-up. *Journal of Applied Behavior Analysis*, 26, 435–450.

Stark, L.J., Powers, S.W., Jelalian, E., Rape, R.N., & Miller, D.L. (1994). Modifying problematic mealtime interactions of children with cystic fibrosis and their parents via behavioral parent training. *Journal of Pediatric Psychology*, 19, 751–768.

Stark, L.J., Jelalian, E., & Miller, D.L. (1995a). Cystic fibrosis. In: M.C. Roberts (Ed.), *Handbook of pediatric psychology*, 2nd edn (pp. 241–262). New York: Guilford Press.

Stark, L.J., Jelalian, E., Mulvihill, M.M. *et al.* (1995b). Eating in preschool children with cystic fibrosis and healthy peers: behavioral analysis. *Pediatrics*, 95, 210–215.

Thompson, R.J., Jr. & Gustafson, K.E. (1996). *Adaptation to chronic childhood illness.* Washington, DC: American Psychological Association.

Thompson, R.J., Jr., Kronenberger, W., & Curry, J.F. (1989). Behavior classification system for children with developmental, psychiatric, and chronic medical problems. *Journal of Pediatric Psychology*, 14, 559–575.

Thompson, R.J., Jr., Hodges, K., & Hamlet, K.W. (1990). A matched comparison of adjustment in children with cystic fibrosis and psychiatrically referred and nonreferred children. *Journal of Pediatric Psychology*, 15, 745–759.

Thompson, R.J., Jr., Gustafson, K.E., Hamlett, K.W., & Spock, A. (1992a). Psychological adjustment of children with cystic fibrosis: the role of child cognitive processes and maternal adjustment. *Journal of Pediatric Psychology*, 17, 741–755.

Thompson, R.J., Jr., Gustafson, K.E., Hamlett, K.W., & Spock, A. (1992b). Stress, coping, and family functioning in the psychological adjustment of mothers of children with cystic fibrosis. *Journal of Pediatric Psychology*, 17, 573–585.

Thompson, R.J., Jr., Gil, K.M., Gustafson, K.E., *et al.* (1994a). Stability and change in the psychological adjustment of mothers of children and adolescents with cystic fibrosis and sickle cell disease: stability and change over a 10 month period. *Journal of Consulting and Clinical Psychology*, 62, 856–860.

Thompson, R.J., Jr., Gustafson, K.E., George, L.K., & Spock, A. (1994b). Change over a 12-month period in the psychological adjustment of children and adolescents with cystic fibrosis. *Journal of Pediatric Psychology*, 19, 189–203.

Thompson, R.J., Jr., Gustafson, K.E., & Gil, K.M. (1995). Psychological adjustment of adolescents with cystic fibrosis or sickle cell disease and their mothers. In: J. Wallander & L. Siegel (Eds), *Advances in pediatric psychology II. Behavioral perspectives on adolescent health* (pp. 232–247). New York: Guilford Press.

Thompson, R.J., Jr., Gustafson, K.E., Gil, K.M., Kinney, T.R., & Spock, A. (1999). Change in the psychological adjustment of children with cystic fibrosis or sickle cell disease and their mothers. *Journal of Clinical Psychology in Medical Settings*, 6, 373–392.

Walker, L.S., Ford, M.B., & Donald, W.D. (1987). Cystic fibrosis and family stress: effects of age and severity of illness. *Pediatrics*, 79, 239–246.

Wallis, C. (1996). Cystic fibrosis: paediatric aspects. *British Journal of Hospital Medicine*, 55, 241–247.

Wysocki, T., Meinhold, P., Cox, D.J., & Clarke, W.L. (1990). Survey of diabetes professionals regarding developmental changes in self-care. *Diabetes Care*, 13, 63–68.

11
Respiratory disorders and their treatment

Thomas L. Creer and John A. Winder

Editors' note—*A plethora of new treatments for asthma, COPD (chronic obstructive pulmonary disease), tuberculosis, and cystic fibrosis has emerged in the past two decades. Their use has been described throughout the book and in clinical treatment guidelines issued for specific disorders. The treatments, based upon the administration of new and more potent drugs, promise greater control over respiratory conditions than has ever been the case. If taken as directed, the treatments not only control flare-ups of respiratory disorders but also can prevent exacerbations from occurring. It is a far cry from when, just a few decades ago, the only weapons for preventing asthma episodes were large doses of oral corticosteroids, with their attendant side effects and, with asthma exacerbations, the administration of epinephrine. Little wonder that in those bygone days, many physicians received regular on-the-job training in reversing status asthmaticus or steadily worsening asthma.*

The newer treatments for respiratory disorders are a double-edged sword, however. On the one hand, they provide hope that these conditions can be controlled: as noted, such hope is a far cry from the situation that existed a few decades ago. On the other hand, however, more potent medications can generate more problems both for health care providers and patients. Health care providers must teach patients the correct way to use these drugs. There is evidence, however, that teaching these skills often does not occur. Despite the constant warnings that inhaled drugs are only effective when taken as directed, many health care professionals fail to convey both the purpose and technique of inhaler use. In fact, they themselves fail to demonstrate that they know the correct way to take inhaled drugs (Creer & Levstek, 1996).

A second, perhaps more dangerous, trend is the describing of several medications to be taken simultaneously (Creer et al., 1999). Before drugs are approved for public use, they are investigated over time in a three-stage manner that commences with tests on animals and proceeds through tests on patients with the condition the drug is designed to control. When a medication has shown proven value in treating a particular condition without generating serious side effects, the drug is likely to be approved for use on patients. Note that the topic of investigation is the medication itself; no attempt is made to study how the drug interacts with other medications that may be given concurrently. It would be impossible, from both economic and logistical standpoints, to do so. Yet, prescribing up to four preventive or controller medications to be taken concomitantly for treatment of asthma is precisely the problem described by Creer and his colleagues. The practice leads to paradoxical reactions. On one hand, the multidrug regimen does not improve the control of asthma in many patients; rather than adhering to such a complex regimen, patients often stop taking controller drugs and use only their short-acting beta-agonist medication as needed. On the other hand, sometimes too much control is established over a patient's asthma. There are cases in asthma, for example, when given combinations of preventive drugs mask the onset of an asthma exacerbation. By doing so, the regimen defeats the very purpose of taking preventive or controller drugs: helping to control asthma.

The above problems can be avoided when, as suggested in treatment guidelines for the condition (e.g., National Institutes of Health, 1995), patients actually become allies with their health care providers in management of the asthma. Such a partnership not only enhances any treatment provided to patients, but yields invaluable information, some subtle, about medication regimens. Both goals are worthy of pursuit.

Introduction

This book is replete with illustrations of the many ways medical and behavioral scientists are involved in the treatment of chronic respiratory disorders, particularly asthma and chronic obstructive pulmonary disease (COPD). Besides applying behavioral change techniques that impact the disease process itself – e.g., smoking cessation programs for COPD patients – behavioral and medical scientists have attempted to synthesize their competencies with the skills of patients to effectively manage chronic respiratory disorders. Terms such as self-care, collaborative treatment, self-regulation, and self-management have been used to describe strategies whereby patients have become empowered to be active partners with their health care personnel in the control of a respiratory disorder. In addition, knowledge of the pathology of asthma and COPD has led to the recognition that, in many cases, environmental and behavioral factors rival in importance the medical treatments used to control these chronic respiratory disorders. The prevention of pulmonary exacerbations, based upon behavioral actions of patients, is increasingly viewed as a major way of lessening the morbidity and mortality burden related to COPD and asthma (Creer & Levstek, 1998).

There is a third type of respiratory disorder – tuberculosis (TB) – where little effort has been made to apply behavioral knowledge and techniques to permit patients to become allies in the management of their disorder. If anything, as Hindi-Alexander and her colleagues (Chapter 13) note, the prevalent treatment approach of direct observed therapy (DOT) actively discourages the use of self-initiated behavioral action to help control TB. Given the magnitude of the problem, as well as the need to prevent the TB epidemic from running roughshod over the world, the practice constitutes ignorance on the part of those treating TB and a tragedy for those with the disease.

The range of respiratory disorders is expansive; it includes patients with airflow limitations who exhibit a variety of symptoms that require a broad array of treatment techniques. Two types of chronic respiratory disorders, asthma and COPD, are the most apt candidates for collaboration by medical and behavioral scientists. The third disease, TB, represents a candidate for future cooperation of scientists and patients. Optimal success of any behavioral change technique, however, requires a basic knowledge of these respiratory disorders and their management.

Definitions of COPD, Asthma, and Tuberculosis

Asthma, emphysema, and chronic bronchitis are chronic respiratory disorders that involve airflow obstruction, resulting from a narrowing of the airways. Until two decades ago, the three conditions were subsumed under the title of chronic obstructive pulmonary disease or COPD. In 1987, however, the American Thoracic Society (1987, p. 225) defined COPD

> *as a disorder characterized by abnormal tests of expiratory flow that do not change over several months observation.*

The definition emphasized that reversibility of lung function was unlikely in COPD, and distinguished the condition from asthma, where reversibility was more apt to occur. Recently, however, the American Thoracic Society (1995, p. 578) has revised the definition of COPD by describing it as a

> *disease state characterized by the presence of airway obstruction due to chronic bronchitis or emphysema; the airflow obstruction is generally progressive, may be accompanied by airway hyperreactivity, and may be partially reversible.*

Symptoms that signal acute or chronic obstruction, such as wheeze, cough, and dyspnea, are not in themselves diagnostic, as they occur in many types of pulmonary disease, including both COPD and asthma (Petty, 1990). It is not surprising, therefore, that differences between chronic bronchitis and late-onset asthma in adults are subtle and by no means clear-cut (Bernstein, 1988). And, as noted, the aspect of variable, reversibility characterizes either asthma or COPD. Considering the ambiguity between the disorders, the major difference between COPD and asthma is the salience of inflammation, involving complex cellular and chemical mediators, that is characteristic of asthma but not of COPD. Other features that distinguish COPD from asthma are described in the excellent chapter by Kaplan and Ries (Chapter 4).

Asthma

The National Asthma Education Program (National Institutes of Health, 1991, p. 1) defined asthma:

> *as a lung disease with the following characteristics: (1) airway obstruction that is reversible (but not completely in some patients) either spontaneously or with treatment; (2) airway inflammation; and (3) airway hyperreactivity to a variety of stimuli.*

Slightly different definitions of asthma are found in the International Consensus Report on the Diagnosis and Treatment of Asthma (National Institutes of Health, 1992) and the Global Initiative for Asthma (National Institutes of Health, 1995). Despite the fact that each successive definition of asthma seems increasingly comprehensive and complex, the three reports established sets of treatment guidelines that can be followed by practitioners around the world to treat asthma. Indeed, there are indications that when guidelines presented by the National Asthma Education Program (National Institutes of Health, 1991) are followed, improvement in the treatment of patients with asthma occurs (e.g., Lantner & Ros, 1995). It is strongly recommended that a set of guidelines be adopted by medical and behavioral scientists who work with asthma. Unfortunately, as Marwick (1995) pointed out, only 1 of 10 physicians surveyed in the United States was familiar with or knew that the National Asthma Education Program guidelines had been issued. Furthermore, even when physicians professed knowledge of the guidelines, particularly those issued by the National Institutes of Health (1991, 1997) in the United States, there was little indication that they had been fully integrated into the practice of the majority of health care providers (Creer *et al.*, 1999; Taylor *et al.*, 1999). A salient failing was the lack of involvement of asthma patients as partners in controlling their disorder. This finding not only has implications for the control of asthma but also suggests potential problems for medical and behavioral scientists who investigate asthma (Creer *et al.*, 1998).

Three aspects of current definitions of asthma merit discussion – reversibility of airway obstruction, airway inflammation, and airway hyperreactivity.

Reversibility

The term refers to the degree to which airway obstruction reverses either spontaneously or with appropriate treatment. Reversibility was long considered as a distinguishing feature of asthma; as noted, however, thought regarding the characteristic has changed as researchers learn more about COPD and its underlying pathology (American Thoracic Society, 1995; Spector & Nicklas, 1995; Sanford *et al.*, 1996). Current thought suggests airway reversibility, like severity, must be perceived as a continuum: while most patients show complete reversibility of airway obstruction when treated appropriately, others experience a significant degree of airway obstruction even with intensive medical treatment (Loren *et al.*, 1978). The fact that reversibility of airway obstruction occurs either in response to therapy or spontaneously presents a challenge when attempting to show cause–effect relationships between treatment and remission of asthma symptoms (Creer, 1982; Creer & Levstek, 1998).

Airway Inflammation

As described in the definition, asthma is a chronic inflammatory disorder of the airways. While the role of inflammation in asthma is still evolving, there is a scientific basis to support the concept that the disorder results from complex interactions among inflammatory cells, mediators, and cells and tissues that reside in the airways. Particular elements thought to play a role include mast cells, eosinophils, T lymphocytes, neutrophils, and epithelial cells (National Institutes of Health, 1997). Inflammation plays a pivotal role in the development of asthma, as indicated by recurrent exacerbations of airways swelling and narrowing. Specifically, airway limitation in asthma is due to airway bronchoconstriction, edema, mucous plug formation, and airway wall remodeling (Lemanske & Busse, 1997). Inflammation may last for a period following an episode or attack, although there are indications – based on evidence supporting variable reversibility (e.g., Loren *et al.*, 1978) – that many people with asthma have some degree of inflammation all of the time. As a chronic inflammatory disorder of the airways, there are major implications for the diagnosis, prevention, and management of asthma (Lemanske & Busse, 1997).

Airway Hyperresponsiveness or Hypersensitivity

Airway inflammation is associated with a number of factors, including airway hypersensitivity, airflow limitation, respiratory symptoms, and disease chronicity (Lemanske & Busse, 1997). Airway reactivity means that stimuli that fail to affect people without asthma are apt to trigger symptoms, such as wheezing, breathlessness, chest tightness, and cough, particularly at night and in the early morning, in people with asthma (National Institutes of Health, 1997). The airways become more sensitive to a host of stimuli with inflammation, increasing the probability of asthma symptoms over what might occur if inflammation was not present.

Over the years, two other characteristics of asthma – the intermittent and variable occurrence of airway obstruction – have posed a challenge both to those who treat and those who conduct research on the disorder. These features occur as a function of individual differences among patients, and variations in the number of asthma triggers, severity of disease, degree of control, and other mediating variables that influence the asthma of individual patients (Creer, 1979, 1982; Renne & Creer, 1985). Each characteristic will be described and analyzed in order to convey its importance in understanding asthma.

Intermittency

This feature refers to the frequency of asthma episodes. The rate of attacks can range from several episodes occurring in the span of a few days, to the passage of several months or even years between attacks. One patient may experience several asthma episodes within a couple of weeks and then not have any symptoms for a year or longer, whereas another patient may have symptoms most days of the year (which is called perennial asthma). Both medical and behavioral scientists must accept that intermittency of exacerbations is a common characteristic of asthma; otherwise, they and their patients may assume they have established control over asthma when the reduction in episodes is actually due to an absence of attack precipitants in the patient's environment. Patients, in particular, may not anticipate future episodes and be unprepared to deal with them when they occur (Renne & Creer, 1985).

Variability

The severity of asthma varies across patients and, within a given patient, from attack to attack. Both the National Asthma Education Program (National Institutes of Health, 1991) and the International Consensus Report (National Institutes of Health, 1992) proposed criteria for judging both the overall asthma severity of patients and the distinct attacks they experience as mild, moderate, or severe. The latter distinction clarified what is meant by variability of asthma for many patients and health care providers. If you were to interview a patient who was experiencing an attack that day, for example, he or she might say that the attack was severe. The term could be used appropriately by the patient in this instance, even though he or she may not have experienced an attack in the preceding 6 months. The intermittency of attacks would need to be considered along with asthma variability in arriving at a realistic treatment regimen for the patient's asthma.

Given multiple uses of the term, Spector & Nicklas (1995) suggested that severity be rated by analyzing a combination of objective and subjective criteria; these include patient symptoms, hyperactivity of airways, pulmonary function, activity restrictions, health care usage, and medication use. As noted, it is common for asthma severity to be rated as mild, moderate, or severe. The report by Spector and Nicklas (1995, p. 749), however, stressed that

> *asthma severity is a continuum across the population and often within a given individual, and that some characteristics of asthma may be more applicable in defining the severity in one patient, whereas different characteristics may be more applicable in another.*

Patient expectations are influenced by their perceptions of episode severity; if most of their attacks are mild, patients are often unprepared to help control severe episodes when they occur (Renne & Creer, 1985).

A final point should be made about asthma: Leff (1997) suggested that the disorder be characterized as a syndrome rather than a disease, because no single causative mechanism has been isolated for asthma. The lack of a mechanism for the disorder, continued Leff, makes the search for a cure extremely complex and elusive. The lack of a common pathogenic link and varied causes of asthma mean, in turn, that different varieties of asthma may require different therapies.

Chronic Obstructive Pulmonary Disease

As Kaplan and Ries provide a comprehensive portrait of this respiratory syndrome in Chapter 4, we will present only a brief review here. Until recently, there was no commonly accepted definition for COPD (Snider, 1995). This all changed when, as described earlier, the American Thoracic Society (1995) provided an operational definition of chronic obstructive pulmonary disease or COPD. Three features of the definition – airflow obstruction, emphysema, and chronic bronchitis – are important to the present discussion.

Airflow Obstruction

Abnormal tests of expiratory flow or airway obstruction are prominent in COPD patients. They are indicative of airflow obstruction, which is progressive in nature. The airflow obstruction has been attributed to alteration of the small airways and, to some degree, to bronchoconstriction. The American Thoracic Society (1995) however, explicitly stated that inflammation, with the participation of complex chemical and cellular mediators, is particularly reflective of asthma. A separation based on inflammation, they continued, was a practical and prudent way to distinguish asthma from conditions that comprise COPD.

Emphysema

Emphysema is a state of progressive airflow obstruction due to abnormal permanent enlargement of air spaces distal to the terminal bronchioles and alveoli. An accompanying characteristic is destruction of air-space walls without obvious fibrosis. Damaged air sacs trap air; when damage is severe, less oxygen moves from the lungs into the blood. Destruction was defined by the American Thoracic Society (1995, p. S78), 'as a lack of uniformity in the pattern of airspace enlargement; the orderly appearance of the acinus and its components is disturbed and may be lost.' Defining emphysema in terms of pathological changes is emphasized by the American Thoracic Society (1995).

Chronic Bronchitis

Chronic bronchitis was described as the presence of a persistent mucous cough of no known etiology. This is due to airspaces becoming swollen and full of mucus. Specifically, the American Thoracic Society (1995) defined chronic bronchitis clinically as the presence of a chronic productive cough for 3 months or more in each of 2 successive years in patients in whom other causes of chronic cough have been ruled out. The American Thoracic Society definition excludes patients with either chronic bronchitis or emphysema who do not exhibit persistent airflow obstruction, and includes a subset of asthma patients in whom airflow obstruction is not totally reversible (Snider, 1995). The symptom configuration for COPD patients and their treatment varies according to the severity and progression of the disease state. COPD normally follows a progressive course, in that patients exhibit a rapid decline in lung function (measured by lung volume), symptoms of cough and dyspnea, more acute chest illness and, later in the disease, hypoxemia (American Thoracic Society, 1995).

Tuberculosis

Tuberculosis is an infectious disease caused by two species of *Mycobacterium* – *M. tuberculosis* and *M. bovis*. The latter causes illness in cattle that can be transmitted to humans, but it is extremely rare that it does so. Currently, the tubercle bacillus and *M. tuberculosis* are considered as synonymous for all intents and purposes (Broughton & Bass, 1999). Broughton & Bass point out that the tubercle bacillus is a hearty organism and survives concentration and digestion techniques that would kill lesser organisms. An infectious particle that reaches the alveoli of the lungs is most apt to cause infection after macrophage ingestion of the bacterium. Depending upon the virulence of the bacillus and the killing activity of the macrophage, Broughton & Bass continue, the tubercle bacillus may or may not survive to create infection or disease. In their chapter, Hindi-Alexander and her colleagues (Chapter 13) describe the current epidemic of TB in which almost a third of the world's population are infected with the tubercle bacillus. Approximately 1 in 10 of those infected with the bacillus will develop active TB; the worldwide death toll from the disease hovers around 2 and 3 million people each year (Broughton & Bass, 1999).

Risk Factors Associated with COPD, Asthma, and Tuberculosis

Environmental Risks for COPD and Asthma

The greatest risk factor for developing COPD is cigarette smoking. Approximately 80–90% of the risk for COPD is accounted for by tobacco smoke (American Thoracic Society, 1995). About 15% of all smokers develop COPD; approximately 15% of one-pack-per-day and 25% of two-pack-per-day cigarette smokers will develop COPD if they continue smoking (Fletcher *et al.*, 1976). There is no direct link between smoking and asthma. Maternal and paternal smoking, however, have been correlated with severe asthma and, in some cases, with early onset of asthma (Kaplan & Mascie-Taylor, 1989; Sherrill *et al.*, 1990; Evans, 1993). Passive smoking has also been implicated as a potential risk factor for the development of asthma; there is little doubt that a worsening of asthma symptoms may occur in the presence of tobacco smoke (Spector & Nicklas, 1995).

Air pollution is an irritant that may exacerbate COPD and asthma (Creer & Levstek, 1998). However, it is unknown whether air pollutants are causative stimuli for the onset of respiratory disease. Air pollutants include smoke, particulate matter, acid rain, reactive gases, and ozone. The negative effects of these airborne pollutants can be damaging to the structure and functional capabilities of the lung, especially with prolonged exposure and exposure during exercise. Asthma patients appear to be hypersensitive to pollutants; in addition, exposure to pollutants increases the patient's sensitivity to other triggers for asthma. The relationship of asthma to air pollution is complicated by the fact that both asthma and pollution also vary according to weather and outdoor temperature. Temperature-adjusted rates for air pollution, however, were still significantly related to increases in asthma attacks (Creer & Levstek, 1998).

Occupational factors are associated with increased prevalence of chronic airway obstruction, quicker rates of lung-function decline, and higher mortality from COPD. One subset of emphysema, centriacinar emphysema, is linked to long-term exposure to ambient particles such as coal dust; as might be expected, centriacinar emphysema is widespread among coal workers (American Thoracic Society, 1995).

Personal Factors Associated with COPD and Asthma

A major difference between COPD and asthma is the occurrence of the disorders at different ages. About one-quarter of childhood asthma cases persist into childhood; in addition, more adult women than men are diagnosed with asthma (Burrows, 1991; Spector & Nicklas, 1995). Gender differences in childhood asthma generate higher prevalence rates in boys, and, as described in the comprehensive review by Gergen and Mitchell (Chapter 2), racial differences are clear-cut for childhood asthma in that black children are 2.5 times more likely than white children to be diagnosed with asthma. Racial differences are also noted in the COPD population, with a lower prevalence of COPD in blacks (3.2%) and other minorities than in whites (6.2%).

The relationship of allergic disease to asthma has been well documented (Sherrill *et al.*, 1990; Evans, 1993; Lemanske & Busse, 1997). Studies have repeatedly demonstrated that asthma prevalence is closely tied to immunoglobulin levels associated with allergy (Sherrill *et al.*, 1990). Asthma has been shown to be, in many cases, allergy-based, and induced by environmental agents and allergens, including pollens, fumes, smoke, weeds, grasses, and hay (Kaplan & Mascie-Taylor, 1989; Spector & Nicklas, 1995). Other risk factors found to predict childhood asthma include residential regions, home environment, parental smoking, low birthrate, young maternal age, low family income, and urban environments (Coultas *et al.*, 1993; Kaplan & Mascie-Taylor, 1989).

Genetic Contributions to Asthma and COPD

There exists an hereditary predisposition for both asthma and COPD. As early as the 1800s, hereditary factors were implicated in the onset of COPD, especially emphysema (Sherrill *et al.*, 1990). In this century, researchers found a hereditary defect, α_1-antitrypsin deficiency, which occurs in about 1% of COPD cases. Alpha$_1$-antitrypsin deficiency is suspected in early-onset cases of COPD where there is a family history of lung disease and the patient is a nonsmoker.

Studies of monozygotic and dyzygotic twins demonstrated there is some degree of family aggregation for COPD, pulmonary function, asthma, and allergic disease (Sherrill *et al.*, 1990; American Thoracic Society, 1995). In households where one parent has a history of an obstructive lung disease, there is a significantly higher prevalence of asthma and bronchitis compared with households where no adult members have respiratory disease (Sherrill *et al.*, 1990). A report by Sanford *et al.* (1996) on the genetics of asthma outlined the heritability of asthma, and suggested that individuals are genetically susceptible for allergic airway inflammation, but that asthma will only occur if the individual is exposed to the correct allergens. Important in this equation are the timing, intensity, and mode of exposure (Creer & Levstek, 1998). Two common viral agents, respiratory syncytial virus (RSV) and the parinfluenza virus, are particularly prominent in the onset of childhood asthma (Ellis, 1993). Ellis described that the risk of a child's developing asthma was related to the presence of asthma in the youngster's parents. If one parent has asthma, there is a 25% chance that the child will develop asthma; with two asthmatic parents, the risk of asthma in the child increases to 50%.

Risk Factors for Tuberculosis

Broughton & Bass (1999) stated that almost all cases of TB are acquired through person-to-person contact via droplet nuclei. These particles, continue Broughton & Bass, are originally tiny droplets of saliva that contain acid-fast bacilli (AFB) formed when individuals have tuberculosis phonate, cough, or sneeze. When the droplets of spit dry to the appropriate size, the can be held aloft by air currents and infect others. At diameters of 1–5 μm, they may contain two or three tubercle bacilli. Broughton & Bass (1999, 29.2) emphasize that this particular diameter

> *is important because the inhalation of larger particles results in impaction of the droplet on the mucosal airway. Impaction on the airway allows removal by the mucociliary system before infection can occur. Smaller particles reach the alveoli where infection begins.*

With effective therapy, the incidence of TB declined in the United States until around 1985. At that time, note Broughton & Bass, HIV infection became common and cases related to it, as well as cases related to the increasing numbers of foreign-born and homeless, brought an approximate 20% increase in the incidence of TB. The trend, in turn, led to a renewal of public health resources directed toward TB. Broughton & Bass point out that, in the United States, risk factors for TB include:

- HIV-positive status (such patients are 200 times more likely to contract TB than HIV-negative individuals)
- lower income strata
- alcoholism
- homelessness
- crowded living conditions
- past gastrectomies
- immunodeficiency
- immigration from a high-prevalence country.

Health care workers are also said to be at an increased risk. Cantwell *et al.* (1998) found that six indicators of socioeconomic status (SES) in the United States – crowding, income, poverty, public assistance, unemployment, and education – account for much of the increased risk of TB previously associated with race and ethnicity.

Recently, outbreaks of multidrug-resistant TB (MDR-TB) were described as emerging epidemic by the Program in Infectious Disease and Social Change (1999) at Harvard University. Features of MDR-TB were summarized:

- MDR-TB is caused by strains of *M. tuberculosis* that are resistant to isoniazid and rifampin, the most powerful anti-TB drugs available.
- MDR-TB results from inappropriate, incomplete, or erratic therapy by selecting naturally occurring drug-resistant mutants of *M. tuberculosis*.
- MDR-TB was ubiquitous throughout the world by 1999 in that it was reported in over 100 countries or territories.
- MDR-TB is a man-made epidemic and was unknown five decades ago.
- Patients with MDR-TB are not curable with short-course therapy, but requires second-line drugs.

Prevention of Asthma, COPD, and Tuberculosis

The Centers for Disease Control (1992) declared that prevention and control of known risk factors must be addressed as part of an overall plan to reduce the morbidity and mortality associated with respiratory disease. Prevention efforts for people with asthma have been twofold:

- to control the symptoms of asthma
- to prevent the occurrence of asthma attacks (Spector & Nicklas, 1995).

Factors identified as triggers for specific asthma attacks include:

1 viral respiratory infections;
2 allergens, such as mold, animal dander, cockroaches, dust mites, and airborne pollens;
3 environmental irritants, such as fumes and strong odors, air pollutants, and tobacco smoke;
4 ingested chemicals, such as aspirin and food additives;
5 exercise or inhalation of cold air;
6 weather changes; and
7 emotional reactions, especially laughing, crying, and shouting.

Despite a general knowledge of risk factors, patients and health care personnel are limited in their ability to identify the onset and precipitating factors of a given asthma attack. There is not only great variation in the interactions produced by trigger variables in a given individual but also in the matrix of stimuli that impinge upon that patient at a given moment. In addition, the immediate or late-onset asthma that may follow exposure to a stimulus further limits the ability to determine what produced a given asthma episode (Creer & Levstek, 1998).

Sherrill *et al.* (1990) derived a statistical model for risk prediction of COPD by looking at low lung function over time and how it related to certain risk factors. Their initial formulations included initial lung function, age, gender, and smoking as the major determinants of COPD. However, these risk factors are likely to occur with the same variability as they do for asthma patients, leaving researchers and clinicians alike still searching for an understanding of the preclinical determinants of COPD (Burrows, 1991).

In recent years, attempts have been made to control the spread of TB in at-risk populations in correctional facilities, hospitals, and homeless shelters. Preventing the transmission of TB is concentrated around reducing person-to-person contacts via droplet nuclei of those afflicted with TB with those who do not have the infection. With recognition of TB, effective therapy can rapidly decrease the number of organisms shed as droplet nuclei (Broughton & Bass, 1999). Ultraviolet radiation in the rooms of patients reduces the number of mycobacterium in the air; additional reduction can occur by covering the mouth and nose of patients with tissues or by having them wear a fine-pore mask. There is no need, Broughton & Bass suggest, for extreme measures to be taken with personal items used by infected patients. Gloves and gowns are not needed unless dictated by other concurrent illnesses. Fortunately, patients with TB who are HIV positive do not transmit their disease at a higher rate than HIV-negative patients with TB.

Diagnostic Evaluation of Asthma, COPD, and Tuberculosis

Asthma

In diagnosing asthma, it is imperative that practitioners (a) conduct a comprehensive evaluation of the individual patient, his or her history and symptoms, and the course of the disease; (b) perform tests of pulmonary function; and (c) establish a treatment regimen based both on the information obtained and the needs of the individual patient. For example, recognition that inflammation plays a significant role in the pathogenesis of asthma has led to the use of different medications to prevent asthma exacerbations (Creer & Levstek, 1998). A diagnosis of asthma is warranted when episodic symptoms of airflow obstruction are present, airflow is at least partially reversible, and alternative diagnoses – particularly COPD and vocal cord dysfunction in adults, and aspiration and cystic fibrosis in children – are excluded (National Institutes of Health, 1997).

Evaluation of the patient suspected of having asthma consists of a complete medical and environmental history that includes delineation of the potential triggers for a patient's asthma attacks. Most asthma experts believe that the patient's history is a significant part of the evaluation (National Institutes of Health, 1991; Ellis, 1993). An approach to obtaining a history in either children or adults suspected of having asthma is depicted in Table 11.1. The table is modified from a history outline presented in the treatment guidelines described by the National Institutes of Health (1991). As shown, it covers a number of topics, including possible triggers of asthma, symptoms, and the impact of asthma upon a patient and his or her family. While primarily developed to assure that health care providers cover relevant topics in determining the diagnosis of asthma, the entire history or sections of it may be useful to behavioral scientists who need a screening instrument in their work or research.

Pulmonary tests aid in differentiating asthma from other respiratory disease. These are typically gathered with a spirometer, and include tests of pulmonary function, such as forced expiratory volume (FEV_1) and peak expiratory flow (PEF) rates. FEV_1 is the total amount of air a patient can exhale in 1 second; it is often measured before and after an inhaled bronchodilator is given to a patient. Significant reversibility of lung function is indicated by an increase of $\geq$12% and 200 ml in FEV_1; such reversibility is used to confirm the diagnosis of asthma. When a spirometric reading is normal but asthma-like symptoms are still exhibited, the individual may be monitored with a peak flow meter for 1–2 weeks, with flow rates obtained on rising and in the afternoon before and after taking an inhaled bronchodilator. Asthma is suggested if there is a difference of at least 20% between high and low readings obtained on the same day (National Institutes of Health, 1997).

Pulmonary function data may also be used to differentiate restrictive from obstructive airways. If given a bronchodilator, patients with asthma often exhibit complete reversibility of the obstruction, whereas lung function may remain impaired for patients with irreversible damage. In addition, measurements of pulmonary function are useful in determining the severity of the airflow difficulties; while they should not be ignored, subjective patient perceptions of their symptoms usually correlate poorly with the more objective pulmonary function tests (Spector & Nicklas, 1995).

Another tool used to diagnose asthma is with a standard form of bronchoprovocation challenge, such as having patients inhale methacholine or cold air, or exercise. This process helps the clinician diagnose and understand the specific nature of the patient's symptoms. At one time, a 15–20% decrease in the pulmonary test data when a patient received a bronchial challenge was the accepted diagnosis of asthma. While provocation challenges are still used to determine precipitants of a patient's asthma, the diagnosis of asthma is generally based upon a 15–20% improvement in pulmonary function in response to the patient inhaling a bronchodilator medication.

Peak flow rates, obtained with a simple, portable, and inexpensive peak

Table 11.1 Asthma questionnaire. (Modified from guidelines presented by National Institutes of Health, 1991.)

I. *Symptoms*
   A. Cough, wheezing, shortness of breath, chest tightness, and sputum production of a modest degree
   B. Conditions associated with asthma, such as rhinitis, sinusitis, nasal polyposis, or atopic dermatitis

II. *Pattern of symptoms*
   A. Perennial, seasonal, or perennial symptoms with seasonal exacerbations
   B. Continuous, episodic, or continuous symptoms with acute exacerbations
   C. Onset, duration, and frequency of symptoms (days per week or month)
   D. Diurnal variation with special reference to nocturnal symptoms

III. *Precipitating and/or aggravating factors*
   A. Viral respiratory infections
   B. Exposure to environmental allergens, such as pollen, mold, house dust mite, cockroach, animal dander, or secretory products, e.g., cat saliva
   C. Environmental change, such as moving, going on vacation, etc.
   D. Exposure to irritants, including tobacco smoke, strong odors, and air pollution
   E. Emotional reactions, such as crying or laughing hard, shouting, etc.
   F. Family dysfunction, such as parent separation, divorce, alcoholism, etc.
   G. Drugs, such as aspirin
   H. Food additives, such as sulfites or yellow food coloring
   I. Changes in weather or exposure to cold air
   J. Exercise
   K. Endocrine factors, such as menses

IV. *Development of disorder*
   A. Age of onset and age at diagnosis
   B. Progress of disorder, e.g., whether asthma is better or worse
   C. Previous evaluation, treatment, and response
   D. Present management and response, including plans for managing acute episodes
      1. Preventative measures taken to avoid symptoms
         a. Degree of adherence to preventative measures
      2. Stepwise regimen taken to manage acute episodes
         a. Degree of adherence to management regimen

V. *Profile of typical exacerbation*
   A. Prodromal signs and symptoms (e.g., itching of neck, nasal allergy symptoms)
   B. Temporal progression
      1. Typical sequence of events taken during an acute episode
   C. Usual management
      1. Strategies taken by patient and family
      2. Degree of confidence in management strategies

VI. *Living situation*
   A. Home age, location, cooling and heating systems, such as central with oil, electric and/or wood-burning stove or fireplace
   B. Carpeting over a concrete slab
   C. Humidifier

continued

Table 11.1 *contd.*

- D. Description of patient's room with special attention to pillow, bed, floor covering, and other items that collect dust
- E. Animals in home
- F. Exposure to cigarette smoke in home
- G. Day care, school, or work environment

VII. *Impact of disorder*
- A. Impact on patient
  1. Number of emergency room visits and hospitalizations
  2. History of life-threatening acute exacerbations, intubation, or oral steroid therapy
  3. Number of days absent from school or work and academic or work performance
  4. Limitation of activity, especially sports
  5. History of nocturnal awakening
  6. Effect on growth, development, behavior, peer relationships, school or work, achievement, and lifestyle
- B. Impact on family
  1. Disruption of family
  2. Effect on siblings
  3. Economic impact

VIII. *Assessment of patient's and family's perception of illness*
- A. Patient, parental, and family knowledge of asthma and belief in the chronicity of asthma and in the efficacy of treatment
- B. Ability of patient and parents to cope with asthma
- C. Level of family support and parent's capacity to recognize severity of an exacerbation
- D. Economic resources

IX. *Family history*
- A. Allergy in close relatives
- B. Asthma in close relatives

X. *Medical history*
- A. General medical history and history of other allergic disorder, history of injury to the airways, viral bronchiolitis, recurrent croup, gastroesophageal reflux, or passive exposure to smoke
- B. Review of symptoms

---

flow meter, are widely used in the management of asthma. When obtained correctly, PEF rates correlate highly with those obtained with the spirometer. PEF values are useful for assessing the degree and severity of airway obstruction, for monitoring response to treatment, for diagnosing exercise-induced asthma, and for detecting asymptomatic deterioration. When patients learn to take PEF rates at home, the clinician's ability to establish effective treatment is enhanced (National Institutes of Health, 1991).

Attempts to classify asthma severity involve a formula based on the interaction between symptom frequency and intensity, activity impairment, pulmonary function, and response to treatment. It is easily determined by using a 4×4 matrix where, on the *x* axis, the severity of asthma is classified prior to the initiation of therapy into four categories – mild intermittent, mild persistent, moderate persistent, and severe persistent – asthma. Four indices of asthma – symptoms, nighttime symptoms, lung function, and peak flow variability – fall along the *y* axis of the matrix. Comparing values obtained from a given patient with those entered in the 16 cells of the matrix permits easy determination of the severity of that patient's asthma (National Institutes of Health, 1991, 1992; Spector & Nicklas, 1995).

Chronic Obstructive Pulmonary Disease

Making the diagnosis as to whether a patient has COPD involves several steps. A thorough physical examination and a complete history of the patient, particularly regarding his or her smoking history, is essential. A physical examination is helpful in revealing signs of dyspnea and airway hyperinflation; chest radiography provides the most direct evidence for COPD because of the known anatomical changes that occur in the disease. A comprehensive history questionnaire for COPD is shown in Table 11.2. Sophisticated pulmonary testing is required for patients suspected of having COPD to determine pathology and disease state. Pulmonary function tests are also useful in determining the rate of decline in pulmonary function for patients with COPD. If chronic bronchitis is indicated, sputum culture tests are performed; in addition, oxygen levels and exercise tests may be given to a patient thought to have COPD (American Thoracic Society, 1995).

Rating systems for severity of COPD are different from those used to gauge asthma severity. Severity of COPD is based on the interrelationship between the degree of airflow obstruction, the subjective sensation of breathlessness (dyspnea), and the impairment of gas exchange (especially oxygen levels). Most patients are in a category of stage I where there is minimal interference of COPD with daily activities; medical care is provided on an outpatient basis and is modest in nature. At stage II, impairment in daily life is more significant, and patients are usually required to seek the ongoing support of a respiratory therapist. Stage III includes a minority of patients; it is the late stage of COPD where quality of life is greatly diminished. Constant care by a respiratory therapist is required. At each stage of the disease process, treatment is guided by the needs of the individual patient, and includes consideration of medical, functional, and psychological factors (American Thoracic Society, 1995).

Tuberculosis

Tuberculosis passes through two phases. In the first or primary phase, the body's natural defenses resist the disease by destroying or walling off

Table 11.2 COPD questionnaire

I. *Symptoms*
   A. Chronic cough
   B. Coughing up mucus
   C. Shortness of breath during activity
   D. Occasional wheezing

II. *Pattern of symptoms*
   A. Continuous, episodic, or continuous symptoms with acute exacerbations
   B. Daily variation in coughing
      1. Smoker's cough in the morning

III. *Precipitating and/or aggravating factors*
   A. Smoking
   B. Respiratory infections
   C. Daily activities
   D. When exercising or engaging in physical activities

IV. *Development of symptoms*
   A. Age patient noticed change
   B. Progress of symptoms, e.g., whether they are ever better or worse
   C. Any recent changes in breathing

V. *Duration of symptoms or related symptoms*
   A. Coughing with mucus
   B. Bouts of bronchitis
   C. Chest colds each winter
   D. Colds last for weeks rather than days

VI. *Present management*
   A. Any preventative measures, including adherence to medical instructions
   B. Any action plan worked out between patient and health care provider

VII. *Impact of symptoms*
   A. Impact on patient
   B. Impact on those around patient, including spouse, children, etc.
   C. Limitations on activities

VII. *Assessment of patient's and family's perception of illness*
   A. Patient knowledge of smoking consequences
   B. Patient knowledge of COPD
   C. Ability of patient to cope with COPD
   D. Ability of patient to quit smoking
   E. Level of spousal or family support in changing behaviors and following medical advice

VIII. *Medical history*
   A. History of patient and family members
   B. General medical history

most of the bacteria. The primary phase may last several months; often the disease does not develop beyond this point. The second or secondary phase most commonly affects the lungs and produces breathing symptoms. Symptoms of the disease are noted in Table 11.3; their occur-

Table 11.3 Common symptoms of tuberculosis

Respiratory symptoms
- Coughing that lasts more than 2 weeks
- Coughing up blood or blood mucus
- Chest pain
- Difficulty breathing

Other physical symptoms
- Anemia
- Unexplained weight loss
- Feelings of being run down
- Easily fatigued
- Fever and sweating
- Fever and sweating at night
- Loss of appetite

rence often prompts the application of several diagnostic techniques, either to confirm or rule out the diagnosis of TB. Diagnostic procedures include the following:

Chest Radiograph

A common diagnostic test leading to the suspicion of TB is the chest radiograph. The chest radiograph in primary tuberculosis

> *often demonstrates infiltrates of an inflammatory nature in the mid- and lower-lung fields, because most tidal ventilation goes to these areas and, thus, droplet nuclei are more likely to be carried there*
> *(Broughton & Bass, 1999, 29.6)*

Skin Testing

Skin testing for tuberculosis has been used for over a century. Broughton & Bass (1999) suggest that skin testing for TB is the only effective way to identify those with asymptomatic infection from *M. tuberculosis*. A problem with the test, Broughton & Bass noted, is that false-negative results occur in such testing. Efferen (1999) reported that false-negative tests are known to occur in up to 30% of immunocompetent and 60% of immunocompromised persons with active TB. Still, Broughton & Bass (1999) agree with Efferen (1999) in believing that skin testing is invaluable in diagnosing TB when care is taken in administering the procedure.

Sputum Testing

A key to using this technique is to obtain a true sputum specimen from a patient. When copious amounts are present, collection of specimens can be readily accomplished; when production is less active, the collection of three deep sputum specimens in the morning is apt to produce positive smears more than random specimens (Broughton & Bass, 1999). If sputum is unavailable through these methods, fiberoptic bronchoscopy may be used.

Mycobacterial Culture

All specimens should be submitted for culture. Direct microscopy with staining procedures is the most widely used test used to establish the diagnosis of TB (Efferen, 1999). Efferen continued by noting that while the approach is simple and rapid, there are concerns about its sensitivity and specificity. Nevertheless, she concluded (Efferen, 1999, p. 778) 'culture is the diagnostic gold standard and is essential for drug sensitivity testing.' The basic problem with the approach is the delay of time that occurs between obtaining the culture and receiving information back on it (Broughton & Bass, 1999; Efferen, 1999). Broughton & Bass (1999) go so far as to suggest that since active TB is potentially contagious, strong consideration be given to the initiation of antituberculous therapy at the time the culture is obtained.

Direct Identification of the Mycobacterium *spp.*

Polymerase chain reaction (PCR) is a nucleic acid amplification procedure that has proven useful in the detection and identification of *M. tuberculosis*. The techniques split and copy specific portions of DNA until a target area can be detected by a DNA problem. Specificity and sensitivity are good for the PCR when the smear is positive (Broughton & Bass, 1999).

Goals of Treatment of Asthma, COPD, and Tuberculosis

Asthma

The goals of treatment for asthma are spelled out in the Expert Panel Report 2 Guidelines (National Institutes of Health, 1997). These are

- to prevent chronic and troublesome symptoms of asthma, including those occurring during nighttime hours;
- to permit patients to maintain normal or, depending upon variability of reversibility, near-normal pulmonary function;
- to permit patients to maintain normal activity levels, including exercise and other physical activity;
- to prevent recurrent exacerbations or acute episodes of asthma, and minimize the need for emergency room or hospital visits;
- to provide optimal pharmacotherapy with minimal or no adverse effects; and
- to meet patients' and families' expectations of and satisfaction with asthma care; and, a final goal – assisting patients, through teaching and self-management training, to become partners with their physi-

cians in the control of asthma – is strongly interwoven into both sets of asthma treatment guidelines (National Institutes of Health, 1991, 1997).

Optimal management of asthma generally rests upon attaining the latter goal (Creer & Levstek, 1998).

Chronic Obstructive Pulmonary Disease

The goals for the management of COPD are similar, to some extent, to those described for asthma. They are

- to teach patients about COPD, including the need for the patient to quit smoking;
- to teach patients to improve their daily lives by exercising regularly;
- to teach patients to become more active, even if this means carrying a portable oxygen supply when out of the house;
- to decrease the shortness of breath experienced by patients;
- to decrease the anxiety experienced by patients and their families; and
- to improve the mood and overall quality of life of patients and their families.

How these goals are achieved is described in Chapter 4 by Kaplan and Ries.

Tuberculosis

Tuberculosis is a concern both to public health and to patients with the disease; each entity, therefore, has its own set of goals. The report by the Program in Infectious Disease and Social Change (1999) recently suggested several targets for TB control for both public health and individual patients with TB. The public health goals for tuberculosis include the following (Heymann *et al.*, 1999):

- To increase involvement of world governments and international standard-setting bodies to respond to the TB epidemic.
- To promote world control over the forces that unleash multidrug-resistant tuberculosis (MDR-TB).
- To ensure that all people with tuberculosis have access to direct-observed therapy (DOT). This type of treatment requires that patients report to a hospital or clinic to receive, under the direction of health care personnel, medications needed to halt and reverse the patient's TB.
- To closely monitor the course of the tuberculosis epidemic, including morbidity surveillance and monitoring of process and impact.
- To rapidly and effectively intervene with a DOTS-PLUS approach to patients with MDR-TB. The DOTS-PLUS approach features two treatment strategies – individualized treatment and standardized treatment – delivered by specialist units (the two approaches have been found to produce similar outcomes in South Africa).

Toward the end of the report by the Program in Infectious Disease and Social Change, Farmer *et al.* (1999) offer their perspective on the world tuberculosis epidemic. First, they propose what they see as the most important messages they could impart regarding TB; their messages mirror the goals described above. Second, however, Farmer *et al.* (1999, p. 176) summarize what has worked in controlling TB:

> *As with drug-resistant Staphylococcus aureus, disease due to drug resistant M. tuberculosis must be treated with agents to which it is susceptible. Where there was an upsurge in TB in New York, it is not true that a single strategy – DOTS – was responsible for 'turning the tide.' In fact, several interventions were made, including more rapid diagnosis, active case finding in epicenters of transmission, more rapid detection and treatment of MDR-TB and for a minority of patients, directly observed therapy. Enormous resources were required to quell the epidemic, but this ultimately successful investment was regretted by few.*

Many of these steps echo strategies suggested by Brahmer & Small (1998), Broughton & Bass (1999), and Efferen (1999).

Treatments of Asthma, COPD, and Tuberculosis

Asthma and COPD

Two types of medications are widely used in asthma and COPD; they are designed either to provide quick relief for pulmonary exacerbations or to prevent such episodes. How the two types of medications are used is a function both of the disorder, whether asthma or COPD, and of particular characteristics presented by individual patients. How the drugs are used is a cornerstone of treatment guidelines for both disorders (e.g., National Institutes of Health, 1991, 1997; American Thoracic Society, 1995).

Quick-Relief Drugs

These drugs are useful in helping control an asthma attack; a quick-relief drug is the only medicine some patients take for their asthma. COPD patients often take β-agonist, anticholinergic, and theophylline drugs to open airways in the lungs or to decrease shortness of breath by relaxing smooth muscles around the airways. Types of quick-relief drugs are summarized in Table 11.4. They include:

- short-acting β-agonists
- anticholinergic drugs
- systemic or oral corticosteroids

Table 11.4 Medications used to treat asthma and COPD

Generic	Brand names
Short-acting β-agonists	
albuterol	Proventil® metered-dose inhaler Ventolin® metered-dose inhaler
albuterol sulfate	
powder for inhaler	Ventolin Rotocaps®
solution for nebulizer	Airet®, Proventil®, Ventolin Nebules®
tablets, syrup	Proventil®, Ventilin®, Volmax®
bitolterol	
aerosol for inhaler	Tornalate® metered-dose inhaler
isoetharine	
aerosol for inhaler	Bronkometer®
solution for nebulizer	Arm-a-Med Isoetharine® Dey-Lute®, Beta-2®, Bronkosol®
isoproterenol	
aerosol for inhaler	Isupret Mistometer®
solution for nebulizer	Isupret Hydrochloride® Isoproterenol Hydrochloride®
injection	Isoproterenol Hydrochloride®
tablets	Isoproterenol Hydrochloride®, Glossets®
combined with phenylephrine	
aerosol for inhalation	Duo-Medihaler®
isoproterenol sulfate	
aerosol for inhaler	Medihaler-Iso®
metaproterenol sulfate	
aerosol for inhaler	Alupent®, Metaprel®
solution for nebulizer	Alupent®, Arm-a-Med®, Metaroterenol®, Dey-Lute®, Metaprel®
tablets, syrup	AlupentR, MetaprelR
pirbuterol acetate	
aerosol for inhaler	Maxair®
terbutaline sulfate	
aerosol for inhaler	Brethaire®
tablets	Brethine®, Bricanyl®
injection	Brethine®, Bricanyl®
Anticholinergic drugs	
ipratropium	
inhaled	Atrovent®
Systemic or oral corticosteroids	
methylprednisolone	Medrol®, Depo-Medrol®
prednisone	Deltasone®, Prednicon®, Sterapred®
prednisolone	Pecliapred®, Prelone®

Short-acting β-agonists

These medications relax the muscles around the airways. They are the most effective drugs to use for relief of acute asthma symptoms, and can also be taken just before exercise to prevent exercise-induced asthma. Beta-agonist drugs are inhaled directly into the lungs by an inhaler or nebulizer, taken in the mouth as a liquid or tablet, or injected during acute asthma emergencies.

Advantages of short-acting β-agonist drugs are (Barnes, 1997):

- they are the most useful bronchodilators to use in treating asthma, and are also most effective when inhaled;
- nebulized β-agonists are the first choice for acute severe asthma; and
- when inhaled at recommended doses, they have few side effects

Disadvantages of short-acting β-agonists are

- possible side effects of β-agonist drugs are dry mouth, anxiety, shakiness, dizziness, headache, restlessness or sleeplessness, nervousness or irritability, and fast, irregular or pounding heart beat;
- tolerance may developed to inhaled β-agonists, but there is little evidence of bronchodilator effects with short-acting forms (Barnes, 1997);
- concerns about increased asthma morbidity and mortality with high doses of short-term β-agonists; and
- as neither short- nor long-term β-agonists fail to reduce inflammation in airways, in many instances they should be used in conjunction with anti-inflammatory medications.

Three other points regarding the use of β-agonists should be noted: (a) if patients miss a scheduled dose, they should take it as soon as possible unless it is almost time to take their next dose and not double doses; (b) if they use a canister of β-agonists a month or require a β-agonist medicine once or twice a week, patients should inform their health care provider; and (c) if patients have trouble breathing after using their β-agonist drug, they should contact their health care provider immediately.

Anticholinergic Drugs

These medications are more effective when used with COPD than they are with asthma (Barnes, 1997).

Advantages of anticholinergic drugs are

- they help relax muscles surrounding the airways;
- they may provide quick relief for wheezing, coughing, and other symptoms;
- they are often used in combination with other asthma or COPD medicines; and,
- because systemic absorption of inhaled anticholinergic drugs is minimal, they have few side effects (Barnes, 1997).

Disadvantages of anticholinergic medications are

- they should only be used as directed, as overdoses can be serious;
- possible side effects of anticholinergic drugs include dryness of the mouth, headache, dizziness, nervousness, and upset stomach or nausea;
- patients should contact their health care providers if, having taken an anticholinergic drug, symptoms worsen or don't improve in 30 min; and,
- patients should tell their health care provider if they have dryness of the mouth and, if for over 2 weeks, they experience difficulty swallowing, severe eye pain, a skin rash or hives, swelling of the tongue or lips, and ulcers or sores in the mouth or on the lips.

Oral or Systemic Corticosteroids

Oral or systemic corticosteroids are powerful drugs that stop the body from producing chemicals that cause asthma attacks. They may be prescribed on a short-term basis to treat persistent asthma symptoms.

Advantages of these corticosteroids

- oral corticosteroids may head off a severe attack or keep an attack from getting worse;
- systemic corticosteroids may be taken orally, in tablet or liquid forms. In emergencies, they may be administered intravenously.

Disadvantages of oral steroids are

- Side effects of short-term systemic corticosteroid therapy include increased appetite, fluid retention, mood changes, weight gain, and, in children, leg pains. However, these effects are unlikely when 'bursts' of the drug are given to bring an exacerbation under control; serious side effects are only likely if a patient must take such a medication to control his or her asthma or COPD over a prolonged period of time.
- Patients should never stop taking an oral corticosteroid without first discussing such action with their doctor or health care provider. Going off these drugs abruptly, particularly high doses of oral corticosteroids, could lead to adrenal suppression and, in extreme cases, death. For this reason, patients should always clear any actions they take regarding oral corticosteroids with their health care provider.
- Patients can only go off from oral corticosteroids in a gradual manner. This prevents some of the more serious side effects of such drugs.

If patients miss a dose of systemic corticosteroids, they should take it as soon as possible, as directed by their health care provider.

Preventive or Controller Drugs

Preventive, controller, or maintenance drugs are taken daily on a long-term basis to control persistent asthma and to prevent attacks. They are not helpful in reducing the symptoms of an attack. In COPD, the drugs are used to reduce and prevent swelling inside the airways, and to decrease mucus production. Types of preventive asthma and COPD drugs are shown in Table 11.5. They include:

- inhaled corticosteroids
- cromolyn sodium and nedocromil
- long-term β-agonists
- methylxanthines or xanthines
- leukotriene modifiers.

Table 11.5 Types of preventive, controller, or maintenance medications

Generic	Brand names
Inhaled corticosteroids	
beclomethasone	Beclovent®, Vanceril®
flunisolide	AeroBid®
fluticasone	Flovent®, Flonase®, Cutivate®
triamcinolone	Azmacort®
Cromolyn or nedocromil sodium	
cromolyn sodium	Intal®
nedocromil sodium	Tilade®
Long-term β-agonists	
salmeterol	Serevent®
albuterol sulfate prolonged-release tablets	Proventil Repetabs®, Ventolin®, Volmax®
Xanthine drugs	
aminophylline	Phyllocontine®, Truphylline
theophylline	Accubron®, Aquaphyllin®, Bronkodyl®, Elixophyllin®, Quibron-T®, Slo-Phyllin®, Theolair®, Theolate®, Theoclear®, Uniphyl®, Theo-Dur®, Theo-24®, Slo-Bid Gyrocaps®, Theo-X®, Uni-Dur®, Uniphyl®
Leukotriene modifiers	
zafirlukast	Accolate®
zileuton	Zyflo®
montelukast	Singulair®

Inhaled Corticosteroids. Corticosteroids are the most powerful and effective long-term drug for asthma. They reduce inflammation and swelling in the airways. Inhaled corticosteroids are prescribed to prevent or control asthma on a long-term basis, particularly in patients with moderate or severe persistent asthma. They are ineffective in halting asthma attacks.

Advantages of inhaled corticosteroids are that they (Barnes, 1997)

- effectively control asthma;
- reduce airway inflammation, thus keeping airways open;
- prevent asthma attacks or episodes; and,
- side effects are problematic with inhaled steroids.

Disadvantages of inhaled steroids are

- Inhaled corticosteroids have few side effects, but patients may experience some local side effects, such as cough, dry mouth, unpleasant taste, hoarseness, headache, or nausea.
- Inhaled corticosteroids do not work right away. It may take 4 weeks or longer of constant use before the patient notices improvement, and several months before the drug's full effects are felt.
- Because of the slow onset of beneficial effects, compliance to a regimen with inhaled corticosteroids may be poor.
- Patients may also show poor compliance to an inhaled corticosteroid regimen when asymptomatic.

If patients miss a dose, they should take it as soon as possible; they should then put themselves back on schedule for the rest of the day. Patients should contact their doctor or health care provider if they have trouble breathing, feel tight, or wheeze right after using an inhaled corticosteroid. Asthma patients should also contact their physician or health care provider if they take inhaled corticosteroids on a regular basis, but experience an attack that does not improve when taking a quick-relief drug.

Cromolyn or Nedocromil Sodium. These drugs prevent airway swelling and inflammation by making the airways less sensitive to irritants. Cromolyn and nedocromil are inhaled directly into the lungs by a metered-dose inhaler or by a nebulizer.

Advantages of cromolyn or nedocromil sodium are that they

- control symptoms of asthma in some patients;
- have few side effects – those reported include temporary bad taste, irritation of the throat, coughing, and headache;
- prevent induced bronchospasm, including exercise-induced asthma; and
- are frequently useful in the control of pediatric asthma.

Disadvantages of cromolyn or nedocromil sodium are that they

- are only effective for some cases of mild asthma;
- do not reduce airway inflammation as occurs with inhaled corticosteroids;
- do not work right away – cromolyn and nedocromil may take 2–5 weeks of regular use before patients obtain the full benefits of the drugs;
- may prompt patient nonadherence because of their slow onset of action;
- require four times a day administration; and,
- are relatively expensive compared with other drugs (Barnes, 1997).

If patients miss a dose, they should take it as soon as possible and resume taking the drug as prescribed. When taking cromolyn or nedocromil sodium, patients should contact their doctor or health care provider if they don't get better by taking a quick-relief medication for an attack.

Long-Term β-Agonists. These drugs relax airway muscles. Long-acting β-agonists are used with anti-inflammatory drugs for long-term control of asthma symptoms, especially those that occur at night. The drugs are sometimes prescribed to prevent exercise-induced asthma.

Advantages of long-term β-agonists are that

- a long-lasting β-agonist can be used with nocturnal asthma;
- they can be taken by an inhaler or orally; and
- they more effectively prevent exercise-induced bronchoconstriction than equivalent doses of β-agonists (Barnes, 1997).

Disadvantages of long-term β-agonists are that:

- unlike short-acting β-agonist preparations, long-term β-agonists cannot be used to treat acute symptoms of asthma;
- side effects of long-term β-agonists include dry mouth, anxiety, shakiness, dizziness, headache, restlessness or sleeplessness, nervousness or irritability, and fast, irregular or pounding heart beat.

If patients miss a dose, they should take it as soon as possible, and return to the schedule prescribed by their doctor or health care provider. Asthma patients should contact their doctor or health care provider if they have trouble breathing after taking a long-term β-agonist or if there is an increase in the weekly use of the drug.

Xanthine Drugs. Xanthine medications relax the muscles around the airways, and may have a mild anti-inflammatory effect. The drugs are prescribed to control both nighttime and moderate-to-severe asthma.

Advantages of xanthine preparations are that

- They open the airways by relaxing the smooth muscle around the airways.
- Xanthine drugs are usually taken by mouth, but they are available as syrup, capsules, or sprinkles. In emergencies, xanthines may be given intravenously.
- Xanthines are a relatively weak bronchodilator.
- They are sometimes useful in the management of nocturnal asthma.

Disadvantages of xanthine drugs are that:

- Xanthines are effective only if taken as directed. If patients take a xanthine drug, their doctor or health care provider must regularly check the amount of the drug they have in their bloodstream to be certain it is at a therapeutic level.
- Xanthine medications have a number of side effects, including nausea, restlessness, sleeplessness, nervousness, and heartburn. Overdose may cause life-threatening side effects.
- Xanthine preparations interact with a number of substances that may decrease or increase the potency of the drug; these substances may include other drugs.
- Monitoring blood levels of patients taking xanthines is inconvenient and expensive (Barnes, 1997).
- Xanthine drugs are usually less effective than inhaled corticosteroids.

If patients miss a dose, they should take it as soon as possible. They should never double up on doses, but return to their regular schedule of taking the drug. Patients should call their doctor or health care provider if they have diarrhea or black, tarry stools; rapid breathing; vomiting; fast, pounding, or irregular heart beat; confusion; increased urination or difficulty urinating; convulsions or seizures; muscle twitching; or chronic headaches.

Leukotriene Modifier. These drugs are relatively new to asthma treatment; they are thought to reduce the effect of leukotrienes, a powerful bronchoconstrictor.

Advantages of leukotriene medications are that

- they are thought to diminish asthma symptoms, improve lung function, and reduce the need for short-term β-agonists;
- they appear effective when used with patients with mild-to-moderate asthma; and
- they are tablets that are taken orally.

Disadvantages of leukotriene medications are that

- they have not been used enough to determine any long-term side effects;
- they have been used primarily in asthma patients 12 years old and older; and

- as the drugs are new, leukotriene modifiers should be carefully monitored by patients and their health care provider.

Two other treatments are often provided to patients with COPD: antibiotics and oxygen therapy.

Antibiotics
These drugs are used to fight bacterial infections that can occur with COPD. Those commonly used include amoxicillin (Amoxil®, Polymox®, Tvimox®, Wymox®) trimethoprim/sulfamethoxazole (Bactrim® and Septra®), and cephalexin (Keflex®). Less commonly used antibiotics are clarithromycin (Biaxin®), cefuroxime axetil (Ceftin®), and ciprofloxacin (Cipro®).

Oxygen therapy
Some patients with COPD need oxygen therapy to ensure there is enough oxygen in their blood. It is often difficult to determine when oxygen therapy is required, although patients with such symptoms as shortness of breath, irritability, ankle swelling, or morning headache may be candidates for oxygen therapy. Oxygen levels can be determined by two methods: oximetry and arterial blood gases.

Tuberculosis

There are currently 13 agents available in the United States for the treatment of tuberculosis (Brahmer & Small, 1998). Broughton & Bass (1999), Brahmer & Small (1998), and Efferen (1999) divide the drugs into two categories: first-line (or primary) and second-line (or secondary) medications. As Brahmer & Small (1998, p. 1631) explain:

> *Agents in the primary group are those used in the initial treatment of tuberculosis. They represent the first choice because of their effectiveness, relatively low toxicity, and relatively low cost. The secondary agents are generally reserved for use in treating disease caused by organisms that are resistant to one or more of the primary drugs or in cases in which hypersensitivity or toxicity is caused by the primary drug. In general, the second-line drugs are less effective, more toxic, and more expensive than the primary agents.*

Five primary (or first-line) drugs are used for TB therapy (Brahmer & Small, 1998; Broughton & Bass, 1999; Efferen, 1999). Brahmer & Small (1998) describe each drug:

- isoniazid, the major bactericidal drug used in any initial treatment regimen;
- rifampin, a potent bactericidal agent especially effective in eradicating

organisms that grow in spurts;
- streptomycin, a bactericidal probably most effective in its early effect on rapidly proliferating organisms;
- pyrazinamide, a drug most efficient in an acid environment; and
- ethambutol, 'effective as a companion to more potent agents because it diminishes the likelihood of proliferation of drug-resistant strains' (Brahmer & Small, p. 1631).

Secondary (or second-line) anti-TB drugs include capreomycin, kanamycin, amikacin, ethionamide, para-aminosalicylic acid, cycloserine, ofloxacin, and ciprofloxacin. Broughton & Bass (1999) caution that secondary (or second-line) drugs are reserved for difficult situations in the treatment of TB and are more complicated to use than primary agents. In addition, Broughton & Bass continue, the advice of a tuberculosis expert is recommended when second-line anti-TB drugs are used.

Brahmer & Small (1998) describe six factors to consider in selecting an antituberculosis drug regimen:

- *History of previous therapy.* Patients treated with nonrifampin-containing regimens who have subsequent recurrent TB, for example, have a higher probability of having organisms that are resistant to the anti-TB regimen taken earlier. Brahmer & Small (1998) suggest these patients are candidates for a regimen of rifampin–ethambutol for 12 months.
- *Probability of primary isoniazid resistance. There are specific circumstances where primary resistance is common; in general, these occur in developing countries in Southeast Asia, the Philippines, and Africa (Brahmer & Small, 1998).*
- *Assessment of patient compliance.* The major reason for treatment failure in TB is noncompliance. Patients who exhibit nonadherent behaviors are candidates for behavioral intervention or for referral for direct observed therapy (DOT).
- *Presence of coexisting diseases.* A general rule, note Brahmer & Small (1998), is that drugs having toxicities that may add to the effects of coexisting diseases should not be used.
- *Results of drug susceptibility studies.* Treatment of TB caused by organisms that are resistant to traditional antituberculosis drugs require modification and tailoring to the individual patient. Brahmer & Small (1998) recommend that susceptibility studies should be obtained for all patients previously treated for TB and for patients with a high probability of primary drug resistance.
- *History of untoward reactions to antituberculosis drugs.* If there is a clear history of a toxic or allergic reaction to a previously administered drug, the drug should be avoided and another agent substituted in its place (Brahmer & Small, 1998).

Discussion

Creer (Chapter 14) describes two factors that have contributed to the synergistic treatment model currently used by medical and behavioral scientists in treating respiratory disorders. First, there has been the gradual evolution away from a multidisciplinary mode of treatment – whereby each member of the treatment team knew only his or her area of expertise and how it could be applied – toward an interdisciplinary model of treatment, where each member of the team has a working knowledge of the other members' skills and specialties. Knowing well one's own discipline is a major strength, but not when the price is knowing nothing about problems faced by other team members and how they might be resolved. Too often, the multidisciplinarian model resulted in patients being treated in an uncoordinated fashion that left gaps in an individual patient's treatment regimen. Physicians, for example, often viewed patients only within the realm of medicine. If they anticipated that taking medications alone would bring control over a patient's asthma, they played the role as they had been taught in medical school. In this scenario, however, little thought is given to the need to alter behavior to reduce environmental precipitants of attacks or to promote adherence on the part of patients. The interdisciplinarian model, in contrast, expects physicians, nurses, physical therapists, social workers, psychologists, and other members of a treatment team to have a working knowledge of the other team members' expertise and skills. Such an approach is synergistic in that the knowledge and skills from various disciplines are integrated into a coordinated plan for patient care (Varni, 1983).

The second factor concerns the need for a working knowledge by all members of a treatment team of the variables involved in a respiratory disorder and its treatment. Of particular importance is the need to be knowledgeable as regards the physiological aspects that characterize a chronic respiratory disorder and how they are managed. This means that everyone on the team needs a basic knowledge of the medications used to manage a disorder. Given the potency of medications used in respiratory disorders, it is no longer the sole responsibility of medical scientists to understand the parameters of these drugs; all members of a treatment team, as well as the patients they treat, must be aware of the effects, side effects, and dosing requirements of each medication. Creer & Levstek (1998) cautioned that without possessing such a background, any member of a treatment team could do more harm than good. Specifically, it was pointed out that without knowledge of the parameters of a prescribed drug, a behavioral scientist might improve adherence to what is a potentially dangerous regimen of a medication. This would violate a cardinal rule in the treatment of patients: above all, do no harm.

At the beginning of the chapter, it was noted that this book is filled with examples of the many ways that medical and behavioral scientists have worked together to develop and test procedures to produce better health for those with asthma, COPD, and TB. By both medical and behavioral scientists understanding the physiological basis of a disorder, as well as how it might be controlled or modified, the consequence should be a more roseate future for the treatment of patients with these respiratory disorders.

References

American Thoracic Society (1987). Standards for the diagnosis and care of patients with chronic obstructive pulmonary disease (COPD) and asthma. *American Review of Respiratory Diseases*, 136, 225–244.

American Thoracic Society (1995). Standards for the diagnosis and care of patients with chronic obstructive pulmonary disease. *American Journal of Respiratory and Critical Care Medicine*, 152, S77–S120.

Barnes, P.J. (1997). Current therapies for asthma: promise and limitations. *Chest*, 111, 17S–26S.

Bernstein, I.L. (1988). Asthma in adults: diagnosis and treatment. In: E. Middleton Jr, C.E. Reed & E.F. Ellis (Eds), *Allergy: principles and practice*, 4th edn (pp. 901–934). St. Louis: C.V. Mosby.

Brahmer, J.R. & Small, P.M. (1998). Tuberculosis and nontuberculous mycobacterial infections. In: J.H. Stein (Editor-in-chief) *Internal medicine*, 5th edn (pp. 1625–1639). St. Louis: C.V. Mosby.

Broughton, W.A. & Bass, J.B., Jr. (1999). Tuberculosis and diseases caused by atypical mycobacterium. In: R.K. Albert, S.G. Spiro, & J.R. Jett (Eds), *Comprehensive respiratory medicine* (pp. 29.1–29.16). St. Louis: C.V. Mosby Co.

Burrows, B. (1991). Epidemiologic evidence for different types of chronic airflow obstruction. *American Review of Respiratory Diseases*, 143, 1452–1455.

Cantwell, M.F., McKenna, M.T., McCray, E., & Onorato, I.M. (1998). Tuberculosis and race/ethnicity in the United States: impact of socioeconomic status. *American Journal of Respiratory and Critical Care Medicine*, 157, 1016–1020.

Centers for Disease Control (1992). Asthma – United States, 1980–1990. *Morbidity and Mortality Weekly Report*, 45, 733–735.

Coultas, D.B., Gong, H., Grad, R., *et al.* (1993). Respiratory diseases in minorities of the United States. *American Journal of Respiratory and Critical Care Medicine*, 149, S93–S131.

Creer, T.L. (1979). *Asthma therapy. A behavioral health care system for respiratory disorders.* New York: Springer.

Creer, T.L. (1982). Asthma. *Journal of Consulting and Clinical Psychology*, 72, 912–921.

Creer, T.L. & Levstek, D. (1996). Medication compliance and asthma: overlooking the trees because of the forest. *Journal of Asthma*, 33, 203–211.

Creer, T.L. & Levstek, D. (1998). Respiratory disorders. In: A.S. Bellack & M. Hersen (Eds), *Comprehensive clinical psychology* (pp. 339–359). New York: Pergamon.

Creer, T.L., Levstek, D., & Reynolds, R.V.C. (1998). History and conclusions. In: H. Kotses & A. Harver (Eds), *The self-management of asthma* (pp. 379–405). New York: Marcel Dekker.

Creer, T.L., Winder, J.A., & Tinkelman, D. (1999). Guidelines for the diagnosis and management of asthma: accepting the challenge. *Journal of Asthma*, 36, 391–407.

Efferen, L.S. (1999). Tuberculosis: practical solutions to meet the challenge. *Journal of Respiratory Disease*, 20, 772–785.

Ellis, E.F. (1993). Asthma in infancy and childhood. In: E. Middleton Jr., C.E. Reed, E.F. Ellis, N.F. Adkinson Jr., J.W. Yunginger, & W.W. Busse (Eds), *Allergy: principles and practice*, 4th edn (pp. 1225–1262). St. Louis: C.V. Mosby.

Evans, R. III (1993). Epidemiology and natural history of asthma, allergic rhinitis, and atopic dermatitis. In: E. Middleton Jr., C.E. Reed, E.F. Ellis, N.F. Adkinson Jr., J.W. Yunginger, & W.W. Busse (Eds), *Allergy, principles and practice*, 4th edn (pp. 1109–1136). St. Louis: C.V. Mosby.

Farmer, P.E., Becerra, M.C., & Kim, J.Y. (1999). Conclusions and recommendations. In: *The global impact of drug-resistant tuberculosis* (pp. 169–177). Harvard University, Cambridge, MA: Program in Infectious Disease and Social Change.

Fletcher, C.M., Peto, R., Tinker, C.M., & Speizer, F.E. (1976). *The natural history of chronic bronchitis and emphysema.* Oxford: Oxford University Press.

Heymann, D.L., Kochi, A., & Raviglione, M.C. (1999). Foreword. *The global impact of drug-resistant tuberculosis* (pp. i–iii). Harvard University, Cambridge, MA: Program in Infectious Disease and Social Change.

Kaplan, B.A. & Mascie-Taylor, C.G. (1989). Biosocial correlates of asthma in a national sample of young adults. *Journal of Science*, 21, 475–482.

Lantner, R.R. & Ros, S.P. (1995). Emergency management of asthma in children: impact of NIH guidelines. *Annals of Allergy, Asthma, & Immunology*, 74, 188–190.

Leff, A.R. (1997). Future directions in asthma therapy. Is a cure possible? *Chest*, 111, 61S–68S.

Lemanske, R.F., Jr. & Busse, W.W. (1997). Asthma. *Journal of the American Medical Association*, 278, 1855–1873.

Loren, M.L., Leung, P.K., Cooley, R.L., Chai, H., Bell, T.D., & Buck, V.M. (1978). Irreversibility of obstructive changes in severe asthma in children. *Chest*, 74, 126–129.

Marwick, C. (1995). Inner-city asthma control campaign under way. *Journal of the American Medical Association*, 274, 1004.

National Institutes of Health (1992). *International consensus report on diagnosis and treatment of asthma (Publication No. 92-3091). Bethesda, MD: National Institutes of Health.*

National Institutes of Health (1995). Global initiative for asthma (National Heart, Lung, and Blood Institute Publication No. 95-3659). Bethesda MD: National Institutes of Health.

National Institutes of Health (1995). *Global strategy for asthma management and prevention* (NIH Publication No. 96-3659). Bethesda MD: National Heart, Lung & Blood Institute.

National Institutes of Health (1997). *Highlights of the expert panel 2 report: guidelines for the diagnosis and management of asthma* (Publication No. 97-4051A). Washington, DC: US Department of Health and Human Services.

Petty, T.L. (1990). Definitions in chronic obstructive pulmonary disease. *Clinics in Chest Medicine*, 11, 363–373.

Program in Infectious Disease and Social Change (1999). *The global impact of drug-resistant tuberculosis.* Harvard University, Cambridge, MA: Program in Infectious Disease and Social Change.

Renne, C.M. & Creer, T.L. (1985). Asthmatic children and their families. In: M.L. Walraich & D.K. Routh (Eds), *Advances in developmental and behavioral pediatrics, Volume 6* (pp. 41–81). Greenwich, CN: Jai Press.

Sanford, A., Weir, T., & Pare, P. (1996). The genetics of asthma. *American Journal of Respiratory and Critical Care Medicine*, 153, 1749–1765.

Sherrill, D.L., Lebowitz, M.D., & Burrows, B. (1990). Epidemiology of chronic obstructive pulmonary disease. *Clinics in Chest Medicine*, 11, 375–387.

Snider, G.L. (1995). What's in a name? Names, definitions, descriptions, and diagnostic criteria of diseases with emphasis on chronic obstructive pulmonary disease. *Respiration*, 62, 297–301.

Spector, S.L. & Nicklas, R.A. (Eds) (1995). Practice parameters for the diagnosis and treatment of asthma. *Journal of Allergy and Clinical Immunology*, 96, 707–870.

Taylor, D.M., Auble, T.E., Calhoun, W.J., & Mosesso, V.N. (1999). Current outpatient management of asthma shows poor compliance with international consensus guidelines. *Chest*, 116, 1638–1645.

Varni, J.W. (1983). *Clinical behavioral pediatrics.* New York: Pergamon Press.

12
Smoking cessation and chronic pulmonary disease

Russ VanCott Reynolds

Editors' note—*In his chapter, Russ Reynolds describes a topic of interest to all of us: smoking prevention and cessation. Cigarette smoking is the single most preventable cause of disease and death in the United States. It results in more deaths each year in the United States than AIDS, alcohol, cocaine, heroin, homicide, suicide, motor vehicle crashes, and fires – combined. Tobacco-related deaths number more than 430,000 per year among US adults, representing more than 5 million years of potential life lost (US Department of Health & Human Services, 2000). By no means is the impact of smoking limited to the United States: WHO Director-General Dr. Gro Harlem Brundtland (2000) recently pointed out that, with current smoking patterns, some 500 million people alive today will eventually be killed by smoking. Worldwide mortality from tobacco is expected to rise from about 4 million deaths a year in 1998 to about 10 million deaths in 2030, with over 70% in the developing world. In just 20 years, it is anticipated that smoking will cause about one of three of all adult deaths in the world, up from one in six adult deaths in 1990.*

In his chapter, Russ describes the limited research conducted on halting smoking in patients already diagnosed as having chronic obstructive pulmonary disease (COPD). He points out that despite deaths from COPD rising throughout the world, little research has been directed specifically at this population. This is a lamentable state, given that while ceasing to smoke may not reverse damage done by the habit, it may still prolong a patient's life.

Equally important is the need to determine ways to reduce the exposure of patients with asthma, particularly children (e.g., Schwartz et al., 2000), to tobacco smoke. This is another topic that seemingly has eluded direct study. Our hope is that the limited research described by Russ Reynolds will stimulate others to apply what we know to help control all types of respiratory disorders linked to smoking. Attaining such a goal would be a worthy pursuit by anyone, including medical and behavioral scientists, no matter where they are in the world.

Introduction

Chronic obstructive pulmonary disease (COPD), including chronic bronchitis and emphysema, is the fourth leading cause of death in the United

States (Wise, 1997). More than 25 years ago, the Surgeon General unequivocally stated that the primary risk factor for COPD is cigarette smoking (US Department of Health & Human Services, 1984). Establishing the connection between smoking and COPD, as well as other smoking-related disease, has led to enormous interest in studying the prevention of smoking onset and the cessation of smoking in otherwise healthy smokers. Although the prevalence of smoking among US adults has leveled off at around 25% of the population (Centers for Disease Control, 1999), we have made modest progress in the areas of smoking prevention and smoking cessation. (See Ockene *et al.* [2000] and Lantz *et al.* (2000) for reviews of the smoking cessation and prevention literatures, respectively.)

Because of our ability to achieve some level of success at both smoking cessation and prevention, we have been able to quantify the impact of smoking cessation on the onset and progression of respiratory symptoms and lung-function decline. For example, we know that if smokers quit prior to the development of chronic lung disease, their respiratory symptoms and rate of decline in lung function will begin to normalize within 5 years after cessation and, in some cases, will approximate that of someone who has never smoked (e.g., Leeder *et al.*, 1977; Camilli *et al.*, 1987; Brown *et al.*, 1991; Townsend *et al.*, 1991).

The landmark Lung Health Study demonstrated a similar effect for individuals with mild-to-moderate COPD (Anthonisen *et al.*, 1994; Kanner *et al.*, 1999; Scanlon *et al.*, 2000), although lost lung function cannot be restored. Specifically, Scanlon *et al.*, (2000) demonstrated that the lung-function benefits of cessation were evident in elderly patients with a history of heavy smoking, poor baseline lung function, or hyperresponsive airways. Thus, even those with mild-to-moderate COPD showed clinically and statistically significant improvement following smoking cessation.

Further, smokers who made multiple attempts to quit smoking during the course of the 5-year trial, and ultimately relapsed, showed less decline in lung function than those who made no attempts to quit (Murray et al., 1998). This finding indicates that even for smokers who quit and eventually relapse, there are some lung-function benefits. There exists, therefore, scientific support for the vigorous pursuit of smoking cessation for healthy smokers and for those with demonstrated airway disease. Unfortunately, there is a dearth of literature on smoking cessation with COPD patients. For example, a MEDLINE search, using the search terms smoking cessation and COPD or chronic obstructive pulmonary disease, produced fewer than 5 smoking cessation studies that were published in the past 25 years.

There are several reasons for this state, although one factor is perhaps pre-eminent: to date, we have been much less successful in promoting smoking cessation for COPD patients than for the general smoking population. It is safe to conclude that behavioral scientists are less apt to pursue areas of research that are unlikely to lead to successful programs of research. For example, longitudinal research with COPD patients is complicated by a high mortality rate; one early study of smoking rates following hospitalization had more than a 30% mortality rate during the 5-year follow-up period (Daughton *et al.*, 1980). In addition to reviewing the relevant smoking cessation literature, this chapter explores the possible reasons for our limited impact on the smoking of individuals with COPD. When considering nicotine addiction, psychiatric co-morbidity, demographic factors, and the cognitive–behavioral process of cessation, it becomes clear why we have been less successful in promoting smoking cessation for COPD patients. Taking these factors into consideration, this chapter concludes with a proposed model for conducting smoking cessation with this population.

Smoking Cessation and the Medical Management of COPD

Hays *et al.* (1998) refer to smoking cessation as the best medicine for combating current trends in the development of smoking-related disease, including COPD. Further, smoking cessation is consistently identified as the most important intervention with the potential for slowing or arresting the course of COPD (Celli, 1998; Heath & Mongia, 1998; Owens *et al.*, 1999). (See Chapter 4 for more information on the medical management of COPD.) The Clinical Practice Guidelines for Smoking Cessation, developed by a panel of experts convened by the Agency for Health Care Policy and Research (AHCPR), advocate that physicians carry out the following steps with each patient contact: ask and record tobacco-use status; provide smoking cessation advice; and promote smoking cessation (US Department of Health & Human Services, 1996). Reviews of the physician advice literature suggest that the approach alone can produce a 5–10% 1-year point prevalence abstinence rate (PPA), while the addition of a brief behavioral or pharmacological intervention can produce 20% or better PPA rates at 1 year (e.g., Richmond, 1999). (See Velicer *et al.* [1992] for a discussion of point prevalence and continuous abstinence smoking cessation outcome measures.) It is important to note that most of this work has been done with patients who do not have a chronic smoking-related illness, COPD or otherwise.

Despite limited empirical support, there are recurrent calls for the use of lung-function testing as a part of all outpatient office visits for smokers (e.g., Ferguson & Petty, 1998). It is suggested that asymptomatic smokers will become more motivated for smoking cessation if they are presented with evidence that their lung functioning has been impaired. Unfortunately, tests of this hypothesis have produced limited and mixed findings. The most convincing trial to date determined that a motivational package, including expiratory carbon monoxide (CO) as well as spirometry and respiratory symptom feedback, improved 1-year continuous abstinence rates from 7% (for usual care) to 20% (Risser & Belcher, 1990). However, another study revealed no incremental benefit for spirometric feedback along with smoking cessation counseling over the impact of counseling alone (Segnan *et al.*, 1991). Perhaps the most promising screening technique identified to date is the use of a methacholine challenge; the results of this test predict future lung-function decline independent of the current or baseline level of airway obstruction (Tashkin *et al.*, 1996).

While the use of measures of lung function and CO levels, as well as other indicators of current or future lung-function impairment, may prove to be reliable motivational aids for the general smoking population, it is unlikely that they will be of benefit to patients with confirmed COPD. The use of this sort of health risk or health impact feedback is designed to create a teachable moment. While there is no operational definition of what constitutes a teachable moment, a review of work that utilizes this concept suggests the following: a teachable moment constitutes clinical contact that either creates or occurs within the context of heightened motivation and receptivity for acting on health information (e.g., Stevens *et al.*, 1995; McBride *et al.*, 1999).

It is suggested that when we are able to produce information that individuals cannot assimilate into their old schemas (e.g., smoking does not affect me, there is no need to quit), then we have a chance to create new schemas (e.g., I am vulnerable) that will allow and improve the assimilation of new information that may lead to health behavior change. However, the opportunity to create this sort of effective teachable moment with COPD patients has long since passed. They have already experienced years of worsening respiratory symptoms, and been repeatedly advised by their physicians, friends, and family members that they should quit smoking. They have become seemingly impervious to additional health and health risk information. The hypothesized reasons for this include the interplay of psychological, psychiatric, and socioeconomic factors discussed below.

Can hospitalization create a teachable moment for patients with COPD? There is evidence that it does for other smokers. For example, Taylor *et al.* (1990) were among the first to use an intensive, multicomponent hospital-based smoking cessation program. Their work with patients hospitalized with acute myocardial infarction (MI) produced impressive outcomes, with the treatment program achieving 1-year PPA rates of 61% compared with 32% for patients receiving usual care (Taylor *et al.*, 1990). In follow-up research, these investigators extended the delivery of their program to other groups of hospitalized smokers. While the abstinence rates produced by this intervention remained superior to usual care, the outcomes did not match those of the initial work with acute MI patients, with 1-year PPA rates ranging from 27 to 31% (Taylor *et al.*, 1996; Miller *et al.*, 1997; Simon *et al.*, 1997).

Only one study has been completed that provided smoking cessation programming to hospitalized COPD patients. Investigators reported a 33.3% 6-month PPA rate for patients receiving a behavioral counseling, self-help guide; however, they acknowledged that they were able to conduct limited validation of participants' self-reported smoking status and had a 21.6% attrition rate (Pederson *et al.*, 1991). Little can be gleaned from the results of this trial, other than it appears that smoking cessation for hospitalized COPD patients is worthy of more study.

Taken together, the work of Taylor and colleagues, and others, e.g., the work of Rigotti *et al.* (1997, 1999) discussed below, suggests that hospitalization can produce a teachable moment for some smokers. However, it appears that the patients who are most receptive are those with an acute medical crisis (e.g., acute MI) associated with little forewarning. Patients with COPD do occasionally have medical crises; however, these acute events have an overlay of a gradually worsening respiratory, physical, and medical status (George, 1999). Thus, the average hospitalization for a patient with moderate-to-severe COPD would be unlikely to create the sort of attention-getting experience that an acute MI does, thereby minimizing the chance for a teachable moment.

Programmatic Smoking Cessation Efforts for Smokers with COPD

Other than research associated with the Lung Health Study, there have only been a handful of smoking cessation projects conducted for or including patients with COPD. Only two small pilot studies evaluated the impact of behavioral interventions. Turner *et al.* (1985) piloted an intervention incorporating nicotine fading (through brand changes) and stimulus control. This early trial produced one abstinent smoker out of four smokers at 3- and 6-month follow-up. Another pilot study by Tobin & Reynolds (1997) tested the use of a computer-delivered multicomponent, behavioral smoking cessation program. They achieved 3-month PPA for one of the eight patients in their study. However, several of the remaining participants registered large reductions in cigarettes smoked, suggesting that smokers with COPD can potentially benefit from a dynamic, interactive, and personalized smoking cessation program that is delivered via computer. (Further discussion of the possible merits of integrating such an approach within an overall smoking cessation program for COPD patients is described later in the chapter.)

Crowley *et al.* (1995) combined smoking cessation programming with home health care, an important part of COPD management once respiratory impairment becomes severe. The multicomponent intervention included smoking self-monitoring, nicotine gum, setting of quit dates, and monetary reinforcement of abstinence. At the end of the 12-week study, subjects in the experimental condition, who were rewarded with lottery tickets for obtaining CO levels consistent with abstinence, achieved 30-day continuous abstinence rates of 25%. This was encouraging given the late stage of these patients' COPD.

Another study evaluated the impact of a brief smoking cessation intervention for patients referred to an outpatient lung clinic (Tonnesen *et al.*, 1996). Using a brief motivational interview paired with educational brochures, the investigators achieved 1 year 30-day CO verified PPA rates of 5.2% (compared with 1.9% for usual care) for smokers who were smoking more than 10 cigarettes per day at the time of referral. (Inclusion in this trial was dependent on their already having refused participation in a nicotine replacement therapy study.) It is difficult to determine, however, how many of the participants had actually been diagnosed with COPD, as the patients were referred to the clinic for either a lung X-ray or lung-function testing.

The most comprehensive smoking cessation trial for patients with verifiable airway obstruction was conducted as part of the Lung Health Study. This multicenter North American trial, lasting from 1986 through 1994, randomly assigned smokers with mild-to-moderate airways obstruction to one of two smoking cessation intervention packages or to usual care. The study compared use of a multicomponent cognitive–behavioral smoking cessation program with inhaled ipratropium bromide (anticholinergic bronchodilator) versus the same program with a placebo inhaler (Anthonisen *et al.*, 1994). Since there was no demonstrated effect of the bronchodilator use either on smoking cessation or long-term function, reports from this project focus on a comparison of the multicomponent program versus usual care (e.g., Scanlon *et al.*, 2000). The Lung Health Study smoking cessation program produced encouraging results, with a 38.2% verified PPA rate at 5-year follow-up, compared with a 20% rate for those receiving usual care (Anthonisen *et al.*, 1994).

There appear to be at least two reasons why the Lung Health Study achieved more encouraging results. First, the project used an inclusion/exclusion criteria that excluded smokers with more advanced COPD ($FEV_1 \leqslant 90\%$ and $> 55\%$ of predicted and a ratio of FEV_1 to $FVC \leqslant 70\%$; Nides *et al.*, 1995). Secondly, they provided one of the most intensive, long-term, and comprehensive smoking cessation programs offered in any smoking cessation trial to date. (The components of the Lung Health Study smoking cessation intervention are discussed in more detail below.) Thus, the Lung Health Study treated smokers with less advanced COPD and provided them with more intensive and long-term cessation programming, both of which should lead to better outcomes (US Department of Health & Human Services, 1996).

Smoking Cessation and COPD: the Impact of Multiple Risk Factors

Smoking cessation trials have consistently identified the same variables associated with failed smoking cessation or relapse. These include less confidence in quitting (weak sense of self-efficacy), higher levels of nicotine dependence or heavier smoking rates, greater use of alcohol, greater respiratory impairment, limited education, lack of social support, the presence of other smokers in the house, fewer prior attempts to quit, higher numbers of stressful life events, and greater dysphoria or depression (Secker-Walker *et al.*, 1990; Hymowitz *et al.*, 1991; Nides *et al.*, 1995; Benowitz, 1999; Killen *et al.*, 1999; Smith *et al.*, 1999; Ockene *et al.*, 2000).

Unfortunately, these risk factors are more prevalent for patients showing moderate-to-severe COPD. For example, Kennedy *et al.* (1994) found that 52% of a sample of smokers with COPD had a lifetime prevalence of alcohol dependence. Further, a study of lung transplant survival rates found that 50% of their patient population had a pretransplant history of anxiety or mood disorder (Woodman *et al.*, 1999). Also, in a study noted earlier, a pilot study of smoking cessation for COPD patients found that 75% of the participants had past or current mood disorder or other psychiatric problems (Tobin & Reynolds, 1997). The following is no surprise: the majority of patients with moderate-to-severe COPD are chronic, heavy smokers with high levels of nicotine addiction (e.g., Kennedy *et al.*, 1994). Population-based research suggests that there is dynamic interplay of chronic illness, such as COPD, with increases in the frequency of stressful life events; these are associated with increased smoking, and ultimately, increased COPD-related mortality (Colby *et al.*, 1994). Common sense suggests that the remaining risk factors that predict continued smoking would also be over-represented in patients with moderate-to-severe COPD; these factors include poor confidence in their ability to quit smoking, greater respiratory impairment, limited education, lack of social support (e.g., individuals with a chronic illness often lose the support of family or friends due to compassion fatigue), presence of other smokers in the house, fewer attempts to quit smoking, and greater daily life stress (if only that occurring because of their worsening physical health).

In a hypothetical case, Fig. 12.1 follows the progression of COPD from the onset of smoking at age 18 through death from multiple system failure at age 72. By age 45, when the individual has already developed moderate disease, he has already smoked for 27 years, and he has ignored or disregarded his symptoms, as well as the pleas of his family and physician, for many years. Early in his smoking years he worked hard to ignore the health facts related to smoking, and possessed the common self-exempting beliefs that allow smokers to begin and continue to smoke:

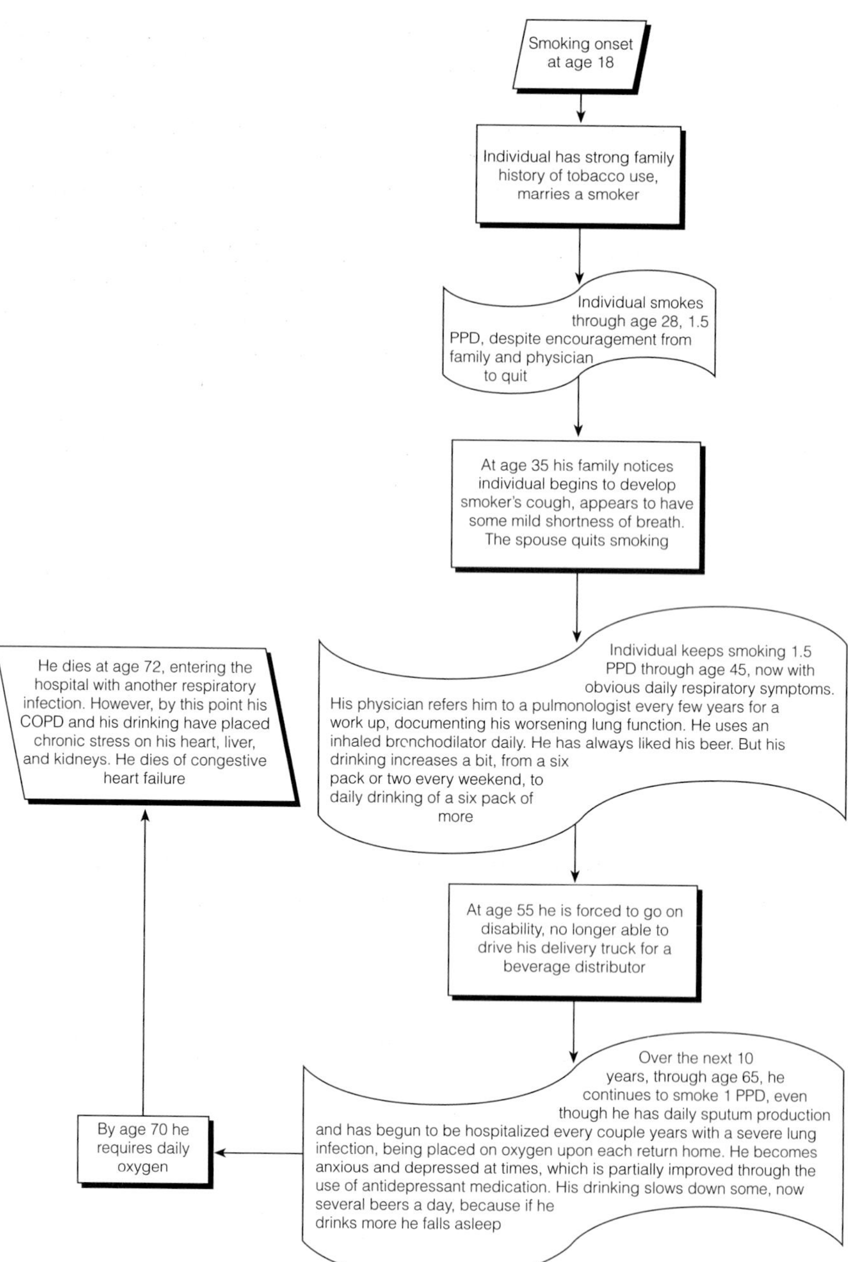

Figure 12.1

Progression of chronic obstructive pulmonary disease (COPD) from smoking onset through mortality. PPD = packs per day.

e.g., it won't happen to me, most smokers continue to smoke, the risk of smoking are overstated, etc. (Chapman et al., 1993; Williams & Clarke, 1997). By the time he experiences impairment in activities of daily living, he has developed an anxiety or depressive disorder, some degree of alcohol abuse, yet is still smoking. While the case is fictitious, any pulmonologist or pulmonary rehabilitation specialist will recognize the history. It would have been ideal to prevent this person's COPD through avoiding smoking onset. Secondary prevention of his COPD would have been possible through about the age of 40 by smoking cessation. Lastly, tertiary prevention of the worsening of his COPD might have been possible through age 65 or 70, probably slowing the decline of his lung functioning and improving his quality of life, if he had quit smoking later in his life. Sadly, this sort of progression is typical of many smokers with COPD. So the question remains: 'How should we approach smoking cessation with patients who already have developed COPD?'

The Ideal Smoking Cessation Program for a COPD Patient

The following program content represents our best scientific guess at what would constitute the most effective smoking cessation program for patients with moderate-to-severe COPD. Table 12.1 presents an overview of this proposed program. Each component will be reviewed briefly.

Pharmacotherapy

Given that patients with COPD are likely to be chronic, heavy, and strongly addicted smokers, use of any pharmacotherapy that would minimize the impact of nicotine withdrawal would be indicated. Recent

Table 12.1 Smoking cessation program components for COPD patients

Intervention class	Components
Pharmacotherapy	Nicotine replacement Bupropion
Multicomponent behavioral program	Group support Weekly or more frequent contact Long-term program, 1–2 years 1:1 contact with a clinician Stage-matched programming Maintenance program Weight management Ongoing medical monitoring Promotion of ongoing self-help

research has shown that withdrawal of nicotine for nicotine-dependent smokers can have physiological and mood-related effects that last for weeks or months (Gilbert *et al.*, 1999). As with other areas of smoking cessation research, there is a dearth of literature in this area for COPD patients. Nonetheless, existing research is encouraging. For example, Glover *et al.* (1997) completed an open-label pilot study of the use of a nicotine nasal spray by heavy smokers with COPD. They found that 31% of the 32 smokers in the study had verified PPA at 12-week follow-up. Also, the Lung Health Study included nicotine gum as part of its smoking cessation program, and achieved encouraging 1–5-year abstinence rates for smokers with mild-to-moderate airway obstruction (e.g., Anthonisen *et al.*, 1994). However, no attempt was made to separate the impact of the behavioral program from the pharmacotherapeutic effect in this study; thus, it is difficult to determine the relative contribution of the various components of the Lung Health Study cessation program. The work of Lewis *et al.* (1998) also suggests that nicotine replacement therapy (NRT) has a place in the treatment regimens for smokers with COPD. They found that in a study of a brief smoking cessation intervention for hospitalized patients, including use of a nicotine patch, patients admitted with respiratory disease had among the best 6-month follow-up PPA rates (46%). However, the study exclusion criteria included active substance abuse and psychiatric illness, both common co-morbid conditions for COPD patients, which suggests that these results cannot be generalized to the general population of patients with advanced COPD.

Findings from the general smoking cessation literature again suggest that inclusion of NRT and other pharmacotherapy options will be important when facilitating smoking cessation for COPD patients. For example, the successful hospital-based cessation program developed and tested by Taylor *et al.* (1996) resulted in increased prescription and correct use of NRT for patients in the treatment group. Further, the relative lack of success of other hospital-based programs has been attributed to the underuse of NRT (Rigotti *et al.*, 1997, 1999). Certainly the use of antidepressant medication (e.g., bupropion, nortriptyline) to ease nictone withdrawal has shown great promise in the general smoking population, including when they are used in combination with NRT (Prochaszka *et al.*, 1998; Jorenby *et al.*, 1999). In addition, research with these medications demonstrates that they ease withdrawal separately from an antidepressant effect, as they decrease withdrawal symptoms and improve cessation rates even in smokers who do not demonstrate clinical depression (e.g., Shiffman *et al.*, 2000).

Multicomponent behavioral program

The smoking cessation intervention package provided as part of the Lung Health Study is perhaps the most comprehensive and intensive smoking cessation program offered as part of any clinical trial to date. The program's smoking cessation specific and nonspecific treatment components included:

- ongoing comprehensive medical and lung-function monitoring;
- a 12-week cognitive behavioral group program containing education in stimulus control, role-playing, assertiveness training, weight management, relaxation training, and relapse prevention;
- 6 months or more of NRT (2 mg gum) for participants and significant others also trying to quit;
- monthly maintenance sessions; and
- unlimited extended intensive intervention for anyone who relapses (Murray *et al.*, 1997).

While it is difficult to identify which components of this program were most important in achieving long-term behavior change, it is likely that the higher dose of therapeutic contact, both in terms of number of contacts and the longitudinal nature of these contacts (several years in many cases), were among the most important aspects of the program. Meta-analyses of the smoking cessation literature has shown that programs that provide longer-term treatment, including more treatment sessions, tend to produce better outcomes (US Department of Health & Human Services, 1996).

While we do not as yet have a precise understanding of the dose–response relationship of density and number of therapeutic contacts and smoking cessation outcomes, it is possible that research will demonstrate a similar relationship to that found in the general psychotherapy literature. This latter area of research suggests that to achieve incremental improvements in outcomes, an intervention must exponentially increase the number of sessions. For example, approximately 25% of patients are found to demonstrate significant improvement after one psychotherapy session. To achieve similar improvement for 50% of the patient sample, one must increase contacts to 8 sessions, and to produce similar improvements for a total of 75% of the original sample, the session count must increase to 26 (Howard *et al.*, 1986). This is similar to individuals who desire to quit smoking: some quit on their own, some quit following brief advice from their physician, and others require more extensive therapeutic support. Smokers with COPD have proven to be among those individuals who require more intensive and frequent doses of cessation services.

It is likely that most patients with moderate or more severe COPD would be classified as Pre-Contemplators in terms of the Transtheoretical or Stage of Change model of health behavior change (e.g., Prochaska & DiClemente, 1992). It appears that it would be particularly important to match the intervention content, including the nature of physician advice (Reynolds & Myers, 1999), to the individual's current stage of change.

Given that most smokers with COPD are likely to be in the Pre-Contemplation or Contemplation stages of change, it will be important to engage them in change processes that match these stages (Velicer *et al.*, 1995). For example, Pre-Contemplators or Contemplators are unlikely to benefit from attempting active behavior change efforts because they are filled with doubt about their ability to change and/or are unmotivated to change. Therefore, most of the early work with smokers with COPD will be to engage them in a process where they can frequently consider what might motivate them to quit smoking, the advantages of quitting that are personally relevant to them, and why there is hope that they could quit.

To maximize the odds of quitting, it appears important to provide COPD patients with multiple forms of intervention, including a group-based multicomponent behavioral program, 1:1 contact with a clinician (physician, nurse, or other ancillary health care provider), and a self-help program that is integrated with the former two modalities to promote engagement in their behavior change efforts. There is a growing number of self-help smoking cessation programs that can be personalized yet efficiently delivered to entire populations, including print (e.g., Velicer *et al.*, 1999), audio (Reynolds *et al.*, 1998), and Internet delivered programs (Jordan *et al.*, 1999). The integration of such self-help methods with traditional smoking cessation efforts may accelerate or otherwise enhance the efficacy of traditional clinician-provided programs. It appears vital that this be tested with a population of patients with COPD. As noted above, Tobin & Reynolds (1997) have demonstrated that patients with chronic lung disease can be engaged in a computer-based self-help program to impact their smoking.

Weight Management Focus and Ongoing Medical Monitoring

Investigators and clinicians agree that the health benefits of smoking cessation are far greater than the risks associated with the average weight gain that can follow quitting. However, the already compromised health status of COPD patients merits great attention to this issue during and following nicotine abstinence (e.g., Wise *et al.*, 1998). The issue of weight gain was addressed by the Lung Health Study, which found that 33% of their sample of smokers, again with mild-to-moderate COPD, gained 10 kg or more of weight (O'Hara *et al.*, 1998). Further, 19.1% of the women who sustained abstinence for 1 year gained 20% of baseline weight. Weight gain was associated with lower FEV1 and FVC at 5-year follow-up for continuous smokers, intermittent smokers, and sustained quitters (Wise *et al.*, 1998). Sustained quitters showed a weight-gain-related reduction in FVC of 17.4 ml/kg for men and 10.6 ml/kg for women.

Frequent medical monitoring of smoking cessation efforts appears essential for this patient population, not only to closely monitor vital information such as lung function and weight but also to engage the patient in the collaborative self-management of their disease (Make, 1994). As noted earlier, empirically supported pharamacotherapies for smoking cessation are strongly indicated for smokers with COPD (unless contraindicated by other factors). Further, regular contact with their health care provider can only reinforce the importance of patients' smoking cessation efforts. Such ongoing monitoring was a component of the Lung Health Study intervention (e.g., Nides *et al.*, 1995).

Conclusions

Scientific evidence shows that smoking cessation produces health benefits even for patients with moderate COPD. To date, however, there has been limited research focused on smoking cessation with these patients. Perhaps this is due to the multiple number of psychosocial risk factors for continued smoking that are prevalent in this population of smokers. However, it is time that we engage smokers with COPD in multisystem, intensive, and long-term programs designed to facilitate smoking cessation. This would involve the integration of contemporary multicomponent behavioral group programs, empirically supported pharmacotherapies such as NRT and bupropion, and self-help programs (manual, audio, or computer-based) that can extend the therapeutic contact with the smoker into their daily lives. As yet, we do not know what dose of behavioral therapies, or what combinations of the above components, are going to prove most effective for patients with COPD. Future trials, however, should first work under the assumption that more is better.

One final challenge involves the payment for such intensive services for patients with COPD: unless health care systems cover the cost or third-party reimbursement is provided, our research efforts will not impact the general health and well-being of this population. Therefore, it is incumbent on investigators to conduct both cost-effectiveness and cost–benefit analyses associated with clinical trials (Warner, 1998). Unless smoking cessation coverage – including coverage of intensive and prolonged services for those already medically compromised – is mandated by state or federal governments, convincing cost–benefit analyses may be the only argument that will compel managed care organizations and insurance companies to provide coverage for these services.

Acknowledgment

I wish to thank Tom Creer, as well as Mark VanderWeg and Barbara Bolin, my wife, for their support and assistance in the preparation of this chapter.

References

Anthonisen, N.R., Connett, J.E., Kiley, J.P., *et al.* (1994). Effects of smoking intervention and the use of an inhaled anticholinergic bronchodilator on the rate of decline of FEV1. The Lung Health Study. *Journal of the American Medical Association*, 272, 1497–1505.

Benowitz, N.L. (1999). Nicotine addiction. *Primary Care*, 26, 611–631.

Brown, C.A., Crombie, I.K., Smith, W.C., & Tunstall-Pedoe, H. (1991). The impact of quitting smoking on symptoms of chronic bronchitis: results of the Scottish Heart Health Study. *Thorax*, 46, 112–116.

Brundtland, G.H. (2000). *Opening address.* International Policy Conference on Children and Tobacco, Washington, DC, March 18, 2000.

Camilli, A.I., Burrows, B., Knudson, R.J. Lyle, S.K., & Lebowitz, M.D. (1987). Longitudinal changes in forced expiratory volume in one second in adults. Effects of smoking and smoking cessation. *American Review of Respiratory Disease*, 135, 794–799.

Celli, B.R. (1998). Standards for the optimal management of COPD: a summary. *Chest*, 113(Suppl.), 283s–287s.

Centers for Disease Control (1999). Cigarette smoking among adults in the United States, 1997. *Morbidity & Mortality Weekly Report*, 48, 993–996.

Chapman, S., Wong, W.L., & Smith, W. (1993). Self-exempting beliefs about smoking and health: differences between smokers and ex-smokers. *American Journal of Public Health*, 83, 215–219.

Colby, J.P., Linsky, A.S., & Straus, M.A. (1994). Social stress and state-to-state differences in smoking and smoking related mortality in the United States. *Social Science & Medicine*, 38, 373–381.

Crowley, T.J., MacDonald, M.J., & Walter, M.I. (1995). Behavioral anti-smoking trial in chronic obstructive pulmonary disease patients. *Psychopharmacology*, 119, 193–204.

Daughton, D.M., Fix, A.J., Kass, I., & Patil, K.D. (1980). Smoking cessation among patients with chronic obstructive pulmonary disease (COPD). *Addictive Behavior*, 5, 125–128.

Ferguson, G.T. & Petty, T.L. (1998). Screening and early intervention for COPD. *Hospital Practice*, 33, 67–72, 79–80, 83–84.

George, R.B. (1999). Course and prognosis of chronic obstructive pulmonary disease. *American Journal of Medical Science*, 318, 103–106.

Gilbert, D.G., McClernon, F.J., Rabinovich, N.E., *et al.* (1999). EEG, physiology, and task-related mood fail to resolve across 31 days of smoking abstinence: relations to depressive traits, nicotine exposure, and dependence. *Experimental and Clinical Psychopharmacology*, 7, 427–443.

Glover, E.D., Glover, P.N., Abrons, J.L., & Franzon, M. (1997). Smoking cessation among COPD and chronic bronchitis patients using the nicotine nasal spray. *American Journal of Health Behavior*, 21, 310–317.

Hays, J.T., Dale, L.C., Hurt, R.D., & Croghan, I.T. (1998). Trends in smoking-related diseases. Why smoking cessation is still the beset medicine. *Postgraduate Medicine*, 104, 56–62, 65–66, 71.

Heath, J.M. & Mongia, R. (1998). Chronic bronchitis: primary care management. *American Family Physician*, 57, 2365–2372, 2376–2378.

Howard, K.I., Kopta, S.M., Krause, M.S., & Orlinsky, D.E. (1986). The dose response relationship in psychotherapy. *American Psychologist*, 41, 159–164.

Hymowitz, N., Sexton, M., Ockene, J., & Grandits, G. (1991). Baseline factors associated with smoking cessation and relapse. MRFIT Research Group. *Preventive Medicine*, 20, 590–601.

Jordan, J.C., Reynolds, R.V., Myers, D.L., *et al.* (1999). *Comparison of Internet delivered and printed self-help smoking cessation programs with hospital employees.* Presented at the meeting of the Society for Research on Nicotine/Tobacco, San Diego, CA, March 6, 1999.

Jorenby, D.E., Leischow, S.J., Nides, M.A., *et al.* (1999). A controlled trial of sustained-release bupropion, a nicotine patch, or both for smoking cessation. *New England Journal of Medicine*, 340, 685–691.

Kanner, R.E., Connett, J.E., Williams, D.E., & Buist, A.S. (1999). Effects of randomized assignment to a smoking cessation intervention and changes in smoking habits on respiratory symptoms in smokers with early chronic obstructive pulmonary disease: the Lung Health Study. *American Journal of Medicine*, 106, 410–416.

Kennedy, J.A., Crowley, T.J., Cottler, L.B., & Mager, D.E. (1994). Substance use diagnoses in smokers with lung disease. *American Journal on Addictions*, 2, 126–130.

Killen, J.D., Fortmann, S.P., Davis, L., Strausberg, L., & Varady, A. (1999). Do heavy smokers benefit from higher dose nicotine patch therapy? *Experimental and Clinical Psychopharmacology*, 7, 226–233.

Lantz, P.M., Jacobson, P.D., Warner, K.E., *et al.* (2000). Investing in youth tobacco control: a review of smoking prevention and control strategies. *Tobacco Control*, 9, 47–63.

Leeder, S.R., Colley, J.R., Corkhill, R., & Holland, W.W. (1977). Change in respiratory symptom prevalence in adults who alter their smoking habits. *American Journal of Epidemiology*, 105, 522–529.

Lewis, S.F., Piasecki, T.M., Fiore, M.C., Anderson, J.E., & Baker, T.B. (1998). Transdermal nicotine replacement for hospitalized patients: a randomized clinical trial. *Preventive Medicine*, 27, 296–303.

McBride, C.M., Scholes, D., Grothaus, L.C., Curry, S.J., Ludman, E., & Albright, J. (1999). Evaluation of a minimal self-help smoking cessation intervention following cervical cancer screening. *Preventive Medicine*, 29, 133–138.

Make, B. (1994). Collaborative self-management strategies for patients with respiratory disease. *Respiratory Care*, 39, 566–579.

Miller, N.H., Smith, P.M., DeBusk, R.F., Sobel, D.S., & Taylor, C.B. (1997). Smoking cessation in hospitalized patients. Results of a randomized trial. *Archives of Internal Medicine*, 157, 409–415.

Murray, R.P., Voelker, H.T., Rakos, R.F., Nides, M.A., McCutcheon, V.J., & Bjornson, W. (1997). Intervention for relapse to smoking: the Lung Health Study restart programs. *Addictive Behavior*, 22, 281–286.

Murray, R.P., Anthonisen, N.R., Connett, J.E., *et al.* (1998). Effects of multiple attempts to quit smoking and relapses to smoking on pulmonary function. Lung Health Study Research Group. *Journal of Clinical Epidemiology*, 51, 1317–1326.

Nides, M.A., Rakos, R.F., Gonzales, D., *et al.* (1995). Predictors of initial smoking cessation and relapse through the first 2 years of the Lung Health Study. *Journal of Consulting and Clinical Psychology*, 63, 60–69.

O'Hara, P., Connett, J.E., Lee, W.W., Nides, M., Murray, R., & Wise, R. (1998). Early and late weight gain following smoking cessation in the Lung Health Study. *American Journal of Epidemiology*, 148, 821–830.

Ockene, J.K., Emmons, K.M., Mermelstein, R.J., *et al.* (2000). Relapse and maintenance issues for smoking cessation. *Health Psychology*, 19(Suppl.), 17–31.

Owens, M.W., Markewitz, B.A., & Payne, D.K. (1999). Outpatient management of chronic obstructive pulmonary disease. *American Journal of Medical Science*, 318, 79–83.

Pederson, L.L., Wanklin, J.M., & Lefcoe, N.M. (1991). The effects of counseling on smoking cessation among patients hospitalized with chronic obstructive pulmonary disease: a randomized clinical trial. *International Journal of Addictions*, 26, 107–119.

Prochaska, J.O. & DiClemente, C.C. (1992). Stages of change in the modification of problem behaviors. In: M. Herson, R.M. Eisler, & P.M. Miller (Eds), *Progress in behavior modification* (pp. 184–214). Sycamore, IL: Sycamore Press.

Prochazka, A.V., Weaver, J.M., Keller, R.T., Fryer, G.E., Licari, P.A., & Lofaso, D. (1998). A randomized trial of nortriptyline for smoking cessation. *Archives of Internal Medicine*, 158, 2035–2039.

Reynolds, R.V. & Myers, D. (1999). *An information management approach for smoking cessation.* SBIR/NHLBI Phase I grant proposal, pending review.

Reynolds, R.V., Relyea, G., Thompson, F., & Berger, P. (1998). *Individualized and personalized self-help smoking cessation: a serial case study evaluation.* Presented at the meeting of the Society of Behavioral Medicine, New Orleans, LA, March 1998.

Richmond, R.L. (1999). Physicians can make a difference with smokers: evidence-based clinical approaches. *International Journal of Tuberculosis and Lung Disease*, 3, 100–112.

Rigotti, N.A., Arnsten, J.H., McKool, K.M., Wood-Reid, K.M., Pasternak, R.C., & Singer, D.E. (1997). Efficacy of a smoking cessation program for hospital patients. *Archives of Internal Medicine*, 157, 2653–2660.

Rigotti, N.A., Arnsten, J.H., McKool, K.M., Wood-Reid, K.M., Singer, D.E., & Pasternak, R.C. (1999). The use of nicotine-replacement therapy by hospitalized smokers. *American Journal of Preventive Medicine*, 17, 255–259.

Risser, N.L. & Belcher, D.W. (1990). Adding spirometry, carbon monoxide, and pulmonary symptom results to smoking cessation counseling: a randomized trial. *Journal of General Internal Medicine*, 5, 16–22.

Scanlon, P.D., Connett, J.E., Waller, L.A., *et al.* (2000). Smoking cessation and lung function in mild-to-moderate chronic obstructive pulmonary disease. *American Journal of Respiratory & Critical Care Medicine*, 161, 381–390.

Schwartz, J., Timonen, K.L. & Pekkanen, J. (2000). Respiratory effects of environmental tobacco smoke in a panel study of asthmatics and symptomatic children. *American Journal of Respiratory and Critical Care Medicine*, 161, 802–806.

Secker-Walker, R.H., Flynn, B.S., Solomon, L.J., Vacek, P.M., & Bronson, D.L. (1990). Predictors of smoking behavior change 6 and 18 months after individual counseling during periodic health examinations. *Preventive Medicine*, 19, 675–685.

Segnan, N., Ponti, A., Battista, R.N., *et al.* (1991). A randomized trial of smoking cessation interventions in general practice in Italy. *Cancer Causes and Control*, 2, 239–246.

Shiffman, S., Johnston, J.A., Khayrallah, M., *et al.* (2000). The effect of bupropion on nicotine craving and withdrawal. *Psychopharmacology*, 148, 33–40.

Simon, J.A., Solkowitz, S.N., Carmody, T.P., & Browner, W.S. (1997). Smoking cessation after surgery. A randomized trial. *Archives of Internal Medicine*, 157, 1371–1376.

Smith, P.M., Kraemer, H.C., Miller, N.H., DeBusk, R.F., & Taylor, C.B. (1999). In-hospital smoking cessation programs: Who responds, who doesn't? *Journal of Consulting and Clinical Psychology*, 67, 19–27.

Stevens, V.J., Severson, J., Lichtenstein, E., Little, S.J., & Leben, J. (1995). Making the most of a teachable moment: a smokeless-tobacco cessation intervention in the dental office. *American Journal of Public Health*, 85, 231–235.

Tashkin, D.P., Altose, M.D., Connett, J.E., Kanner, R.E., Lee, W.W., & Wise, R.A. (1996). Methacholine reactivity predicts changes in lung function over time in smokers with early chronic obstructive pulmonary disease. The Lung Health Study Research Group. *American Journal of Respiratory & Critical Care Medicine*, 153, 1802–1811.

Taylor, C.B., Miller, N.H., Killen, J.D., & DeBusk, R.F. (1990). Smoking cessation after acute myocardial infarction: effects of a nurse-managed intervention. *Annals of Internal Medicine*, 113, 118–123.

Taylor, C.B., Miller, N.H., Herman, S., *et al.* (1996). A nurse-managed smoking cessation program for hospitalized smokers. *American Journal of Public Health*, 86, 1557–1560.

Tobin, D.L. & Reynolds, R.V. (1997). Computer delivered smoking self-management for smokers with chronic respiratory disease. *The Health Psychologist*, 19, 20–23, 27.

Tonnesen, P., Mikkelsen, K., Markholst, C., *et al.* (1996). Nurse-conducted smoking cessation with minimal intervention in a lung clinic: a randomized controlled study. *European Respiratory Journal*, 9, 2351–2355.

Townsend, M.C., DuChene, A.G., Morgan, J., & Browner, W.S. (1991). Pulmonary function in relation to cigarette smoking and smoking cessation. MRFIT Research Group. *Preventive Medicine*, 20, 621–637.

Turner, S.A., Daniels, J.L., & Hollandsworth, J.G. (1985). The effects of a multicomponent smoking cessation program with chronic obstructive pulmonary disease outpatients. *Addictive Behaviors*, 10, 87–90.

US Department of Health and Human Services. (1984). *The health consequences of smoking in chronic obstructive lung disease: a report of the surgeon general.* Washington, DC: US Government Printing Office.

US Department of Health and Human Services. (1996). *Smoking cessation: clinical practice guideline.* (AHCPR Publication No. 96-0692). Washington, DC: US Government Printing Office.

US Department of Health & Human Services (2000). *Healthy people* (conference edition in two volumes). Washington, DC: US Department of Health and Human Services.

Velicer, W.F., Prochaska, J.O., Rossi, J.S., & Snow, M.G. (1992). Assessing outcome in smoking cessation studies. *Psychological Bulletin*, 111, 23–41.

Velicer, W.F., Fava, J.L., Prochaska, J.O., Abrams, D.B., Emmons, K.M., & Pierce, J. (1995). Distribution of smokers by stage in three representative samples. *Preventive Medicine*, 24, 401–411.

Velicer, W.F., Prochaska, J.O., Fava, J.L., Laforge, R.G., & Rossi, J.S. (1999). Interactive versus noninteractive interventions and dose-response relationships for stage-matched smoking cessation programs in a managed care setting. *Health Psychology*, 18, 21–28.

Warner, K.E. (1998). Smoking out the incentives for tobacco control in managed care settings. *Tobacco Control*, 7(Suppl. 1), s50–s54.

Williams, T. & Clarke, V.A. (1997). Optimistic bias in beliefs about smoking. *Australian Journal of Psychology*, 49(2), 106–112.

Wise, R.A. (1997). Changing smoking patterns and mortality from chronic obstructive pulmonary disease. *Preventive Medicine*, 26, 418–421.

Wise, R.A., Enright, P.L., Connett, J.E., *et al.* (1998). Effect of weight gain on pulmonary function after smoking cessation in the Lung Health Study. *American Journal of Respiratory and Critical Care Medicine*, 157, 866–872.

13
Future issues in behavioral science research with respiratory disorders

Michele Hindi-Alexander, Gregory Fritz, and Thomas L. Creer

Editors' note—*In the chapter that follows, Michelle Hindi-Alexander and her colleagues describe policies regarding the management and control of respiratory disorders. In doing so, their conclusions are Dickensonian in that they echo the phrase, 'It was the best of times, it was the worst of times, it was the age of wisdom, it was the age of foolishness. . . .' Given advances in the treatment and management of asthma and chronic obstructive pulmonary disease (COPD), patients can make the critical difference in helping to control their condition. By integrating current medical knowledge and advice with the self-management skills they perform, patients can control asthma and, in many instances, COPD. Achieving this goal is, to a large measure, the responsibility of patients themselves; attaining the goal, in turn, is reflective of the 'best of times.'*

The treatment of the worldwide epidemic of tuberculosis, on the other hand, can only be considered as the 'worst of times' or 'the age of foolishness. . . .' As Alexander and colleagues note, the approach to treatment ignores much of the knowledge and research regarding TB that was accumulated in the first half of the 20th century. The current approaches place an undeserved amount of emphasis on direct observed therapy – a procedure that produces significantly better results only when compared to hypothetical data – while ignoring the potential role of patients in both treating their disease and preventing its spread to others. The lack of prevention effort is perplexing: prevention of tuberculosis was the major reason the disease was controlled throughout the world in the first half of the last century. The lack of a preventive strategies has, in addition, resulted in a prevalence rate where almost one-third of the world's population are infected with MTB or Mycobacterium tuberculosis (Dye et al., 1999). Preventive measures in countries such as Russia are nonexistent (e.g., Program in Infectious Disease and Social Change, 1999). This has permitted the TB bacterium to not only explode in prison populations but also to be spread in surrounding communities by unprotected guards and other prison personnel. The overall conclusion is that if tuberculosis is ever to be conquered, it will require a cooperative effort by health care personnel and the population they are asked to serve. Unfortunately, there are no indications of this trend throughout the world.

The Role of Behavior in Health and Disease

Behavior is a major intervening variable in both health and disease. Directly or indirectly, behavior is implicated in the 10 leading causes of death: heart disease, cancer, cerebrovascular disease, accidents, chronic obstructive pulmonary disease (COPD), pneumonia and influenza, diabetes mellitus, suicide, chronic liver disease, and atherosclerosis (Centers for Disease Control, 1990). In fact, it can be argued that the leading contributor to death in both developed and developing countries is risky behavior (Blumenthal *et al.*, 1994; World Health Organization, 1999).

Behavior may be defined as a wide range of observable actions (e.g., Bourne & Russo, 1998); it includes actions and reactions that occur in response to internal or external stimuli. Ford (1987) provided a broader definition by referring to behavior as all life processes or functions. The broader term is more applicable in the present context in that it recognizes that all human responses and functions are made possible by a biological structure. Its diversity provides the 'constituents of the stream of life' (Ford, 1987, p. 5). Behavior interacts with biological and environmental factors; the interactions, in turn, generate major determinants of health and disease. Recognition of the significance of these interactions spawned the fields of behavioral medicine, health psychology, health education, and both pediatric psychology and behavioral pediatrics; we will use the term behavioral medicine as encompassing these areas.

The first conference regarding behavioral aspects of disease was held in 1969 at the University of Kentucky. Since then research in behavioral sciences in general, and behavioral medicine in particular, has become a significant part of biomedical research. Findings from this research have been shown to be relevant to the prevention, diagnosis, and treatment of disease or illness. The magnitude of growth and maturity occurring in behavioral sciences in the past three decades has been impressive. This is certainly true with respect to behavioral science and respiratory diseases. The inextricable linkage of behavior to respiratory disorders is, as reflected in the chapters of this book, paramount to our understanding of all respiratory diseases and how they are treated. The content of the chapters indicate that we have started on the road towards fulfilling a comment made by Sir William Osler who, in referring to a patient with tuberculosis, remarked that: 'It is just as important to know what is going on in man's head as in his chest' (Blumenthal *et al.*, 1994).

Reflecting the importance of the interaction between behavior and health, the areas subsumed under the term behavioral medicine have evolved to integrate physical, environmental, emotional, and mental aspects of health and illness in both research and practice. It is widely accepted that decreasing behavioral risk factors will result in a lower incidence of disease, and that behavior changes influence the course of a variety of diseases and their response to treatment (World Health Organization, 1999). During the last three decades, there has been considerable research directed at the development and implementation of behavioral strategies that effectively encourage people to adopt health-promoting behaviors. These efforts are important in unraveling the intricate and interacting roles that poverty, culture, education, gender, age, and ethnicity play in health behavior; the findings, in turn, have implications for disease progression and remission. The successful implementation of behavioral medicine methods in health care requires knowledge about relevant risk factors, how to bring about desired behavioral change, and the most effective way to identify populations likely to benefit from these behavioral interventions (Redline *et al.*, 1996).

Behavioral medicine is more than psychology, education, and physiology combined; it also concerns neurological, immunological, endocrinological, and pharmacological interactions in the body. The hallmark of behavioral medicine is its capacity to foster connections and interactions among basic and applied sciences, and to translate this knowledge into health promotion, disease prevention, improved patient care, and enhanced quality of life. This characterization of the field still faces challenge by parts of the medical community, although an interdisciplinary team approach including behavioral scientists has proven successful with several of the disorders, e.g., asthma, cystic fibrosis, and COPD, described in this book. We expect that continued solid and credible outcomes research will promote the use of behavioral techniques in respiratory diseases. In addition, the challenge in the future will be to determine mechanisms whereby biological, behavioral, and environmental processes act in concert to promote health and reduce the impact of disease (Blumenthal *et al.*, 1994; World Health Organization, 1999).

Biomedical and technological advances are changing disease management. For example, it is known that antibiotics have a broad-spectrum aspect that they can be used to treat an array of conditions, and that combination therapy is often effective where monotherapy fails. This is certainly the case with tuberculosis and HIV. At a more basic level, a polygenetic basis is to be considered when a single gene cannot be identified. This recognizes that generally no single gene, bacterium, or environmental event can completely account for the onset and progression of a specific disease; while interventions at the level of gene expression are promising in the management of a variety of diseases, particularly cystic fibrosis, most diseases are multicausal and thus require complex and interdisciplinary treatments. These interventions are complicated by adherence behavior which, in turn, becomes even more difficult to predict. To further confuse matters, the increased longevity of the population has created a trend away from acute infectious diseases toward chronic illness and co-morbidities (World Health Organization, 1998). All these factors point to a need to broaden our therapeutic approaches, and to move away from a reductionistic stance toward an integrative approach.

In respiratory disorders, as in most other chronic conditions, behavior plays many roles, ranging from being a risk factor or cofactor of the disorder, to that of being a health promoter or facilitator of appropriate change. Traditional lifestyle changes associated with respiratory disorders include smoking prevention, cessation, adherence to treatment regimens, and the change of behaviors to include exercise and/or diet patterns. We will examine some of the interactions between the behavioral and physiological processes that occur at various stages of respiratory disorders. In doing so, we hope to provide some answers to the following questions: How do behavioral and physiological factors interact to achieve prevention? What role do these factors play in the development, management, and rehabilitation of respiratory diseases? How does motivation develop? How can interdisciplinary collaborative research be facilitated? We propose a paradigm – therapeutic behavior analysis – to explore the interaction between physiology and behavior as it relates to respiratory disorders (Boner *et al.*, 1992; Eakin *et al.*, 1996; Nguyen *et al.*, 1996). We summarize progress made in using the model in respiratory illnesses, as well as identifying opportunities for future research.

The Anatomy of Behavior Change

The disease framework often utilized assumes that the risk behaviors that contributed to the development of disease can be easily modified. For this to occur, the culprit needs to be replaced by a new 'healthy' behavior. Behavior change is usually the first intervention, as exemplified by smoking cessation (Blumenthal, *et al.* 1994; see also Chapter 12). The inherent expectation is that some strategy to either adapt to the changes neces-sitated by the disease process, or to implement a therapeutic plan to counteract those processes is needed.

To modify behavior, we need to refine our understanding of the principles governing behavior change. With that in mind, Redd (1994) proposes five questions for future research:

1 What common behavioral effects are associated with specific disease and treatment modes?
2 How do such effects vary between individuals and what are their determinants?
3 How do the behavioral sequelae of respiratory diseases and treatment affect activities of daily life?
4 What are the psychological and physiological mechanisms underlying change in health behavior?
5 What prognostic implications do such lifestyle changes have for the course of disease?

To provide answers for these questions, we must analyze a large set of behaviors. We must then bring some semblance of order out of the myriad array of potential behaviors; out of individualized inventories of common behavioral profiles associated with specific disorders, treatments, or sequelae. These subsets of behaviors need to be categorized. As some profiles emerge, a common mechanism of action pointing to some common intervention may materialize.

An appreciation that behavior may be as much a state as it is a trait leads to the realization that adherence to a specific recommendation or treatment cannot be expected to reoccur reliably or to generalize to other conditions. To propel the field forward, a better grasp of the *contexts* which drive behavior change is necessary. The point is based on the assumption that people are complex, open systems that exist and develop only in transaction with these contexts. In this model, we each construct our own developmental pathway and functional patterns, within changing and variable conditions, provided by our bodies and these contexts (Ford & Urban, 1998). These interactive pathways predicate that the cataloguing of individual barriers and facilitators are the essential elements for beginning to understand the long-term retention of newly acquired behaviors, may be the next necessary step. Much of this has been accomplished already, as noted in earlier chapters. Just as dissection and knowledge of anatomy and physiology was basic to the progress of medicine in general, so is the understanding of the 'anatomy and physiology' of behavior change essential to the success of behavioral medicine.

Behavior change relevant to respiratory disorders can be voluntary or involuntary. It is involuntary when a disease process insidiously imposes changes in someone's behavior. Almost surreptitiously, a person with COPD may gradually adapt to a loss of the ability to walk as fast or as far as usual, to climb stairs, or to participate in a favorite sport. Children with asthma begin to state that they do not like sports because they think they are not as good at these activities as their nonasthmatic peers; adults with respiratory disorders also tend to rationalize alterations in their abilities. Only when one becomes cognizant of these subtle changes, can motivation develop. One can then voluntarily exercise a measure of control over the effects of the disease by instituting changes. Such actions might include smoking cessation for pulmonary disease in general or, in the case of asthma in particular, premedicating before exercise if this is a trigger of asthma.

The willingness to institute change is, as noted, a dynamic and complex process that may include psychological, physiological, environmental, sociocultural, religious, economic, and political variables. These factors may act alone or in combination; they may directly or indirectly encourage or discourage the process of behavior change. The salient motivating factor for behavior change is a need or gap – either perceived or real – between where one is and where one wants or wishes to be physically, emotionally, or environmentally. For individuals with respiratory disease, the need or wish may be to participate in sports or to sleep through the night. As is well known, these needs and desires become goals that, depending on their strength, provide an impetus for modifying one's behavior.

As noted earlier, it is understood that behavior patterns and changes develop over time through interactive activities such as reading, listening, observing, speaking, and performing. Thus, behavior is an open, dynamic state influenced by continuous input from and interaction with new information, environmental changes, and both physiological and psychological contexts. Because of this continuous input/interaction, behavior change is impermanent. If behavior is to be appropriate, it has to be adaptive, with ongoing feedback obtained from evaluating and re-evaluating its effects on oneself, on one's environment, and on other individuals (Ford & Urban, 1998). This dynamic, interactive process underlies all behaviors, including those affecting respiratory health. Because of the complexity of this process, the efficacy of a behavioral intervention often cannot be measured for years; hence, longitudinal studies are needed to gain a better grasp of these interactions. As aptly described by McGinnis (1994, p. 217): 'this labyrinth of interconnectedness' adds to the 'paradox of behavioral medicine that is unlike other branches of science: the more enlightened we become, the more complex are our solutions.'

The critical path to behavior change begins with new information, which can take the form of a health care provider's advice, news, a pamphlet, or a hand-out. New information alone does not constitute education. Furthermore, although a necessary condition, education alone is not sufficient to induce behavior change. Education of everyone, patients or health care professionals alike, requires mastering the information so that it can be translated into action. To achieve both the acquisition of information and the performance of new behaviors, information content must be appropriate in terms of language and vocabulary level; in addition, contextual variables must be culture, age, and gender sensitive. The extent to which these requirements are met provides the basis for acceptance or rejection of the information. If the new information is tailored to fit the needs of the individual, it will be accepted; if it does not fit, it will probably be rejected. If accepted, the information can be integrated into one's pool of knowledge; the process, in turn, may allow a new behavior to evolve. Knowledge calling for the performance of a new or novel skill, such as using an inhaler correctly, must be strengthened both through practice by the individual and by reinforcement by others.

Clearly, the long-term maintenance of behavior change needs supportive feedback, and a commitment to consistent and continuous effort. Motivation is the key element; without it, the whole process is undermined. Even the best of intentions cannot guarantee that the expected change will develop nor, if it occurs, that it will endure without further reinforcement. A challenge for future research is to develop a knowledge base that informs us on ways to predictably modify behavior and to sustain motivation to maintain the performance of that behavior. Understanding human behavior and experience will, as pointed out by Borkevec (1997, p. 145), 'necessarily involve an integrated view of all relevant human systems.' We have attempted to describe such an integrated view.

Without regular and repeated practice, new behaviors and skills tend to deteriorate over time (Bender *et al.*, 1997). The problem is especially relevant to asthma because periods of quiescence are interspersed between attacks and exacerbations. In addition, frequent treatment changes may be dictated both by new drugs for treatment of the disorder and by changes in the course of a patient's asthma. Because such factors affect the long-term maintenance of behavior change, updates in treatment regimens need to be provided on a regular basis. Skills, such as inhaler use or peak flow measurement, deteriorate; to make certain a patient's skills remain at a optimal level, booster sessions on use of the devices, coupling demonstration by health care personnel with performance by users, needs to occur on a regular basis.

Therapeutic Behavior Analysis

In order to generate appropriate behavior change, we propose a construct – *therapeutic behavior analysis*. The construct details the specific skills and behaviors necessary to maintain health, prevent the development of a disease, manage a disease, or successfully rehabilitate patients. Results from such a situation-specific, tailored analysis would be expected to facilitate the development of effective interventions targeted to meet the needs of individuals in various situations. Identifying the skills and behaviors needed to control the disease process would suggest novel areas for biobehavioral research.

Therapeutic behavior analysis could be prescriptive of the skills and resources needed to maximize healthy outcomes. The approach reflects a synthesis between therapy and behavior; it involves interdisciplinary and collaborative efforts among patients, providers, family, and community. The five stages prominent to such an analysis are considered below.

Setting Goals

Establishing goals occurs in the initial stage. The goals should be specific to each patient and would involve disease prevention, management, or rehabilitation. Whatever goals are set, they should be jointly established by patients and health care providers.

Determining Specific Skills

The second stage involves determining the specific skills required to achieve the goals. These might include knowledge development, communication skills, adherence to instructions, smoking cessation, exercise, or diet. Some skills could be general, such as monitoring one's performance; other skills, however, would be specific to either given patients or their disorders. An example would be the correct use of a peak flow meter by an asthma patient to determine if a relief medication should be taken.

Determining Resources

This stage of the analysis is more difficult to determine. For example, it might be relatively easy to determine resources for persons in a developed country, but less easy to do so for persons in a developing nation. It would involve a detailed analysis of patient variables, including environmental factors, developmental determinants, cognitive abilities, motivation, sociocultural variables, perception of risk factors, and disease variables. In short, the aim of this stage is to determine what variables are likely to interact together to form the context leading to the patient's behavior.

Matching Skills to Resources

Once the required skills to achieve the agreed upon goals are identified, the critical step of matching these skills to the resources of individual patients can take place. For example, most patients, need to receive education about their disorder and its management. This is the basic component of this stage, as it is a necessary step to determine the needed skills and the resources available to the patient.

Tailoring Action Plan

The action plan is a set of written procedures jointly developed and agreed upon by patients and health care providers. This prescription for action consists of specific referrals for skills development, education, or support. Therapeutic behavior analysis is an evolving, progressive process that, to be effective, must be open, dynamic, and adaptive to the situation at hand. It requires a cognitive–behavioral process that progresses according to individual motivation, environmental factors and abilities. The state of the physical disorder needs to be assessed regularly by medical and behavioral scientists to nurture and enhance the progress patients make toward reaching the jointly set goals.

Therapeutic Behavior Analysis of Respiratory Illnesses or Conditions

The framework of therapeutic behavior analysis is applicable across respiratory illness or conditions. We would like to expand our argument by spending the remainder of the chapter to provide a brief and general therapeutic analysis of several respiratory illnesses or conditions. In doing so, we have selected three conditions – asthma, COPD, and cystic fibrosis (CF) – where, as described in other chapters of the book, progress has occurred. We would then like to briefly review a disease – tuberculosis – and a behavior – smoking – where less progress has occurred.

Asthma

The chapter by Gergen and Mitchell (Chapter 2) thoroughly examines the epidemiology of asthma. It is apparent that this disorder has received the bulk of attention from behavioral scientists, as shown in other chapters in the book. As a result, any treatment behavior analysis will be more advanced with asthma than with any other respiratory disorder. This uniqueness illuminates other problems and challenges, that occur when an intradisciplinary team works together in an attempt to control a respiratory disorder. These can be illustrated by using the model applied to analyze asthma.

Setting Goals

After patients acquire the necessary knowledge about asthma and its management, they should begin to perform the skills they have been taught to help control their condition. It is at this juncture where it is imperative that patients sit down with their health care providers and establish goals for controlling asthma. Indeed, asthma is one of the few chronic illnesses where such a process is clearly stated in treatment guidelines as central to management of the disorder (National Institutes of Health, 1997). The guidelines expressly say that patients and health care personnel should 'Jointly develop treatment goals' (p. 48). Such a process is regarded as fundamental to the success of any treatment plan.

What evidence is there that such joint plans are developed and implemented? Not much, unfortunately. From the perspective of health care providers, there are at least three barriers. First, many health care personnel have not read the guidelines; therefore, they cannot incorporate the directives into their practice. Marwick (1995), for example, pointed out that only 1 in 10 physicians knew about the initial set of treatment guidelines issued in the United States for asthma, including the fact they had been published (National Institutes of Health, 1991). Secondly, Creer *et al.* (1999) recently observed that even when physicians did read the guidelines, there was little evidence that they jointly developed treatment guidelines with their patients. Rather, they continued their regular practice and followed treatment guidelines of their own. Finally, Cabana *et al.* (1999) found another reason why physicians don't follow clinical guidelines: lack of self-efficacy and lack of positive expectancies. Self-efficacy is a judgment of one's ability to organize and execute different types of performance, while outcome expectations are judgments of the likely consequence one's performance will produce (Bandura, 1997). If physicians lack confidence that their performance will produce positive outcomes, they are less likely to adopt new guidelines, but will continue to do what they have been doing regardless of outcomes. This finding by Cabana and his colleagues (1999) has major implications for both the preparation and adoption of any set of treatment guidelines.

The culpability for this situation should not be laid totally at the feet of health care providers. Patients are often no better prepared to assume some responsibility for managing their disease, particularly a chronic illness; they are used to relying upon medical advice for everything, from how to care for asthma to whether they should diet (Creer, 2000). From both perspectives – that of the patient and that of the health provider – there is need for change. How and when it can occur depends, in a large degree, upon what behavioral strategies are taken in the future to rectify the stalemate. As it is the one activity where there is a true collaboration between patients and their health care providers (Creer & Holroyd, 1997), it is imperative that we determine how to achieve the most success from goal-setting activities.

Determining Specific Skills

Establishing the skills of the patient occurs during this stage; that is why that process is so significant. Health care providers can attempt to determine exactly how much knowledge and abilities patients have to attain whatever goals are set. Patients, on their part, have the opportunity to describe their abilities and skills, as well as to express any concerns they have.

While a broad range of skills are required to manage asthma, we would like to reiterate the need for successful discrimination of asthma symptoms, a topic covered in detail by Rietveld and Everaerd (Chapter 5). This is not only a topic that, along with Rietveld and Everaerd, we have investigated (e.g., Fritz *et al.*, 1990, 1996; Klein *et al.*, 1995), but one that has piqued the interest of the National Institutes of Health. This is indicated by separate statements made on dyspnea (Statement: American Thoracic Society, 1999) and symptom discrimination (Banzett *et al.*, 2000). We concur with Rietveld and Everaerd (Chapter 5) that this is a significant area for research by medical and behavioral scientists.

Thanks to governmental and private initiatives, many asthma patients have had the opportunity to learn about asthma and how it can be managed through patient education and self-management programs. In fact, providing education and self-management training to asthma patients is probably the greatest contribution made by behavioral scientists in the past three decades. A wide gamut of programs exist for teaching patients educational and self-management skills; in the future, research will be directed at refining, disseminating and extending these programs.

Determining Resources

Earlier, we pointed out that this stage of the analysis would be more difficult to determine. Part of the problem is that we often do not know what resources are available or how they can be used until we have initiated an intervention program. Perhaps this is best illustrated by attempts to change environmental triggers of asthma in the inner city. A number of attempts have been made to achieve this goal. The results have been mixed: on the one hand, innovative techniques have been developed both to retain participation (Senturia *et al.*, 1998) and to provide effective intervention (Evans *et al.*, 1999) in these programs. On the other hand, despite some positive findings (Evans *et al.*, 1999), attempts to reduce cockroaches, a significant allergen in the inner city, have proved short-lived (Gergen *et al.*, 1999). While the findings were characterized as mixed, all were positive with respect to delineating resources available for asthma patients in the inner city; consequently, they provide the stimulus for further research.

Matching Skills to Resources

This stage is a critical step in the treatment behavior analysis. The emphasis until now has been upon describing the need to train patients to perform self-management skills to help control their asthma. This is but one area where patients may need training; there may also be the need to alter their philosophy of health care toward their accepting a shared responsibility for their health care, improving their communication skills, and teaching them to proactively seek information about their asthma (Creer, 2000). They may need training, such as that described by James and Sheeler (1997), to learn and practice communication skills required to interact in an appropriate manner with health care providers. Our discussion of determining resources, however, shows that there is still the need to determine what resources are available for patients, no matter what the context, for them to manage their asthma successfully.

Tailoring Action Plan

Each patient, regardless of illness, requires a treatment action plan that is tailored to his or her specific needs. This was emphatically stated in the asthma guidelines issued in 1997 by the directive to 'teach asthma self-management, tailoring the approach to the needs of each patient' (National Institutes of Health, 1997, p. 48). Tailoring such a plan requires not only a thorough knowledge of a patient's skills and resources but also how to integrate them into a workable set of guidelines for that patient alone. Obtaining such information to tailor a treatment plan, in turn, entails a far more intensive treatment behavior analysis than typically occurs.

The future challenge will be to obtain, and effectively use, information about patients' cultural beliefs and practices within the structure and confines of managed care. As these programs emphasize the importance of outcome data, particularly morbidity information, better techniques of assessing and gathering such data will continue to improve.

Chronic Obstructive Pulmonary Disease

In chapter 4, Kaplan and Ries succinctly describe the behavioral model as applied to patients with COPD. As they point out, it is becoming more common to apply comprehensive behavioral programs to rehabilitate these patients. The programs contain many components similar to those incorporated into self-management programs for asthma, including self-initiated actions, exercise, and compliance to agreed upon treatment regimens. There is a major departure in the rehabilitation of COPD patients that differs from self-management programs for asthma: the emphasis upon smoking cessation. As smoking is usually the most prominent ingredient in the pathogenesis of COPD, it is necessary that patients quit smoking. This, as noted by Reynolds (Chapter 12), is much easier said than done.

Although there are components unique to COPD, rehabilitation programs are amenable to dissection via therapeutic behavior analysis.

Setting Goals

While is may not be spelled out as precisely as it is in guidelines for the treatment of asthma (National Institutes of Health, 1997), it is likely that health care personnel and patients jointly set many goals in rehabilitation. Patients with COPD must reach the point where they recognize the need to become an active partner in the management of their disease. Other goals that are apt to be reached by health care personnel and their patients include helping the patient become more active; decreasing his or her shortness of breath, perhaps through breathing retraining; and improving the patient's mood.

Determining Specific Skills

As with any disease, patients with COPD have varying levels of skills. However, the educational components added to rehabilitation programs are designed to teach patients skills that they can perform to help manage their COPD. Skills would include learning more about COPD, how to avoid infections, ways to exercise more, and medications for the disease and how to use them. By the time patients finish an educational programs for COPD, they should know how and when to perform self-help skills to help control their condition.

Determining Resources

Kaplan and Ries (Chapter 4) emphasize the need for social support. As the patient begins to make changes in his or her life, such as quitting smoking, social support is imperative. Such assistance is also invaluable as the patient attempts to establish a regular exercise routine.

Matching Skills to Resources

Following the acquisition of skills to help manage their COPD, patients need to put together what they know with the skills they can perform. By synthesizing skills with resources, they can start on the road to better health. How persistent they are in matching skills to resources is, as Kaplan and Ries (Chapter 4) highlight, a function of the level of self-efficacy they have in believing that the actions they take will lead to a particular goal. The perceived self-efficacy patients have is not based upon the number of skills they can perform, but what they believe they can do with the mixture of skills and resources they have in any given situation. Self-efficacy thus emerges as a major ingredient in the overall success of symptom control.

Tailoring Action Plan

Perhaps more so than with other respiratory diseases, it is necessary to tailor an action plan for each individual patient with COPD. Part of this is because of the heterogeneity of COPD; it does not include one distinct disease, but two – emphysema and bronchitis – along with a variety of hybrid respiratory conditions. As this presents a range of respiratory characteristics and symptoms, a plan for one patient is unlikely to fit the needs of another. Only action plans tailored for the disease, skills, and resources of one individual are likely to produce change. As with asthma, each action plan must be jointly developed to include the cultural beliefs and practices of each individual patient.

Future challenges to the rehabilitation of COPD will be to provide services within the structure of managed care, particularly disease management. As with other chronic conditions, this will mean a greater emphasis upon the gathering of outcome data.

Cystic Fibrosis

Unlike other respiratory diseases, CF is the result of a genetic disorder. Consequently, any major change in the prevalence or course of the disorder will require some sort of genetic breakthrough. In the meantime, as Gustafson and Bonner (Chapter 10) reported, patients require intensive treatment designed to them active and to prolong their lives.

The course of treatment for CF is applicable to description using therapeutic behavior analysis.

Setting Goals

As with other respiratory diseases, CF requires the daily use of a number of treatment procedures. As outlined by Gustafson and Bonner, these include the taking of medications, particularly for the respiratory component of CF; the taking of vitamins and replacement enzymes; the following of a calorie-laden diet; and chest physiotherapy. All of these tasks are discussed when a child is diagnosed with CF; the goals of treatment are set with the youngster and his or her parents at that time.

Determining Specific Skills

Through the repetitive performance of the daily maintenance skills, patients and members of their families learn how to manage CF. The challenge, as noted by Gustafson and Bonner, comes when older adolescents move on to a more independent lifestyle where they need to perform the skills themselves in order to survive. Self-help skills have probably been prominent with these older adolescents and with adults, but self-management components have been specifically added to treatment programs to insure that patients perform the skills they have been taught over the years.

Determining Resources

CF is not a disease that is experienced only by the patient: it is a disease that is experienced by every member of a patient's family. Families provide the major resource to CF patients; in addition, there are increasingly more regional centers, particularly in developed countries, for the medical treatment of CF. Access to these centers needs to be ascertained. Together, these factors offer considerable social support to a patient with CF and his or her family.

Matching Skills to Resources

There are treatment facilities for most patients with CF, at least in developed countries. Patients already have a basic background in the skills needed to control CF; when their knowledge is integrated into the framework of self-management, they acquire a more systematic way of using both their skills and the resources available to them.

Tailoring Action Plan

Cystic fibrosis differs from other respiratory diseases in another manner: there is little leeway for patients to take in managing their disease. While a patient with COPD may continue to smoke, patients with CF and their families must engage in the daily tasks of taking medications and vitamins, following specific diets, and chest physiotherapy. Changes can be made to tailor a regimen to fit the characteristics of a patient's disease, but the basic steps of CF management will probably need to continue.

The future for CF treatment is basically a function of progress made in genetic research. In the meantime, treatments for CF will attempt to achieve two goals. First, the challenge of increasing the longevity of CF patients remains. A recent study in Great Britain by Lewis *et al.* (1999) reported that while the trend in the numbers of CF patients surviving into later adulthood is increasing, the mortality rates do not appear to be improving. This is a concern for the patients, their families, and all members of their interdisciplinary treatment teams. Secondly, in the age of managed care, there is concern about the cost of such care. Lieu *et al.* (1999) noted that in one health maintenance organization, costs per year in 1996 averaged US$13,300 per patient, ranging from US$6200 among patients with mild CF to US$43,300 among patients with severe CF. Thus, an attempt to increase the longevity of CF patients, while containing costs of the condition, is likely to be a major policy of the future.

Tuberculosis

Tuberculosis is a disease caused by a potentially deadly form of bacteria. Until the 1940s when the development of antibodies effectively controlled the disease, it was a leading cause of death in both developed and developing countries. It was thought that TB was a thing of the past in developed countries but, it recent years, it returned with a vengeance. A particular strain – multidrug-resistant tuberculosis (MDRTB) – is rapidly increasing on five continents. The four drugs used to treat MDRTB produce high cure rates in areas of low drug resistance; it is more difficult, however, in areas that have high levels of drug resistance. These areas, unfortunately, are found in poorer regions of the world (Centers for Disease Control, 1999; World Health Organization, 1999). In developing countries, it causes 25% of preventable mortality among young people, and is a leading killer of young women worldwide (World Health Organization, 1999).

The World Health Organization estimated that approximately 1.8 billion people were infected with the tuberculosis bacillus; this estimate was supported by Dye *et al.* (1999), who presented data gathered from 212 countries by the WHO Global Surveillance and Monitoring Project in 1997. The data indicated that the global prevalence of TB and *Mycobacterium tuberculosis* (MTB) continues unabated. The MTB infection was found in 32% or 1.86 billion people in the world. While dormant in most patients, approximately 10% of those infected with MTB can be expected to develop active tuberculosis (Broughton & Bass, 1999). Globally, the burden is enormous, mainly because of poor control in Southeast Asia, sub-Sahara Africa, and Eastern Europe, and because of high rates of MTB/HIV co-infection in south African countries.

It is imperative that we, as behavioral scientists, review TB from the perspective of a therapeutic behavior analysis.

Setting Goals

The World Health Organization (1999) described a global initiative – Stop TB – launched by a number of public and private groups to halt the spread of TB. Goals of the group include

- a global action plan to guide and coordinate responses;
- a global drug facility;
- a global research agenda; and
- a global charter for advocacy and commitment.

These goals are appropriate in that TB has only been controlled through aggressive medical treatment. However, the approach of Stop TB is solely aimed at medical control of the disorder; nothing is said about the use of behavioral techniques to assist in either the prevention or management of tuberculosis.

Determining Specific Skills

A universal type of supervised strategy – direct observed therapy (DOT) – is used throughout the world. DOT calls for patients, much like heroin addicts who receive methadone, to report to a medical facility and receive their treatment. It does not ask TB patients to become partners in the management of their disease, thus ignoring their accessibility to the program (Heyman *et al.*, 1998) or willingness to participate.

Determining Resources

A series of studies, many on the cost-effectiveness of DOT, have been conducted. The results, in part because they are often based upon hypothetical data (e.g., Palmer *et al.*, 1998), are mixed. On the one hand, a decision analysis by Burman *et al.* (1997) suggested that DOT is more effective than self-administered therapy (SAT). Other investigators (e.g., Gourevitch *et al.*, 1998; Snyder *et al.*, 1999) have reported similar findings. However, noncompliance to DOT is common, particularly among alcoholics and the homeless (Burman *et al.*, 1997a); it addition, DOT may not be cost-effective in low-risk patients (Snyder & Chin, 1999). And, in perhaps the best study, a randomized controlled trial in two communities in South Africa, Zwarenstein *et al.* (1998) compared direct observation to self-supervision. The results showed that at high rates of treatment interruption, self-supervision achieved equivalent outcomes to clinic direct observation, but at a lower cost. In addition, self-supervision achieved better outcomes for retreatment patients. Other studies (e.g.,

Davidson, 1998) indirectly support self-supervision, in part because of outcomes that were obtained despite major methodological flaws inherent in the research.

Matching Skills to Resources

The World Health Organization (1999) noted that over 100 countries accept DOT as a standard approach, and that over 1 million patients have been treated with it since 1990. The WHO report goes on to note that progress is too slow – the only conclusion when considering 1 million patients treated versus almost 1 billion patients who could end up with TB – and credit this to a lack of political commitment within countries with a high rate of the disease. No mention is made of applying existing behavioral strategies that probably would be effective in both the prevention and management of tuberculosis.

Tailoring Action Plan

The Stop TB initiative is excellent as a way of rallying and coordinating global policies and support for the control of tuberculosis. However, it ignores two components for which behavioral scientists could provide behavioral techniques: prevention of spread of the disease and management of active cases of TB. Almost all cases of tuberculosis are acquired through person-to-person contact via droplets nuclei; prevention occurs by use of ultraviolet radiation in a patient's room, or by covering the mouth and nose of patients by having them wear a mask or cough into a handkerchief (Broughton & Bass, 1999). The latter – behaviors used with some success by TB patients prior to the 1940s – should be refined, reintroduced, and investigated by teams of medical and behavioral scientists. Management of the disease could occur efficiently and effectively by use of behavioral compliance strategies developed and applied by patients themselves. In this manner, patients could make a significant contribution to helping control TB. Given the magnitude of the program, this seems the only possible solution to the increasing problem of tuberculosis.

Smoking

The World Health Organization (1999) reported that, since 1950, more than 70,000 scientific articles have left no doubt that smoking is an important cause of premature mortality and disability worldwide. In developed countries alone, smoking will have caused about 62 million deaths between 1950 and 2000. The WHO estimates that, worldwide, smoking causes about 4 million deaths annually; with current smoking patterns, this number is likely to increase dramatically. Applying the therapeutic behavior analysis to the problem, a realistic perspective of smoking emerges.

Setting Goals

Health care organizations, such as world and national organizations, agree that smoking must be curtailed. The World Health Organization (1999) enumerated such principles of control as

- creating a 'fair information' environment based upon accurate, evidence-based public health information on the risks of tobacco;
- using taxes and regulations to reduce consumption;
- encouraging cessation of tobacco use; and
- building tobacco control coalitions to defuse opposition to control measures.

Behavioral techniques for tobacco control, as described by Reynolds (Chapter 12), are not discussed; rather, the World Health Organization (1999) elected to emphasize the use of patches, tablets, inhalers, or other means for dispensing nicotine as the best practical approach to cessation. As will be pointed out, this is an unconscionable position.

Determining Specific Skills

In the past half century, considerable progress has been made in helping people to stop smoking, at least in developed countries. In the United States alone, for example, the prevalence of smoking increased steadily from the 1930s; it peaked in 1964 when more than 40% of Americans, including 60% of men, smoked. Since then, the smoking prevalence has decreased, falling to 23% by 1997 (World Health Organization, 1999). Such progress would not have occurred had not behavioral smoking cessation progams been developed and made widely available to smokers. These procedures, as outlined by Reynolds (Chapter 12), are based upon behavioral skills, along with information, increasing regulation of tobacco products, and nicotine substitution products.

Determining Resources

These can only be considered on the basis of developed or developing countries. Globally, the World Health Organization (1999) reported that about 6000 billion cigarettes are consumed each year. This is an increase from 3000 billion cigarettes in 1970, despite the fall in countries such as Australia, Canada, Japan, New Zealand, the United Kingdom and the United States, and most northern European countries. This means that the bulk of the increase has occurred in developing countries through such factors as a lack of information on risks, nicotine addiction, and – probably the most significant factor – that tobacco dealers make enormous profits. The tobacco industry continues to expand, noted the WHO, with the world retail market in cigarettes now worth approximately US$300 billion.

Matching Skills to Resources

In developed countries, both governmental and private organizations have cooperated to reduce smoking. In the United States, for example, programs supported by the government through National Institutes of Health and by private groups, such as the American Lung Association and the American Cancer Association, have long been allies in the war against smoking. Other notable examples include programs sponsored by the Asthma Foundation of the Netherlands and VicHealth, the Victoria Health Promotion Foundation, of Australia. Such partnerships epitomize the matching of skills with resources.

In developing countries, a far different picture is seen. Based on current smoking patterns, it is estimated that by the third decade of the 21st century, smoking will kill 10 million people worldwide each year. This will be more than the total number of deaths from malaria, maternal and major childhood conditions, and TB combined. It is estimated that over 70% of these deaths will be in the developing world; by 2020, smoking will cause about one in three of all adult deaths, up from one in six adult deaths in 1960 (World Health Organization, 1999).

The most notable example of deaths from smoking in developing countries is provided by China. The country has the world's highest number of tobacco deaths; smoking, in fact, causes more deaths from chronic respiratory diseases than it does from cardiovascular disease. In addition, smoking causes about 12% of all tuberculosis deaths in the world (World Health Organization, 1999). Liu *et al.* (1998) noted that tobacco caused about 0.6 million deaths in Chinese men in 1990; by the year 2000, it was estimated that this would increase to 0.8 million men, including 0.4 million between the ages of 34 and 69 years. Liu and his colleagues estimated that tobacco will kill about 100 million of the 0.3 billion males, now between the ages of 0 and 29 years, in China.

Tailoring Action Plan

Action plans, based upon past behavioral research coupled with nicotine replacement strategies, are in place in most developed countries. They complement governmental regulations and an expanding base of information disseminated about the health consequences of smoking. Given the broad arrays of strategies, a program can easily be tailored for any individual who smokes. However, the war against tobacco, at least in the United States, is far from over, as a report by the Centers for Disease Control (1998) noted there was an increase in young smokers.

These are minor problems, however, compared with the situation in developing countries. As noted earlier, tobacco is a big business that, faced with resistance in developed countries, has shifted its attention toward developing countries. In 1997, the top tobacco company in the world was the China National Tobacco Corporation; they sold approximately 1700 billion cigarettes in 1997; the next three tobacco companies with a big market niche in developing countries were Philip Morris (947 billion cigarettes), British American Tobacco (712 billion cigarettes), and R.J. Reynolds (316 billion cigarettes). Through the political control they exercise because of the big profits they generate – tobacco taxation has been a major source of revenue in China for many years – the denial of tobacco's health risks, and advertising and promotional tactics, they are likely to continue increasing their sales.

Conclusion and Future Trends

If we had reviewed the treatment of chronic disease a few short decades ago, we would have found a multidisciplinary model strongly entrenched. The model called for professionals from a number of disciplines to treat patients in an uncoordinated discipline-specific fashion. Each professional would have possessed skills specific to his or her area of expertise, but would have been ignorant both of the problems faced by other team members and the knowledge required to manage them. Behavioral scientists, for example, were apt to focus on a narrow range of behaviors – those generally considered as psychopathological – and ignored how the patient was being treated medically. This all changed with the gradual evolution toward adopting an intradisciplinary model of collaborative treatment. The model calls for all who work with patients – behavioral and medical scientists alike – to not only possess knowledge and skills relevant to their specific discipline but also to have a working knowledge of the skills and specialities of other team members. The approach, commented Varni (1983, p. 5), 'is synergistic, integrating the knowledge and skills from the various disciplines into a coordinated plan for patient care.'

The synergistic approach is exemplified by what we have described as behavioral medicine. As discussed, it does not involve any one set of variables, typically categorized as medical or behavioral, but entails the study of the interaction of physical, cognitive, environmental, and behavioral aspects of both a disease and patients with the disease. The approach has fostered progress in several respiratory diseases or illnesses, including those discussed in the book, by taking on questions that can only be resolved in an intradisciplinary manner.

In addition to its application to complex treatment issues, behavioral medicine provides a means of assessing for analyzing problems. We described what we referred to as therapeutic behavior analysis, a technique that calls for breaking down aspects of a problem – permitting the analysis of everything from a disease itself to the behaviors of a patient with a specific disease – by reviewing several processes:

- setting goals;
- determining specific skills;

- determining resources;
- matching skills to resources; and
- tailoring action plans.

The technique was applied to five disorders or behavioral problems – asthma, chronic obstructive pulmonary disease, cystic fibrosis, tuberculosis, and smoking.

Where an interdisciplinary team approach has been applied in behavioral medicine – to such problems as the self-management of asthma (Chapter 6), the rehabilitation of COPD patients (Chapter 4), and the development of coping skills in patients with CF and their families (Chapter 10) – empirical results have been almost immediate. Patients taught to shoulder responsibility for their illness and to become allies with health care personnel have been able to control many aspects of their illness; consequently, they are living fuller and more productive lives. Many aspects of their lives still revolve around a disease, but it is not the all-consuming burden it once was for patients and their families. There is also an optimism emanating from these chapters that interdisciplinarian teams are outlining an evidence-based treatment strategy for altering the course of a disease. This indicates that the best is yet to come.

By contrast, the application of a therapeutic behavior analysis to tuberculosis and smoking reveals snapshots of problems where attempts to solve them have been depressingly ignorant and simplistic. Attempting to treat tuberculosis as if it were a drug addiction has no relevance in the real world. Not only is it devoid of any empirical support but it will also be drowned by the immensity of the problem. With 1.86 billion people afflicted with the tuberculosis infection, their only salvation will come if they can be taught to prevent the spread of the disease and provide treatment to themselves. With the empirical evidence presented in the chapters of this book, we have the capability of producing such personal changes. The picture with respect to smoking is also muddled. When developing countries of the world do decide to take the offensive against smoking, progress will not occur by substituting one form of nicotine addiction for another. Rather, it will come through the commitment of countries to produce this change through stricter regulation of tobacco products and, in particular, by the application of information, the encouragement of cessation, and all of the behavioral techniques found to be effective in helping people to stop smoking (Chapter 12). The empirical basis of behavioral smoking cessation products is well-established; it cannot be ignored if we are to reduce the human toll tobacco extracts in the world.

Dr. Gro Harlem Brundtland, the Director-General of the World Health Organization, offered this advice in the World Health Report of 1999 (World Health Organization, 1999, p. viii):

> *Opportunity brings responsibility. Working together, we have the opportunity to transform lives now debilitated by disease and fear of economic ruin into lives filled with realistic hopes. . . . We must be realistic: there will be setbacks and difficulties. A greater collective effort will generate more demands on each of us individually and on the institutions we represent – national and international, public and private. Compressing the time required to accomplish major and tangible results is the task for leadership in the 21st century. This leadership must be technical. It must be political. And it must be moral.*

Behavioral medicine, pooling the tools of behavioral and medical scientists, has the skills to provide the required synergy needed to produce tangible results with the respiratory diseases that haunt the world.

References

American Thoracic Society (1999). Dyspnea. Mechanisms, assessment, and management: a consensus statement. *American Journal of Respiratory Medicine*, 159, 321–340.

American Thoracic Society (in press). Symptom perception in asthma: a consensus statement. *American Journal of Respiratory and Critical Care Medicine.*

Bandura, A. (1997). *Self-efficacy. The exercise of control.* New York: W.H. Freeman and Company.

Banzett, R.B., Dempsey, J.A., O'Donnell, D.E., & Wamboldt, M.Z. (2000). Symptom perception and respiratory sensation in asthma. *Am J Respiratory and Critical Care Medicine*, 162: 1178–1182.

Bender, B.G., Ikle, D.N., DuHamel, T., & Tinkleman, D. (1997). Retention of asthmatic patients in a longitudinal clinical trial. *Journal of Allergy and Clinical Immunology*, 99, 197–203.

Blumenthal, S.J., Mathews, K., & Weiss, S.M. (1994). New research frontiers in behavioral medicine: proceedings of the national conference. *NIH Publication No.* 94-3772.

Boner, A.L., De Stefano, G., Piacentini, G.L., Bonizzato, C., Sette, L. Banfi, F., & Hindi-Alexander, M.C. (1992). Perception of Bronchoconstriction in Chronic Asthma. *Journal of Asthma*, 29(5), 323–330.

Borkevec, T.D. (1997). On the need for a basic science approach to psychotherapy research. *Psychological Science*, 8, 145–147.

Bourne, L.E., Jr. & Russo, N.F. (1998). *Psychology. Behavior in context.* New York: W.W. Norton.

Broughton, W.A. & Bass, J.B., Jr. (1999). Tuberculosis and diseases caused by atypical mycobacteria. In: R.K. Albert, S.G. Shapiro & J.R. Jett (Eds), *Comprehensive respiratory medicine* (pp. 29.1–29.16). St Louis: C.V. Mosby.

Burman, W.J., Cohn, D.L., Rietmeijer, C.A., *et al.* (1997a). Noncompliance with directly observed therapy for tuberculosis. Epidemiology and effect in the outcome of treatment. *Chest*, 111, 1168–1173.

Burman, W.J., Dalton, C.B., Cohn, D.L., Butler, J.R. & Reves, R.R. (1997b). A cost-effectiveness analysis of directly observed therapy vs self-administered therapy for treatment of tuberculosis. *Chest*, 112, 63–70.

Cabana, M.D., Rand, C.S., Powe, N.R., *et al.* (1999). Why don't physicians follow clinical practice guidelines? A framework for improvement. *Journal of the American Medical Association*, 282, 1458–1465.

Centers for Disease Control (1990). (March 10).

Centers for Disease Control (1998). Incidence of initiation of cigarette smoking – United States, 1965–1996. *Morbidity and Mortality Weekly Report*, 48 (October 9), 837–840.

Centers for Disease Control (1999). Primary multi-resistant tuberculosis – Ivanovo Oblast, Russia, 1999. *Morbidity and Mortality Weekly Report*, 48 (August 6), 661–664.

Creer, T.L. (2000). Self-management and the control of chronic pediatric illness. In: D. Drotar (Ed.), *Promoting adherence to medical treatment in chronic childhood illness.* (pp. 95–129). Mahwah, NJ: Lawrence Erlbaum Associates.

Creer, T.L. & Holroyd, K.A. (1997). Self-management. In: A. Baum, C. McManus, S. Newman, J. Weinman & R. West (Eds), *Cambridge handbook of psychology, health, and behavior* (pp. 255–258). Cambridge: Cambridge University Press.

Creer, T.L., Winder, J.A. & Tinkelman, D. (1999). Guidelines for the diagnosis and management of asthma: accepting the challenge. *Journal of Asthma*, 36, 391–407.

Davidson, B.L. (1998). A controlled comparison of directly-observed therapy vs self-administered therapy for active tuberculosis in the urban United States. *Chest*, 114, 1229–1234.

Dye, C., Scheele, S., Dolin, P., Pathania, V. & Raviglione, M.C. (1999). Global burden of tuberculosis. *Journal of the American Medical Association*, 282, 677–686.

Dye, C., Scheele, S., Dolin, P., Pathania, V. & Raviglione, M.C. (1999). Global burden of tuberculosis. Estimated incidence, prevalence, and mortality by country. *Journal of the American Medical Association*, 282, 677–686.

Eakin, E.G., Kaplan, R.M., Reis, A.L., & Sassi-Dambron, D.E. (1996). Patients' self-report on dyspnea: an important and independent outcome in chronic obstructive pulmonary disease. *Annals of Behavioral Medicine*, 18(2), 87–90.

Evans, R., III, Gergen, P.J., Mitchell, H., *et al.* (1999). A randomized clinical trial to reduce asthma morbidity among inner-city children: results of the National Cooperative Inner-City Asthma Study. *Journal of Pediatrics*, 135,.

Ford, D.H. (1987). *Humans as self-constructing living systems: a developmental perspective on behavior and personality.* Hillsdale, NJ: Lawrence Erlbaum Associates.

Ford, D.H. & Urban, H.B. (1998). *Contemporary models of psychotherapy: a comparative analysis*, 2nd edn. New York: John Wiley & Sons.

Fritz, G.K., Klein, R.B. & Overholser, J.C. (1990). Accuracy of symptom perception in childhood asthma. *Journal of Behavioral Pediatrics*, 11, 69–72.

Fritz, G.K., McQuaid, E.L., Spirito, A. & Klein, R.B. (1996). Symptom perception in pediatric asthma: relationship of functional morbidity and psychological factors. *Journal of American Academy of Child & Adolescent Psychiatry*, 35, 1033–1041.

Gergen, P.S., Mortimer, K.M., Eggleston, P.A., *et al.* (1999). *Journal of Allergy and Clinical Immunology*, 103, 501–506.

Gourevitch, M.N., Alcabes, P., Wasserman, W.C. & Arno, P.S. (1998). Cost-effectiveness of directly observed chemoprophylaxis of tuberculosis among drug users at high risk for tuberculosis. *International Journal of Tuberculosis and Lung Disease*, 2, 531–540.

Heyman, S.J., Sell, R. & Brewer, T.F. (1998). The influence of program acceptability on the effectiveness of public health policy: a study of directly observed therapy for tuberculosis. *American Journal of Public Health*, 88, 442–445.

James, T.C. & Sheeler, R.D. (1997). Open-ended questions may help avoid the dreaded 'hidden agenda' getting the most out of a 15 minute asthma visit. *Journal of Respiratory Disease*, 18(2), 135–141.

Klein, R.B., Fritz, G.K., Yeung, A., McQuaid, E.L. & Mansell, A. (1995). Spirometric patterns in childhood asthma: L Peak flow compared to other indices. *Pediatric Pulmonology*, 20, 372–379.

Lewis, P.A., Morison, S., Dodge, J.A., *et al.* (1999). Survival estimates for adults with cystic fibrosis born in the United Kingdom between 1947 and 1967. *Thorax*, 54, 420–422.

Lieu, T.A., Ray, G.T., Farmer, G. & Shay, G.F. (1999). The cost of medical care for patients with cystic fibrosis in a health maintenance organization. *Pediatrics*, e72, 1–4.

Liu, B-Q, Peto, R., Chen, Z-M., *et al.* (1998). Emerging tobacco hazards in China: 1. retrospective proportional mortality study of one million deaths. *British Medical Journal*, 317, 1411–1422.

Marwick, C. (1995). Inner-city asthma control campaign underway. *Journal of the American Medical Association*, 274, 1004.

McGinnis, M. The role of behavioral research in national health policy. In S. Blumenthal, K. Matthews, & S. Weiss (Eds.), *New research frontiers in behavioral medicine; Proceedings of the National Conference* (pp. 217–222). Washington, DC: NIH Publications.

National Institutes of Health (1991). *Expert panel report executive summary: guidelines for the diagnosis and management of asthma* (Publication No. 91–3042). Washington, DC: US Department of Health and Human Services.

National Institutes of Health (1997). *Expert panel report II, guidelines for the Diagnosis and Management of Asthma* (Publication 97–4051). Washington, DC: US Department of Health and Human Services.

Nguyen, B.P., Wilson, S.R., & German, D.F. (1996). Patients' perceptions compared with objective ratings of asthma severity. *Annals of Allergy Asthma & Immunology*, 77, 488–492.

Palmer, C.S., Miller, B., Halpern, M.T. & Geiter, L.J. (1998). A model of the cost-effectiveness of directly observed therapy for treatment of tuberculosis. *Journal of Public Health Management Practice*, 4, 1–13.

Program in Infectious Disease and Social Change. *The global impact of drug-resistant tuberculosis*. Boston: Harvard University.

Redd, W.H. (1994). Advances in psychosocial oncology in pediatrics. *Cancer* 1994; 74: 1496–1502.

Redline, S., Wright E.C., Kattan, M. & Kercsmar, B. (1996). Short term compliance with peak flow monitoring results from a study of inner city children with asthma. *Pediatric Pulmonary*, 21, 203–210.

Senturia, Y.D., Mortimer, K.M., Baker, D., *et al.* (1998). *Controlled Clinical Trials*, 19, 544–554.

Snyder, D.C. & Chin, D.P. (1999). Cost-effectiveness analysis of directly observed therapy for patients with tuberculosis at low risk for treatment default. *American Journal of Respiratory and Critical Care Medicine*, 160, 582–586.

Snyder, D.C., Paz, E.A., Mohle-Boetaini, J.C., Fallstad, R., Black, R.L. & Chin, D. (1999). Tuberculosis prevention in methadone maintenance clinics. Effectiveness and cost-effectiveness. *American Journal of Respiratory and Critical Care Medicine*, 160, 178–185.

Varni, J.W. (1983). *Clinical behavioral pediatrics: an interdisciplinary biobehavioral approach.* New York: Pergamon Press.

World Health Organization (1998). *The world health report 1998: life in the 21st century – a vision for all.* Geneva, Switzerland: World Health Organization.

World Health Organization (1999). *The world health report 1999: making a difference.* Geneva, Switzerland: World Health Organization.

Zwarenstein, N., Schoeman, J.H., Vudule, C., Lombard, C.J. & Tatley, M. (1998). Randomized controlled trial of self-supervised and directly observed treatment of tuberculosis. *Lancet*, 352, 1340–1343.

14
Future directions of research on respiratory disorders

Thomas L. Creer

Context is everything

Jonathan Letham, Motherless Brooklyn, 1999

A few decades ago, behavioral scientists were included as members of multidisciplinarian teams working with respiratory disorders, particularly pediatric asthma (Renne & Creer, 1985). At two dozen or so residential treatment centers for the disorder in the United States, behavioral scientists attempted to help patients cope with asthma and the problems it spawned. There were few effective medical treatments for the condition; in addition, a number of treatment-related problems were prominent. Perhaps the biggest single problem involved the consequences arising from a reliance on oral corticosteroids for severe asthma. The only way to manage asthma in many children was through a regimen of up to 90 mg of prednisone, a commonly prescribed oral corticosteroid taken on an alternate-day basis. The price of control was steep: the children often experienced a stunting of growth, puffiness of the face, delayed menses, brittle bones, and unwanted facial hair. Even so, it was not uncommon for corticosteroids to fail in controlling a child's asthma.

At what was the Children's Asthma Research Institute and Hospital (CARIH), a residential treatment center for pediatric asthma in Denver, there were often several cases of status asthmaticus – steadily worsening asthma – each week. Without aggressive treatment, the children could have lapsed into cardiac arrest and, perhaps, have died. The situation for the medical staff was similar to that of surgeons working on a battleground; their daily lives were punctuated by episodes where they frantically used the few techniques they had to keep patients alive. It is to their credit that they saved so many lives from asthma-related sequelae; almost all the children survived into adulthood, where they would later be treated with more effective and less intrusive drugs. While not always under the same time pressures, behavioral scientists had their hands full in helping the children live with the disorder and all its ramifications. Given the variety of behavioral problems presented by asthmatic children, we were always challenged (Creer & Christian, 1976; Creer *et al.*, 1976).

The treatment teams at CARIH exemplified the multidisciplinarian model: each member knew his or her area of expertise and how it could be applied, but very little about the problems faced by other team members and how they might be solved. The result, as Varni (1983) described the model, was an uncoordinated approach that generated frustration and, at times, conflict among team members. Physicians and other medical personnel on the team, for example, viewed the patients only within the prism of medicine. Once medical control had been established over a child's asthma, they wanted to set a discharge date and return the child to his or her home. Behavioral scientists, on the other hand, sometimes perceived that the child was not ready to be discharged; many times, these clinicians felt that the youngster lacked the skills to cope effectively with asthma in his or her community. Such divergent views by medical and behavioral scientists often put team members at an impasse from which few were willing to budge. Regular meetings of multidisciplinarian teams were sometimes marked by arguments and recriminations among team members, with little agreement as to how to proceed in treating patients.

The switch from a multidisciplinarian treatment model to an interdisciplinarian model occurred somewhat serendipitously at CARIH beginning in 1967. In what some have referred to as an early illustration of behavioral pediatrics or pediatric psychology (Russo & Varni, 1982), the first component of an interdisciplinary team model emerged when a behavioral scientist approached his medical colleagues and asked them if they were facing behavioral problems that he might help them solve. After they overcame their initial surprise at the suggestion, they blurted out, 'Yeah, we'd like to keep a couple of kids from spending so much time in the hospital. We think they're faking sometimes, but we're afraid not to admit them in case they're telling the truth. And, while you are at it, could you help some of the kids who panic when they have severe attacks?' Both problems proved amenable to change via behavioral techniques. The first problem, in what came to be referred to as the inappropriate overuse of hospitals (Hochstadt *et al.*, 1980), was changed by introducing time-out in that setting. By removing potential reinforcers – comic books, television, and the opportunity for social interactions with other children – the amount of time spent in the hospital dropped from 68% to 7% for one child and from 55% to 5% for the second child (Creer, 1970). These findings were replicated in a larger sample of children with asthma by Hochstadt *et al.* (1980). With the second problem, difficulties were encountered in operationally defining what was meant by panic. The initial focus was on the children themselves when, in actuality, panic could have been operationally defined by referring to the pattern, as any behaviors exhibited by children that frightened attending medical personnel and interfered with treatment of the children's worsening asthma (Creer, 1979). Nevertheless, without arriving at a precise definition of panic, the children were treated through application of systematic desensitization by reciprocal inhibition (Wolpe, 1958). With this procedure, responses incompatible with anxiety or panic – systematic relaxation skills – were taught to the children and they stopped exhibiting what health care personnel referred to as panic during their attacks (Creer & Christian, 1976; Creer *et al.*, 1976). Thus, the first component of an effective interdisciplinarian model – knowledge of the behavioral problems faced by medical personnel and how they might be changed – fell into place.

The second component – acquisition of knowledge of a respiratory condition and how it was treated – became important to other members of the treatment team, particularly behavioral scientists. The incentive at CARIH occurred when the late Elliott Middleton, Jr., a splendid teacher and mentor, and I were on a panel discussion together at a meeting of allergists and chest physicians. The question was asked, 'What is the difference between negative reinforcement and punishment?' Before I could respond, Elliott replied, 'I can answer that.' He then did so in a manner that would have made any behavioral scientist proud. Elliott's response led me to recognize that, as behavioral scientists, my colleagues and I had to emulate Elliott and learn as much as we could about the medical aspects of asthma and other respiratory conditions. This helped put us all on the same page, so to speak, in perceiving asthma and how it was treated. It also permitted us to take a synergistic approach to asthma by integrating the knowledge and skills of various disciplines not only to develop effective treatments for asthma but also to conduct more comprehensive and sophisticated research on the disorder.

The third component was added with the development and introduction of new drugs and treatment strategies for asthma. Perhaps the biggest concern for medical and behavioral scientists was prompted by the use of theophylline to treat asthma. Theophylline is a safe drug when taken correctly; thus, it was widely accepted into the treatment armamentarium for treating asthma. A problem arises in that theophylline is effective only when it is present within a narrow band in the bloodstream. If the theophylline level falls below this band, the drug is ineffective and asthma is not controlled; if the level exceeds the band, however, dire consequences, in the form of seizures and even death, are possible. Medical and behavioral personnel became concerned about how and when patients took their prescribed theophylline; this spurred on the interest in medication compliance to asthma regimens (Creer, 1993). Increased interest in the topic arose because of a study by Sublett *et al.* (1979), who assessed blood theophylline levels in a group of 50 children randomly selected from 500 youngsters admitted to a hospital emergency room because of asthma. The blood level of only one child – 2% of the sample – fell within the therapeutic band of theophylline. The authors, however, expressed concern about this child, because she was not compliant to her physician's prescribed regimen (Creer & Levstek, 1996). Had the child been totally adherent, she would have taken what surely would have been a toxic dose of the drug. This accentuates the point that, as behavioral scientists, only our knowledge of medical treatments, especially those involving drugs, can prevent us from naively doing irreparable harm to patients.

The fourth and final component came with recognition by some medical and behavioral scientists that a more effective model was required for management of a chronic illness such as asthma and other respiratory disorders. It was thought that patients had to accept more responsibility for their condition and become allies with those involved with their treatment. If they were to do so, a different model of health care was needed. Basically, there are three theoretical models – paternalistic, informed, and shared – and derivations of the models used to treat patients (Charles *et al.*, 1999).

Models of Health Care

Paternalistic Model

The most widely used approach is the paternalistic model. Here, physicians and other health care personnel expect patients to agree to a treatment option; patients, in turn, have little input into the decision making process, but acquiesce to the wishes of their health care provider. Because there is no sharing of any steps of decision-making in this model, Charles *et al.* (1999) question whether, by definition, a doctor–patient relationship exists. Therefore, while a pure paternalistic model may be useful for the treatment of acute disease, it is inappropriate in chronic illness.

Informed Model

The informed model involves a partnership, based on a division of labor, between health care providers and patients. In the information exchange stage, for example, the health care provider leads, and communication is one way from the provider to the patient. The provider offers information on all relevant treatment options and their benefits and risks. At a minimum, noted Charles *et al.* (1999), enough information is provided so as to permit patients to make informed treatment decisions.

Shared Model

The essential characteristic of this model is its interactional nature where health care providers and patients concurrently share all stages of the decision-making process (Charles *et al.*, 1999). There is a reciprocal exchange of information in that health care personnel, patients, and behavioral scientists reveal treatment preferences, as well as agree on the best treatment strategy to implement. This approach assumes that patients, health care personnel, and behavioral scientists have a legitimate investment in the treatment decision. Each party states their treatment preferences and the rationale for their choice, while trying to build a consensus on the appropriate treatment to implement. The challenge for health care personnel and, when involved, behavioral scientists is to create an environment in which patients feel comfortable in expressing their treatment preferences, including doing nothing or watchful waiting (Charles *et al.*, 1999).

Intermediate Models

Intermediate approaches may be taken where health care providers do not use a pure model, but a hybrid of elements selected from two or more models. The treatment approach taken with some respiratory diseases reflects an intermediate model. With chronic obstructive pulmonary disorder (COPD), for example, there is little interaction among parties regarding the need to stop smoking; however, how the patient achieves this goal is the result of a reciprocal exchange of information and a consensus on what smoking cessation procedure to use. Thus, elements of both a paternalistic and shared model are integrated into treatment plans for COPD. Cystic fibrosis is another disorder where a mixed paternalistic/shared model would be of value. With asthma, on the other hand, treatment options and goals must be established through interactions among health care personnel, behavioral scientists, and patients. Treatment guidelines for the disorder explicitly outline the role of patients by asking them to jointly develop treatment goals, including asthma action plans, with their health care personnel, and by learning and performing self-management skills tailored for each patient (National Institutes of Health, 1997).

Chronic respiratory disorders represent other challenges to traditional treatment models used by medical and behavioral scientists who treat the conditions. A major challenge occurs because these conditions are of long duration – what Verbrugge & Patrick (1995) consider the defining characteristic of a chronic disease. These conditions do not resolve spontaneously and have no cure. No guarantee can be given that, despite the best efforts of patients and health care providers, markedly improved health will occur as an outcome of whatever model is used. Another challenge is that the ultimate success or failure of any treatment strategy often rests entirely upon the shoulders of patients themselves. Only they know if they have quit smoking or where and when they experience an exacerbation of their condition; in the latter case, only they can often provide whatever action is needed either to prevent or to alleviate the exacerbation (Creer, 2000).

Finally, we face the twofold challenge of having patients, health care personnel, and behavioral scientists accept a shared model of decision making and treatment. For their part, patients are often hesitant to accept responsibility for their condition; they would rather cling to the tattered remnants of the paternalistic model and 'let the doc do it.' A chronic respiratory disorder, however, doesn't permit nonparticipation on the part of patients. Physicians, for their part, are often unwilling or unprepared to discard the paternalistic model and adopt a shared model. Doing so would go against everything they were taught in medical school. Consequently, despite the intentions of the initial set of asthma treatment guidelines in the United States (National Institutes of Health, 1991), there has been a lack of adherence on the part of health care personnel to these directives (Creer *et al.*, 1999).

Where does this leave us as behavioral and medical scientists? The answer is easy: we must develop and apply shared treatment models that, in addition to including the professionals who treat patients, include patients themselves. The mushrooming of sophisticated medical treatments for all respiratory conditions, including asthma, COPD, cystic fibrosis, and tuberculosis, demands nothing less. Techniques for guiding this complex and revolutionary treatment process will continue to evolve with the continued and widespread dissemination of information on disease and health, as well as with the acceptance of medical and behavioral scientists of a shared treatment model.

Equally significant to changes in how patients with a respiratory disease are treated are questions regarding directions of future research. The remainder of the chapter will focus on

- research on respiratory disorders;
- reductionism;
- complexity;
- social cognitive learning theory;
- the integration of complexity and social cognitive learning theory;
- mechanisms for action;
- framing, and
- an analysis of the impact of nonlinear variables on asthma research.

Research on Respiratory Disorders

In working with respiratory disorders, we are often presented with problems that are too complicated to solve by common sense. Therefore, we attempt to solve the problem by strings of mixed inductive and deductive inferences woven back and forth between what we observe and our knowledge of a given respiratory condition. In most instances, what we do is a sophisticated form of problem solving. We use our personal base of knowledge and expertise or, in the case of a problem faced by an interdisciplinary team, the collected knowledge of the team, to try and solve the problem. In other instances, the only correct approach to solving the problem is, as suggested by Pirsig (1974) and Wynn (1997), the scientific method. We usually think of how to examine our problem in terms of linearity, or a system where the whole is precisely equal to the sum of its parts (Waldrop, 1992). This is based, in part, upon the way we think (Goerner, 1995) and, in part, because a lot of nature seems to work that way (Waldrup, 1992). For example, linear thinking and the research it generates underlie much of what we know about physics, mathematics, and chemistry.

Based upon observations, we generate logical statements or theories about what we observe. Scientific theories, noted Wilson (1998), are a product of informed imagination. They reach beyond their ability to predict the existence of unsuspected phenomena. The best theories generate hypotheses about the phenomenon we are observing. What comprises a hypothesis varies somewhat according to different scientists. Wynn (1997) said that hypotheses should be as general as possible in order to deal with other phenomena besides the specific ones observed; Kneller (1978), on the other hand, suggested that a hypothesis should account for known facts, be precise enough to yield testable prediction, and be able to predict some fact or facts hitherto unknown. The best theories generate the most fruitful hypotheses which, Wilson (1998, p. 53) explained, 'translate cleanly into questions that can be answered by observation and experimentation.' Experimentation is conducted to test the hypotheses; we may predict the results of our experiments beforehand or we may be satisfied just to see what happens with manipulation of a specific set of variables. If the results fit our hypotheses, then our predictions have credibility; if they do not, we may discard the results or modify them to accommodate what we found (Wynn, 1992). The real purpose of the scientific method, suggested Pirsig (1974), is to be certain nature hasn't misled us into thinking we know something that we don't actually know.

Science, in the words of Wilson (1998, p. 53), 'is the organized, systematic enterprise that gathers knowledge about the world and condenses the knowledge into testable laws and principles.' The scientific method has served as the skeleton upon which we have draped the reproducible knowledge we have collected about all chronic disorders, including respiratory conditions. Issues arise in using the method, however, particularly in interdisciplinarian research where both physical and behavioral variables are concurrently manipulated and examined.

Reductionism

Given the large number of variables involved with respiratory diseases, as well as the behavioral variables that interact with them, we usually take a reductionistic approach. It is the primary and essential activity of science (Wilson, 1998), and basically 'a doctrine according to which complex phenomena can be explained in terms of something simpler' (Coveney & Highfield, 1995, p. 432). This means we think in a linear manner and design our experiments to simplify the study of a natural phenomena by eliminating all but a few variables; we then base our explanations in terms of the most fundamental units.

Is reductionism the best approach to take in studying respiratory diseases and related behaviors? We'd likely respond that it is if we actually want to carry out a study we've designed; we might otherwise drown in the pool of potential variables we could examine. Does reductionism always yield the most accurate portrait of a respiratory disease and related behaviors? Here we might hesitate, but the answer is no. As Baruch Blumberg, a Nobel Laureate in medicine explained,

> *My experience is that, in medicine, where observational science is crucial, the complexities of a phenomenon can be understood, at least in part, by repeated observations of a whole organism or a population of organisms under a wide range of circumstances; all variables are retained and as many as possible are examined. For example, in the study of disease, it is possible to build up a knowledge of the effects of a large number of variables on the host, genetic susceptibilities to the disease, and outside factors which interact with each other, the host, and the environment.*
>
> *(Blumberg, 1995, p. ix)*

Somehow, perhaps because of a perceived necessity to be reductionistic in designing and executing studies – what Cowan (cited in Waldrop, 1992, p. 60) described as the 'royal road to the Nobel Prize' – we repeatedly design linear studies that are reductionistic in nature. The widespread reverence and use of what are defined as clinical trials leaps to mind. By reducing what we study to the simplest of designs, however, we often miss the complexity of the very phenomenon we wish to explain.

Problems with reductionism can be explained by describing hypotheses testing and how it can lead us to overlook important findings. Before conducting a study, we often generate hypotheses as what we think we will find; either explicitly or implicitly, the hypothese serves as a guide through the remaining processes of the research. The purpose of observation in general, and experimentation in particular, is to test hypotheses in order either to falsify or validate them. This would be an excellent practice if the study had already been conducted and we knew our findings. As this is rarely the case, however, we often let the hypotheses lead us into a tunnel where we look for verification of expected results and overlook what might be more significant findings.

In contrast to this position, Klahr & Simon (1999, p. 529) argued that much of the important empirical research in science is undertaken

> *in the context of discovery rather than the context of verification. That is, a major goal of empirical research in science is to discover new phenomena and generate hypotheses for describing and explaining them and not simply to test hypotheses that have already been generated. Indeed, theories cannot be tested until they have been created, and creation takes place in the context of discovery, not verification.*

This creates a different and more complex context than is usually the case with respect to research in respiratory disorders.

Complexity

Complexity is defined in several ways. To Coveney & Highfield (1995, p. 425), it is 'the study of the behavior of macroscopic collections of simple units (e.g., atoms, molecules, bits, neurons) that are endowed with the potential to evolve in time.' While clearly worded, the definition has only tangential relevance to the medical and behavioral scientists who work with respiratory disorders. Waldrup (1992, p. 11) defines complexity in a manner more akin to our interests when he says a system is complex, 'in the sense that a great many independent agents are interacting with each other in a great many ways.' While this provides a broader definition of complexity, it is still too general for both behavioral and medical scientists. Donald H. Ford attempted to define behavior and psychology in terms of complexity (Ford, 1987; Ford & Ford, 1987; Ford & Urban, 1998). Ford & Urban (1998, p. 674) note that psychologists

> *assume that people are complex, open systems that exist and develop only in transaction with contexts. All people construct their own developmental pathways and functional patterns, within variable and changing facilitating and constraining conditions provided by their bodies and contexts.*

This definition of complexity has greater applicability to medical and behavioral scientists, particularly with respect to our consideration of contextual factors.

In discussing why he did not provide a definition of complexity in his book, Cilliers (1998, p. 2) cautioned that the concept is elusive at both the qualitative and quantitative levels. Instead, Cilliers continued, it would be better to analyze the characteristics of complex systems 'in order to develop a general description that is not constrained by a specific, a priori definition.' Before doing so, however, Cilliers thought it imperative to make two important distinctions. First, he pointed out that the distinction between simple and complex is not as sharp as one might think. Many systems appear simple, but have remarkable complexity when examined closely; other systems, on the other hand, appear complex but can be described simply. To further confound matters, complexity is not located at a specific and identifiable site in the system, but results from interactions taking place between components of a system and manifested at the level of the system itself. Secondly, Cilliers noted, there is the distinction between complex and complicated. A system may have a large number of components and perform sophisticated tasks. If the system can be analyzed accurately, it is complicated. In systems with nonlinear relationships and feedback loops, only certain aspects can be analyzed at a time, often causing distortions. These systems are complex. Such systems are usually associated with living things, such as bacterium, the brain, and social systems. Respiratory disorders can be added to the list of complex systems.

Characteristics of Complexity

In developing a description of a complex system, Cilliers highlighted the following characteristics as integral to such a scheme:

Elements of System

Complex systems have a large number of elements. If the number of elements is small, the behavior of the elements can be given a formal description. However, when sufficiently large, conventional means not only become impractical but also cease to assist in understanding the system.

Necessary but not Sufficient Elements

Cilliers pointed out that it is not the sheer number of elements in a system that is important, but the fact they interact in a dynamic manner. Such a system changes with time. The interactions in the system do not have to be physical; they can also be thought of as significant in the transfer of information. Indeed, Ford (Ford, 1987; Ford & Ford, 1987) views the transfer of information through the interaction of elements as central to the complex behavioral system he outlined.

Interactions are Rich

Cilliers (1998) suggested that the richness of interactions means that any element in the system influences and is influenced by many others. The behavior of the system is not determined by the amount of interactions associated with specific elements. If there are enough elements in the system, a number of sparsely connected elements can perform the same function as that of one richly connected element.

Nonlinearity

Interactions between or among elements are nonlinear. This means that the whole is greater than the sum of parts, and can only be understood by examining global behaviors in addition to a detailed analysis of the individual agents of which the whole is comprised (Blumberg, 1995). Nonlinear systems do not obey the simple laws of addition (Coveney & Highfield, 1995); in addition, a large number of linear elements can usually be collapsed into an equivalent system that is much smaller. Nonlinearity guarantees that small causes can have large results, and vice versa. Nonlinearity is, concluded Cilliers (1998), a precondition for complexity.

Interactions Usually Have a Short Range

Cilliers suggested that interactions usually have a fairly short range in that information is received primarily from immediate neighbors. Long-range interactions are possible, but are limited by practical constraints. This does not preclude the possibility that interactions can have a wide-ranging influence; since the interaction is rich, the route from one element to another can generally be covered in a few steps. As a result, Cilliers proclaimed, the influence is modulated along the way. It can be enhanced, suppressed, or altered in a number of ways.

Loops in the Interaction

Loops exist in interactions. The effect of any activity can feed back on itself, sometimes directly and sometimes after a number of intervening stages. The feedback can be positive (enhancing, stimulating) or negative (detracting, inhibiting). Both types of feedback are necessary in a system of this nature, a point emphasized in the self-regulation model proposed by Carver & Scheier (1998).

Complex System are Open

Closed systems are usually just complicated. Complex systems, however, are open in that they interact with their environment. For this reason it is often difficult to define the border of a complex system. Cilliers (1998) suggested that instead of being a characteristic of the system itself, the scope of the system is determined by the purpose of the description of the system, and is often influenced by the position of the observer. This process, Cilliers continued, is referred to as framing.

Complex Systems Lack Equilibrium

Complex systems require a constant flow of energy to maintain the organization of the system and to insure its environment. Equilibrium, according to Cilliers, is another word for death.

Complex Systems Have History

Not only do systems evolve over time but also their past is co-responsible for their present behavior. Any analysis of a complete system that ignores the dimension of time, suggested Cilliers, is incomplete or, at most, a synchronic snapshot of a diachronic process.

Elements Are Ignorant of Behavior of System as a Whole

Elements in a system respond only to information that is available to them locally; the elements are, therefore, ignorant of the behavior of the system as a whole. This point, emphasized Cilliers, is vitally important. If each element 'knew' what was happening to the system as a whole, all of the complexity would have to be present in that element. Complexity just doesn't happen this way. Rather, concluded Cilliers (1998, p. 4),

> *Complexity is the result of a rich interaction of simple elements that only respond to the limited information each of them is presented with. When we look at the behavior of a complex system as a whole, our focus shifts from the individual element in the system to the complex structure of the system. The complexity emerges as a result of the patterns of interaction between the elements.*

Indispensable Characteristics of Complex Systems

Cilliers described two indispensable characteristics of complex systems: representation and self-organization.

Representation

In order to respond appropriately to its environment, a complex system must be able to gather and store information about that environment. The structure of the system is not a random collection of elements; it must have some meaning or purpose that is not determined by the outside. Meaning is the result of a process, involving elements from inside and outside, as well as historical information.

Self-Organization

A complex system, such as a living organism, has to develop its structure and adapt that structure to cope with environmental changes. The key concept is the notion of self-organization. This does not mean, noted Cilliers, that a complex system contains some sort of internal mechanism that controls the behavior of the system; rather, he continued, the whole nature of central control becomes suspect. What is implied by self-organization is a process whereby a system can develop a complex structure from unstructured beginnings. A working definition of self-organization by Cilliers (1998, p. 90) is

> *The capacity for self-organization is a property of complex systems which enables them to develop or change internal structure spontaneously and adaptively in order to cope with, or manipulate their environment.*

The process changes the relationships between the distributed elements of the system under the influence of both the external environment and the history of the system. As the system has to cope with unpredictable changes in the environment, the development of the structure cannot be contained in a rigid program that controls the behavior of the system.

Social Cognitive Learning Theory

Structure pertains to the internal mechanism developed by the system to receive, encode, transform, and store information on the one hand, and to react to such information by some form of output on the other (Cilliers, 1998). Complexity can emerge from very simple processes; it need not be either represented or controlled centrally (Carver & Scheier, 1998). A model that fits these criteria has been referred to as a social cognitive learning model that features reciprocal determinism (Bandura, 1977, 1986, 1997). This interactive model, depicted in Fig. 14.1, presents a

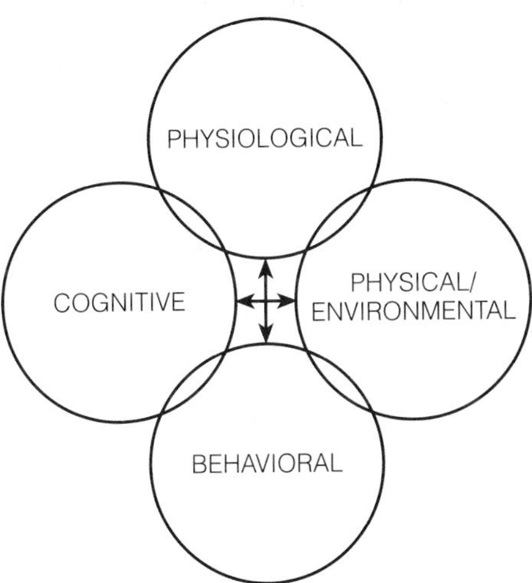

Figure 14.1
Reciprocal determinism model

framework that encompasses the reciprocal influence of external and internal components.

Depending upon how the model is depicted, there are three or four categories of events. Bandura (1997), for example, described a triadic model that includes behavior; personal factors in the form of cognitive, affective, and biological events; and the external environment. Thoresen & Kirmal-Gray (1983) and Creer (1983), however, outlined a model that includes behavior, cognition, physiology, and environment variables. Outside of how components are categorized, there is no difference between models: both models view influence as multidirectional where an event acts and reacts, often modifying the future probability of the prior event as well as other events (Thoresen & Kirmal-Gray, 1983). Depicting a fourth set of interacting determinants, however, highlights the physiological events that characterize a respiratory disease or condition (Creer, 1983).

There are a few points about social cognitive learning theory that merit attention. First, the interactive perspective suggests that cognitive, physiological, environmental, and behavioral sources of influences should be studied in concert (Thoresen & Kirmal-Gray, 1983). Elements of the system never operate in an autonomous manner, and a complete account of the state of the individual requires consideration of all elements. For example, symptom discrimination is a prototypical event to investigate in that it requires a concurrent analysis of all elements of the system (Creer, 1983). Secondly, reciprocity does not mean that sets of interacting determinants are of equal strength; their relative influence varies for different activities and circumstances (Bandura, 1997). This is important with respiratory disease, where our focus shifts between and among sources of influence. Thirdly, mutual influences and their reciprocal effects do not occur simultaneously as a holistic entity (Bandura, 1997). Rather, Bandura continued, it takes time for a causal factor to exert its influence. Because of this time lag in the operation of the sets of factors, it is possible to gain an understanding of how different segments of reciprocal causation operate. Finally, Thoresen & Kirmil-Gray (1983) issued the caveat that the cognitive social learning model includes complexity and some ambiguity. Multidirectional interactive models make for difficult science, they continued, particularly at the levels of empirical assessment and causal explanations. However, Thoresen & Kirmil-Gray (1983, p. 599) concluded,

> *the tradeoff may be worthwhile insofar as the model more closely fits the experience of people. Whether the model endures will depend on its utility in fostering the understanding and treatment of complex human problems.*

Integration of Social Cognitive Learning Theory and Complexity

Both complexity and social cognitive learning have been defined and discussed. The task now is to synthesize these topics and describe their potential importance in respiratory disorders. This process will be illustrated by describing the relationship of components of social cognitive learning – physiological, cognitive, environmental, and behavioral – to respiratory conditions.

Elements of System

Complex systems have a large number of elements. This is particularly true with an interdisciplinarian approach where we concurrently examine, from several perspectives, the elements and processes of a chronic respiratory disorder. The elements do, however, easily fit into the components of the social cognitive learning model. Environmental elements, for example, range from triggers of asthma to spousal support for a COPD patient. The impact environmental elements have on the physiology of a person may result in the avoidance or exacerbation of a respiratory condition. Cognitive elements are reflected in how patients perceive environmental and physiological variables, and in the decisions they make to avoid or to approach them. Finally, whatever overt actions the patient makes in response to the situation are behavioral. The question thus shifts from asking whether the elements of a complex system fit within a social cognitive learning model, to asking whether the sheer number of variables is too large to permit us to conduct research aimed at expanding our understanding of the complex nuances of a given respiratory condition. This is the challenge faced by medical and behavioral scientists.

Necessary but not Sufficient Elements

Bandura's (1997) social cognitive model is unique in that it emphasizes interactions that occur among cognitive, physiological, behavioral, and environmental elements. The system based upon these elements evolves over time. In addition, the interaction of physiological, behavioral, cognitive, and environmental variables permits the transfer of information.

Interactions Are Rich

Any element in a proposed system influences and is influenced by a large number of elements (Cilliers, 1998). This is a strength of the social cognitive learning model. Richness of interactions is necessary given the task of examining the large number of physiological, cognitive, environmental, and behavioral factors involved with any chronic respiratory disorder.

Nonlinearity

Interactions that occur in the social cognitive learning system are often nonlinear. Dealing with nonlinearity presents the greatest barrier to the study of complexity. In part, this is because of our reliance upon linear research designs and our failure to come up with better ways to conduct research on respiratory disorders. However, much of this may change as more powerful and sophisticated computers are developed and integrated into respiratory research. This has occurred in other areas. As Coveney & Highfield (1995, p. 59) explained, 'today people working in all areas of complexity use computers in an experimental capacity for gaining insights where no other routes are feasible.'

Interactions Have a Short Range

At this point, there is no way to determine whether interactions have a short range when a social cognitive learning model is applied to a respiratory disorder. We do know that different elements interact with one another to the extent that particular interactions can have a far-ranging effect. Exposure to a stimulus at work, for example, may trigger asthma several hours later when the person is in a totally different environment. Tracing the steps involved before an element or set of elements have this effect, however, is often beyond the scope of our knowledge of respiratory disorders and their treatment.

Loops in Interactions

Loops are defined in several ways. Ford (1987; Ford & Ford, 1987) described both open systems – functional patterns without self-regulating feedback – and closed systems – functional patterns with closed loops. The former type of loops are a significant component of the self-regulating system he described, but not of the systems proposed by others (e.g., Carver & Scheier, 1998). However, there is agreement that feedback provides information about consequences. Most theorists would concur with Coveney & Highfield (1995), who described both positive feedback – that which reinforces and strengthens a response – and negative feedback – that which dampens a response. Feedforward, considered both as anticipatory output and as creating a change in reference values, is also relevant (Carver & Scheier, 1998). It is central to Ford's (1987) theory in that he proposed that when feedback and feedforward are combined, a dynamic system emerges that combines information from past, present, and projected future events to guide the flow of activity in a variable environment either to maintain or to alter its current steady state.

Feedback and feedforward are important to the control of a chronic respiratory disease. After teaching patients self-management skills for their condition, we later reinforce them for performance of these skills. In doing so, the skills are strengthened. However, given a constant – the flow of time – whether the changes are maintained can only be assessed through a continued examination of a patient's behavior; thus, the importance of anticipatory feedforward on the future activities by patients.

Complex Systems are Open

Ford (1987) stated that systems are open if they exchange material, energy, and/or other information within their environment; they are closed systems if they do not. Living systems, such as humans, are open systems. In the case of respiratory disorders, there is continuous interaction among elements of the system. A patient may be performing appropriate behavior, for example, to control an exacerbation of a respiratory condition. The efforts of that individual, in turn, could have a direct impact on the severity of the exacerbation. A change in breathing would hopefully be detected by the patient who, if the exacerbation is decreasing in intensity, might do nothing or, if the exacerbation is increasing in intensity, perform management behaviors, such as taking an inhaled quick-relief drug.

Complex Systems Lack Equilibrium

There is no equilibrium in breathing, although changes occur in response to everyday events, such as exercising, or with onset of a respiratory exacerbation. The elements involved in social cognitive theory attempt to alter what are perceived as inappropriate breathing patterns and restore breathing to an adaptation level considered as normal by that individual. However, this does not mean that there is a state of equilibrium of breathing. The natural rhythm of breathing is constantly changing; for that reason, breathing is best considered as a phenomenon that exhibits steady-state variability (Creer, 1979).

Complex Systems Have History

The past impinges upon the present in a number of different ways. For example, sight of an approaching cat may cause a child who is allergic to cat dander to move away from the animal. Or, the history of past attacks may serve as a guide for managing an asthma exacerbation experienced by another individual. History plays a role in how we perceive and react to any stimulus we believe could affect our breathing. It is also important in that it determines what we perceive as an adaptation level of breathing.

Elements Are Ignorant of System

There are a number of potential examples of one part of the system being ignorant of the entire system, but symptom discrimination is a good illustration (Chapter 5). As Rietveld and Everaerd noted, a person lacking hypoxic receptors might begin experiencing asthma, but be unaware of the onset of the attack. Only after the attack becomes severe or others point out symptoms of the attack, may the required action be taken by that individual. At CARIH, we admitted children who lacked what was then called hypoxic drive. As they had difficulty discriminating the onset of asthma, they were taught to use other cues, such as information provided by symptoms of asthma, information provided by others, reliance on the use of peak flow meters, and so on, as ways to compensate for the lack of hypoxic feedback.

Representation

Earlier, it was noted that an approaching cat, as witnessed by an asthmatic child allergic to such pets, might serve as a stimulus to initiate action on the part of the youngster to avoid the animal. In this example, environmental and cognitive elements interact so as to produce escape behavior on the part of the child. This illustration reflects the role of cognition in the collection and storage of information regarding the environment, and its relation to possible physiological exacerbation of the child's asthma. The child's action is not random, but the result of a cognitive process involving elements both of memory and the current environment that prompts escape behavior.

Self-Organization

When in the field, youngsters playing baseball may feel a tightening in their chest that signals the onset of asthma. When they sit down when their team is at bat, however, the tightening may decrease and fade away. This might occur in reaction to a change in activities from running in the field to taking a sedentary position in the dugout; however, at least with asthma, it might also indicate the spontaneous remission of the episode. Spontaneous remission of an asthma attack is the prototypical example of self-organization, particularly as no one knows exactly what stimulus or stimuli trigger a given attack or specifically what ameliorates the episode.

Mechanisms for Action

Ball (1999, p. 2) observed that 'the idea of complexity from simplicity has become almost a new scientific paradigm in recent years, and most probably a cliché too.' This connotes that describing components thought to comprise complexity is relatively simple; in doing so, however, we might oversimplify complexity to the point that it becomes a cliché. Describing a mechanism by which complexity occurs or by which it can explain our observations in a practical manner, on the other hand, is difficult. The task requires both knowledge of the phenomenon and the imagination to view it from a different perspective. Michael Hyland (1999) has done this in proposing a connectionist theory of asthma.

Connectionism, parallel distributed processing, or neural networks derive from the idea that humans do not process the world sequentially, but from many different flows that occur in parallel (Carver & Scheier, 1998). Connectionists seek to model thought processes of simple neuron-like units where processing consists of passing activation among units in parallel. While there are several types of connectionist systems, they have four features in common (Hyland, 1999). First, there is a set of units, including a variety of constructed (or simulated patterns) or self-made tapestries (Ball, 1999). The latter include such natural phenomena as flocks of birds, the movement of sand, or the flow of fluids. Secondly, each unit has causal connections with other units. All connectionist systems have excitatory (activation) or inhibitory (deactivation) signals. Third, the processing of signals in a network proceeds entirely by an activation rule that determines how a unit is influenced by others, and does not require any higher-order executive to direct or control the processing. Finally, the system as a whole has an activation pattern that describes the overall inhibitory and excitatory relationships in the network (Hyland, 1999). In a distributed connectionist network, knowledge is not represented in a central way or as nodes of information; rather, concluded Carver & Scheier (1998, p. 324), 'knowledge is represented in terms of the pattern of activation taken by the network as a whole. Thus, knowledge is distributed.' A connectionist system regulates the internal environment and solves the complex problem of internal regulation (Hyland, 1999). Such systems are dynamic and operate in a nonlinear manner.

Properties of connectionist systems are relevant to the present discussion because they are compatible with the social cognitive learning model. Hyland described four such properties:

1 A connectionist network is an effective way of achieving integration in a system that has multiple tasks. Hyland continues by suggesting that the body achieves self-regulation not through a series of independent feedback loops which may be coincidentally connected, but through a recurrent network. Such recurrent networks exist in a social cognitive learning model through both the separate actions and reciprocal determinism of cognitive, physiological, environmental, and behavioral components.
2 Connectionist systems are tolerant of local error. Because information in systems is distributed over the entire network, an error in one part of the system has a comparatively small effect. This undoubtedly occurs in considering the variegated tasks achieved in a social cognitive model of learning.
3 Recurrent networks have the technical property of relaxation in that they may relax over a period of cycles from an initial unstable state into one or more stable states. This is not the same as total equilibrium, however. As pointed out earlier, breathing represents a case of

steady-state variability where corrections occur to reduce the variability, but not to achieve total equilibrium. As a connectionist system, a social cognitive learning model can help control the steady-state variability that defines breathing.

4 A connectionist system provides a theory of learning which, in this case, is the social cognitive learning model. In sum, Hyland concluded, the network responsible for self-regulation has a short-term adaptive response hardwired into the system – consisting here of the basic components of cognition, behavior, physiology, and environment – and a long-term adaptive response involving the system changing, through learning, its activation pattern. In social cognitive learning theory, this could entail the teaching of self-management skills which, through continued performance, results in greater control over a respiratory disorder.

Framing

Hyland proposed a theory of asthma based on the premise that asthma is a particular type of relaxation pattern that results from faulty learning in the body's recurrent network. In other words, Hyland continued, asthma results because there is a breakdown in the efficiency of that part of the network that controls inflammatory self-regulation in the lung. The change in the relaxation pattern, in turn, gives rise to the mediators of inflammation.

Hyland's theory is a thoughtful and imaginative approach to asthma. It not only merits careful study but also should serve as a blueprint for future research. Rather than take such a comprehensive approach, however, I would like to describe how a model of complexity offers unique perspectives to the interpretation of findings in several studies with asthma patients. By doing so, it is hoped that complexity and connectionism can be illustrated. Before proceeding, however, I would like to describe a framework for the discussion.

Direct Observation of Asthmatic Children and Their Families

In a series of studies, Charles M. Renne and his colleagues conducted a complex analysis of the behavior of asthmatic children within the natural environment of their homes and families (e.g., Renne, 1982; Renne & Creer, 1985; Renne *et al.*, 1985). The study was highly complex in that it featured the concurrent analysis of cognitive, behavioral, physiological, and environmental variables. A number of findings emerged from this work, which was conducted over a number of years (Renne & Creer, 1985). First, studying only the flow of behavioral events proved a highly complex task. Developing a reliable and valid system for coding the behavior gathered by observers using handheld computers took 6 years. The overall reliability found in observing such a complex matrix of behaviors and patterns was $r = 0.61$. Secondly, training observers proved equally difficult. Not only did they require intensive training but also they needed regular follow-up training to avoid observer bias or observer drift. Thirdly, breaking up the stream of behavior into segments resulted in a massive amount of information. A major finding from the study was that there was a nonsignificant relationship between the 24 main categories of behavioral events and asthma. These findings were not unexpected and reflect the results of analyzing only linear events, the common procedure used in most of our studies. However, by looking at the correlations of events within each category, a broader and more accurate picture emerges concerning the interactions of behavior to asthma. One finding, for example, was that parents displayed varying degrees of attention to the nonasthma behaviors of children with asthma than they did with their nonasthmatic peers. Only by exhibiting asthma-related behaviors did the children with asthma receive attention; this confirmed a finding reported earlier by Creer and Renne (Creer, 1978) which showed that the context existing within the home often inadvertently reinforces asthma-like responses in children. It offers an alternative explanation for the phenomenon of rapid remission of asthma to be discussed later. Finally, the data analysis of the accumulated data overwhelmed computer facilities of that period. Thus, while the main effects were analyzed, there remains a matrix of 120,000 coefficients that require further analysis. If analyzed in a more detailed manner by modern computers, the array of correlations should create a complex mosaic that will bear witness to the synergistic relationship of behavior, physiology, cognition, and environmental variables. What was captured by Renne and his colleagues is akin to what occurs in genetics with DNA microarrays or an orderly process of DNA strings. The massive amount of data gathered by Renne consists of an orderly process of behavioral samples. Analyzing the data in terms of complexity would undoubtedly show, as has been found in genetics (Collins, 1999), that many of these microallays have macroconsequences with respect to the impact of behavior upon respiratory disorders.

For purposes of framing the discussion of asthma research, three processes emerged as significant in the study by Renne and colleagues (Renne, 1982; Renne *et al.*, 1985): the inexorable forward movement of time, sequences of events, and context.

Irreversible Medium of Time

In their book, Coveney & Highfield (1995) suggested that two features were necessary for complexity to emerge: time and nonlinearity. The latter has been described throughout the chapter; however, note Coveney & Highfield (1995, p. 9), the first and foremost ingredient is 'an irreversible medium in which things can happen: this medium is time, flowing from the past that lies closed behind us toward a future that is open.' It is important to discuss this component because use of the term feedback often leads to the erroneous conclusion that a response that occurred in the past is strengthened. This is not the case; what occurs with positive feedback is a strengthening of a response that is indicated by an increased probability of that response occurring in the future. Negative feedback, on the other hand, weakens a response and often leads to a decreased probability of the response occurring in the future. The work by Renne and his colleagues clearly showed changes in behavior, in both children with asthma and their families, over time.

Time as an irreversible medium is a key ingredient in social cognitive learning theory. Bandura (1997, p. 21) distinguished self-efficacy from an outcome expectation when he noted that,

> *Perceived self-efficacy is a judgment of one's ability to organize and execute given types of performances, whereas an outcome expectation is a judgment of the likely consequences such performances will produce.*

Bandura continued by noting that outcome expectations can take three forms: (a) the positive and negative physical effects that accompany the behavior; (b) positive and negative social effects; and (c) positive and negative self-evaluative reactions to one's own behavior. These outcome expectancies are influential in applying a social cognitive learning model to respiratory disorders.

Sequences of Events

The research by Renne and his colleagues demonstrated that behavioral patterns consist of observable sequences of events. Behavioral nodes or events often consisted of a string of several distinct behaviors, although sequences of one or two events were also observed. The sequences generally involved interactions between the target person, the child with asthma, and members of his or her family. These interactions were initiated by someone making a verbal statement, such as a command by a parent, and terminated when the command was either fulfilled or, as was more prone to happen, ignored. Physiological data, in the form of peak flow values and a daily diary, were obtained in the study; in addition, environmental events were observed and recorded.

Behavioral, physiological, and environmental events are often public acts (Skinner, 1953); they easily lend themselves to public observation. Cognition and most physiological events, however, can only be investigated through overt reactions, particularly verbal behaviors, exhibited by those being observed. However, based upon indirect data, we often can make reliable guesses regarding these cognitive acts; it is important to do so because they often indicate the nonlinear events that occur in a study.

Context

Ford (1987) considered the environment as the context within which behaviors occur. Context, however, can be viewed in a broader sense in that it is consists of cognitive, behavioral, physiological, and environmental events that both operate independently and interact with one another in a given situation. Various patterns of interactions form different contexts; in addition, contexts both set the stage and interact with whatever sequence of behavior we perform or observe. Often, they serve to frame a series of related sequences, as observed by Renne and his colleagues (e.g., Renne & Creer, 1985).

Impact of Nonlinear Variables in Asthma Research

Four types of research regarding asthma will be reviewed in this section. These investigations will be analyzed in order to demonstrate the necessity of considering a dynamic, nonlinear, and complex model in respiratory research. The types of research include studies on suggestion, medication compliance, overuse of hospitals, and rapid remission of asthma.

Suggestion

A former colleague at CARIH, Jon Weiss, and his associates presented several sets of stimuli to a group of 28 children with asthma (Weiss *et al.*, 1976). One stimulus was a film depicting children experiencing severe asthma; the film showed the youngsters coughing, wheezing, and gasping for breath. Weiss and his co-workers found that more subjects exhibited a decrease in maximum expiratory flow rate while watching the film depicting the children having asthma than occurred with presentation of other stimuli. Levenson (1974) found increases in total respiratory resistance occurred in adults shown what were thought to be three stressful films, including the same film used by Weiss *et al.* (1976).

While conducting their study, Jon Weiss reported that twin boys appeared totally unmotivated to participate in the study; they were, therefore, excused from participation. Jon suggested I talk to the twins and find how why they were uncooperative. I did so. During our conversation, one of the twins said, 'Why do they think that watching other children with asthma would cause us to feel anything? We've watched each other have asthma attacks, some bad, all our lives. It just doesn't bother us anymore.' Thus, while their data were discarded from the final analysis, the twins shed an intriguing light on suggestion and asthma: they illuminated nonlinearity, typical of the real world by showing, in a qualitative sense, 'more than was bargained for' in the study (Coveney & Highfield, 1995). First, with respect to suggestion, their comments indicated that to produce respiratory change within a suggestion paradigm, a presented stimulus had to be truly novel. If it is not novel, then any respiratory changes would be unlikely. If the suggestion paradigm was depicted in a sequence, the most simple one would appear as

Context
[E (Stimulus)] → [C (Interpretation)] → [B (Behavioral change), P (Physiological change)]

where the environmental stimulus is the film, the cognitive event is the interpretation of the stimulus, and physiological and behavioral changes that occurred in response to the film. With the twins, however, the following sequence appeared:

Context
[E (Stimulus)] → [C (Interpretation)] → [B/P (No behavioral or physiological changes)]

The twins did not come into the study with a blank tabula rasa. Their comments indicated they had adapted to the sight of someone having severe asthma; it was, therefore, not a novel stimulus to watch a film of others experiencing an asthma attack. The findings indicate that in order for suggestion to change respiratory responses, the stimulus must be truly novel. It also indicates that with repeated presentations of the stimulus, no behavioral or respiratory reactions will occur. A conclusion is that, with or without deceptive instructions presented before presentation of a stimulus (Creer, 1978), the response that occurs is an artifact unique to the suggestion paradigm rather than a genuine respiratory change. In the long run, a nonlinear variable – the adaptation of the twins to the sight of someone having an attack – yielded an equally significant finding with respect to suggestion and asthma as that described by Weiss *et al.* (1976).

Compliance

Earlier, the study by Jim Sublett *et al.* (1979) was described. Their hypothesis was that children who came to a hospital emergency room for treatment of asthma were likely to be noncompliant to their theophylline regimen. Their data fit their hypothesis: only one of 50 children showed compliance, as indicated by the theophylline level in her bloodstream. However, Sublett and his colleagues went beyond their research hypothesis and reviewed the dose levels of theophylline prescribed for each patient. They found that the one child whose theophylline levels were within the appropriate therapeutic range was not really compliant; had she been, she would have been taking a toxic level of the drug. The finding was frightening to Jim and his co-workers (pers. comm., May 11, 1984): while it was possible that any of the 49 children classified as noncompliers could have died from their asthma, the probability of this happening was less than it was for the child to take a toxic and potentially deadly dose of a prescribed drug. This nonlinear variable – the prescribing practice of a physician – provided information that would have been lost had the investigators been blinded to information occurring outside their hypotheses and findings.

Breaking down the study into the sequence of events for the study reveals:

Context
[E (Physician instructions)] → [B/C (Noncompliance)] →
[P (Asthma attack)]

Physician instructions on taking theophylline medication served as an environmental event. The children's behavior indicates that they do not comply with the instructions, here depicted as both cognitive and behavioral events; these events, in turn, lead to a physiological reaction, an asthma attack severe enough to prompt treatment at a hospital emergency room. The context, in this case, was established by the analysis of compliance to medication instructions. The child who had theophylline levels within the therapeutic range exhibited a similar, yet totally different, sequence:

Context
[E (Physician instructions)] → [B/C (Noncompliance)] →
[P (Asthma attack)]

The physician instructions provided the patient were different than those provided to other children in the study. As depicted, the patient complied, both cognitively and behaviorally, to a degree that led her to have the proper amount of theophylline in her bloodstream compliance. However, had she totally adhered to the prescribed regimen, there was a strong likelihood of a toxic reaction. The behavior, noncompliance, was similar across all subjects in the study; in addition, they all experienced asthma attacks although, given the fact that the one child had theophylline within the therapeutic level, the reason for the attack was different. The context in this situation, however, would have been unique, in part because of the physician's instructions and their interactions with behavioral, cognitive, and physiological events.

Recently, Creer *et al.* (1999) described a scenario regarding the taking of controller or maintenance medications. In the last Expert Panel Report 2 (National Institutes of Health, 1997), it was suggested that patients take a controller drug, namely inhaled corticosteroids, if their asthma could not be controlled with relief or as-needed drugs. The scenario would appear as

Context
[E (Physician instructions)] → [B/C (Compliance)] →
[P (Control of asthma)]

Indeed, if patients adhere to this regimen, their asthma will probably be controlled.

A problem in taking prescribed asthma medications was described by Creer *et al.* (1999). The issue was that health care personnel not only prescribed inhaled corticosteroids but also added three other controller drugs to patients' regimens: inhaled cromolyn sodium, a long-lasting β-agonist, and an anti-leukotriene drug. The apparent aim was to provide optimal control over the patient's asthma. The cumulative effect of prescribing the four controller drugs, however, apparently establishes too much control over the patient's asthma. The specific problem, suggested Winder (pers. comm., November 7, 1999), is that the combined regimen seems to blunt signs of an asthma exacerbation, which means that patients fail to recognize the onset of an attack and initiate steps to alleviate the episode. Looking at it in a behavioral manner, it would appear as

Context
[E (Physician instructions)] → [B/C (Compliance)] →
[P (Masking symptoms)]

Patients have reported that only by not adhering to the prescribed controller medications and relying on a relief drug do they know what is happening to their asthma. This is a paradoxical finding that is found when controller drugs, each designed to maintain a patient's breathing in a particular manner, are added together to essentially create an entirely new class of medications that seemingly controls asthma too well, possibly by blunting hypoxic receptors.

Overuse of Hospitals

Two studies looked at how environmental factors controlled the duration of time that children spent in a hospital. Both studies produced information that was of value in other ways. First, in the study by Creer (1970), the amount of time that two children spent in the hospital was reduced by removing reinforcers from the hospital. The initial thought was that time-out had reduced a type of malingering. However, others said the study showed that environmental manipulation controlled asthma per se, as days hospitalized is an important outcome variable of asthma. Which is the correct interpretation of the data? Both are. While my purpose was to limit the unnecessary use of the hospital, the study showed that time-out also influenced what could be considered as a significant outcome measure – time spent in the hospital. Secondly, Hochstadt *et al.* (1980) also reduced the amount of time spent in the hospital in children with asthma by manipulating reinforcers.

The initial sequence that influences the children could be presented in the following manner:

Context
[E (Hospital setting)] → [B/C/E (Reinforcement in hospitals] →
[B/C (Hospital overuse)]

The context of hospital overuse would also have been reinforcing to the patients; hence, they overused the hospitals when their asthma did not require such treatment.

When the behavior was altered through reducing reinforcement in the hospital, the following sequence occurred:

Context
[E (Hospital)] → [B/E (Reinforcement reduced)] →
[B/C (Hospital use decreased)]

The context in this case also changed. Overall, the time-out procedure led one child to remark, 'The hospital's no fun no more' (Creer, 1970).

Hochstadt *et al.* (1980) discovered that a nonlinear variable – the living situation of some children – impinged upon their findings. This was detected when time-out had no effect upon the amount of time these children spent in the hospital. In discussions with the children, it was found that even without the typical hospital reinforcers, they preferred a bed with clean sheets in a safe environment over the housing projects where they lived in inner-city Chicago. In considering this within a social cognitive learning theory, it would appear as

Context
[E (Hospital)] → [B/C/E (Reinforcement reduced)] →
[(B/C (Hospital use unchanged)]

Cognitive and behavioral events, in this case, led the children to believe that they were still better off in the hospital than at home with their families.

Rapid Remission

Asthma has always been regarded as a disorder with no known cure. In his classic work, Osler (1892) implied this when he said that the 'asthmatic pants into old age.' While Osler may not have seen asthma as a potentially deadly condition, he reiterated the writings of many others (e.g., McFadden & Stevens, 1983) concerning the incurable nature of asthma.

Whether or not asthma could be reversed was questioned by Peshkin (1930) with an approach he called 'parentectomy.' He coined the word because of what happened with 41 children with what he called intractable asthma. Based on his findings, 23 of 25 children removed from their homes and parents for periods extending from 2 months to more than 1 year showed improvement or remission of their symptoms;

hence the word parentectomy. No improvements were noted in 16 children who were not removed from their homes or families. Based upon these findings, Peshkin championed the creation of a residential treatment center for children with asthma. His plea was answered in 1940 with the creation of the Jewish National Home for Asthmatic Children, a forerunner to CARIH, in Denver.

The claims of Peshkin were initially supported by findings at CARIH. The change in environment resulted in the remission of asthma for many children admitted to the facility. Peshkin (1959) presented data which indicated that 98% of the youngsters in residence at CARIH between 1953 and 1955, irrespective of age, sex, and duration of illness, experienced a complete remission of their asthma. The duration of such changes was short lived, however, in that from 1958 to 1959, Falliers (1970) noted that complete remission of asthma was found in only 28% of those admitted to CARIH. By 1969, Falliers continued, the percentage of children showing complete remission with admission to CARIH declined to 12%. The number of children showing remission of their asthma symptoms continued to decline, so that by the time CARIH was closed in 1981 the term rapid remitter had disappeared from the vocabulary of the staff at the facility. There simply were no residents who fitted the label (Creer *et al.*, 1983).

What produced the change in the number of rapid remitters? Renne & Creer (1985) cited three factors:

- milder forms of asthma were successfully treated in the communities of children who might have been admitted to CARIH;
- CARIH began accepting more severe cases of asthma, particularly children who were steroid-dependent; and
- the facility began admitting children from all socioeconomic and ethnic groups.

The latter reason merits the closest scrutiny.

In the earliest years of the facility, the majority of residents were from intact families who were first- and second-generation immigrants to the United States (initially, the facility only accepted Jewish children, but it is unknown if this, in and of itself, was a relevant factor). Parents were undoubtedly overprotective of their children, in part because the entire family was in the process of assimilating themselves into a new culture. One result of this overprotectiveness, Renne & Creer noted, was that the children were reinforced for exhibiting asthma-like symptoms. If we break this down into a sequence, it would appear as

Context
[B/P (Asthma-like symptoms)] → [B/C/E (Reinforcement)] →
[(C/B/P (Increased symptoms)]

Here, asthma-like symptoms, as well as accompanying behaviors, were reinforced by environmental and behavioral stimuli. The result was an increase in the asthma-like symptoms and the diagnosis of asthma. The interactions of behavioral, environmental, physiological, and cognitive variables created a context that reinforced and maintained the inappropriate symptoms. When the children were admitted to CARIH, they encountered a totally different context. It would look like this:

Context
[(B/P (Asthma-like symptoms)] → [B/C/E (No reinforcement)] →
[B/C/P (Remission of symptoms)]

With no reinforcement provided for exhibiting asthma-like symptoms, there was a rapid remission of symptoms.

Did the children diagnosed as rapid remitters actually have asthma? No. At that period of time, asthma was diagnosed on the basis of observed symptoms; no challenges were made, such as occurs by inhaling methacholine or by exercising, while pulmonary functions were carefully measured. The latter measures were not uniformly adopted in confirming the diagnosis of asthma until the late 1970s or early 1980s.

There are also three other sets of data that argue against a diagnosis of asthma: the parent separation study, learned respiratory responses, and vocal cord dysfunction. Each set of data will be described.

Parent Separation Study

A question raised about rapid remitters was whether they experienced a major change in environments when they moved from their homes to the Rocky Mountains and CARIH. To determine if this was the case, Purcell *et al.* (1969) decided to do the reverse of parentectomy: they removed the parents from the home and had the children remain with surrogate parents. Based upon parent's response to a structured interview, children were divided into two groups. Half of the parents indicated that emotional precipitants were highly relevant to their child's asthma; Purcell and his colleagues predicted these youngsters would show an improvement in their asthma with removal of the parents. The remaining parents claimed emotional precipitants were not involved to any degree in their children's asthma; no improvement was expected in the asthma of these children. Looking at this from the point of reciprocal determinism, it appears as

Context
[B/C/E (Family)] → [B/C/E/P (Reinforcement)] →
[B/C/P (Respiratory responses)]

The context would be created by the interaction of cognitive, behavioral, physiological, and environmental factors.

After securing baseline data, the separation procedure was introduced for 2 weeks. During this period, the parents moved to a local hotel while the children remained at home with a trained child care worker. A reunion period of 2 weeks followed the end of the separation period.

Purcell and his colleagues gathered information regarding clinical examinations, daily history of asthma, pulmonary physiology, and medication requirements. Results indicated there was a statistically significant improvement of all measures for the children with emotional precipitants when they were separated from their parents. For children with no reported emotional precipitants, on the other hand, only one measure – history of daily asthma – suggested improvement with family separation. This would be depicted in the following manner:

Context
[(B/C/E (Family)] → [B/C/E/P (No reinforcement)] →
[B/C/P (Respiratory responses)]

The context had no effect upon the children who reportedly had no emotional precipitants to their asthma. However, it had a major effect in reducing respiratory responses in the children with emotional triggers.

Although the findings reported by Purcell and his colleagues were, in many instances, statistically significant, Renne & Creer (1985) pointed out that the study had several major flaws. First, there is no evidence of clinical significance, particularly with the all-important respiratory data. Changes in peak flow values, for example, are only clinically significant when there is a low baseline of values to begin with (Creer *et al*, 1998). Secondly, there is the likelihood that the children were more compliant to their medication regimen with the trained child care worker than they were with their parents. This was reflected by a change in the asthma diary data found in both groups of subjects when left at home with a surrogate parent. Finally, as occurred with the phenomenon of rapid remission, the asthma of the children was not confirmed by methacholine or exercise challenges (Renne & Creer, 1985). Nevertheless, the study by Purcell and his colleagues is invaluable in that it yielded insight into the acquisition of learned asthma-like respiratory responses by children.

Learned Respiratory Responses

Besides the acquisition and extinction of asthma-like symptoms, a number of respiratory responses have been exhibited by various patients. All have been ameliorated by the application of behavioral techniques. These responses include sneezing (Kushner, 1968), coughing (Alexander *et al.*, 1973; Creer *et al.*, 1977), and laryngeal wheezing (Rodenstein *et al.*, 1983). These responses can be depicted in the same manner as was shown for participants in the parent separation study:

Context
[B/C/E (Family)] → [B/C/E/P (Reinforcement)] →
[B/C/P (Respiratory responses)]

These respiratory responses lent themselves to change via the application of behavioral techniques, including the application of aversive stimuli. In the study by Creer *et al.* (1977), for example, a 15-year-old boy came to the clinic with a severe cough. It occurred during a cold, but continued long after the cold had ended. The boy was examined; he showed no respiratory changes to a bronchial challenge. Therefore, a harmless and mild electric shock was to be administered with what was to be an A–B–A–B reversal design. After a baseline period of 1 hour during which the subject coughed 22 times, an electric shock was applied to the next cough. What occurred can be depicted as follows:

Context
[B/C/E (Family & school)] → [E/P (Shock)] → [(B/C/P (No coughing)]

One harmless shock totally extinguished the behavior in what Kazdin (1989) has cited as the only known case of one-trial learning.

Vocal Cord Dysfunction
Christopher *et al.* (1983) described a respiratory pattern that they labeled as vocal cord dysfunction. Patients displayed asthma-like symptoms that, upon examinations, proved not to be asthma; the pattern only mimicked asthma. As most of these cases occur in adults, it is difficult to determine exactly how such cases of dysfunction develop. These are cases probably similar to other learned respiratory responses, where patients are reinforced by others in acquiring and maintaining these maladaptive patterns of behavior. However, it could also be that the patients acquire these patterns because a change in breathing initially helps them breathe better. This can be depicted in the following way:

Context
[B/C/E (Problems breathing)] → [B/C/P (Breathing change)] →
[B/C/P (Improvement)]

In these cases, however, the improvement is illusionary; the patients do not breathe better. When they are diagnosed with vocal cord dysfunction, they often require retraining in how to breathe properly. When there is no response to treatment for asthma in these patients at the National Jewish Medical Center in Denver, 20–30% of them are suspected of having vocal cord dysfunction (Bruce Bender, pers. comm., October 4, 1999).

Discussion

This chapter focused on several topics; overall, however, it addressed how we conduct research on respiratory disorders, while suggesting a potential paradigm for future research. The topics of reductionism and complexity were explored as polar points along a continuum. At one end of the spectrum, we reduce the number of variables we investigate to the smallest number we believe we can manipulate and go from there. This linear way of conducting research has many advantages, including that it makes our dependent and independent variables manageable, and often mimics the way we think and conceptualize research. Furthermore, the approach has generated much of the knowledge we have about chronic respiratory conditions. At the other end of the spectrum, it was noted that conducting research in a linear manner extracts a price: mainly, the elimination of information that can only be obtained by conducting complex and nonlinear investigations, where the components of the study are allowed to interact in a dynamic manner.

Social cognitive learning theory was proposed as a model for conducting future research with respiratory disorders. The interaction and synthesis of cognitive, physiological, behavioral, and environmental variables, indigenous to the theory, permits us to make a more refined analysis of the dynamics of a study, including the intrusion of nonlinear variables in an investigation. These analyses often result in more significant information than is found with traditional research. To illustrate this point, four types of studies – suggestion, compliance, hospital overuse, and rapid remitters – were dissected and discussed. The practice was shown to yield a more complex and meaningful interpretation than was originally presented in the studies.

By no means did the chapter attempt to present a simplistic view of complexity and its application. Wilson (1998) pointed out that complexity was born in the 1970s, gathered momentum in the 1980s, and generated controversy in the 1990s. He suggested that the latter occurred because of the way complexity is perceived by scientists. Their perceptions fall along a continuum: one end is anchored by those who, because they are focused on narrowly defined areas, care little for complexity theories. In many instances, in fact, the scientists had never heard of the theory. The opposite end of the continuum, continued Wilson, is anchored by those who not only believe deep laws of complexity exist but also that their discovery is just around the corner. These scientists – abstraction-absorbed, computer-oriented, light on natural history, heavy on nonlinear transformation – seemingly smell success. The third group, of which Wilson claims reluctant membership, is composed of those strung along the continuum from complete rejection to true believers. He places himself here because, he notes, there are currently insufficient facts to support complexity.

Wilson's position is the only prudent stance to take at the present time; it would be foolhardy to disagree with it. However, the aim of the chapter was to review past research and to suggest ways we might proceed with our research in the future. It will not be an easy transition. However, as Baruch Blumberg (1998, p. xii) noted:

> *The continued study of complexity, even if it does not provide totally satisfactory solutions, should make reductionist science aware that*

no matter how many details are uncovered, no matter how comprehensive understanding may be, there will always be unknowns beyond the sum of current knowledge. Each time an experiment is performed to test a hypothesis, more questions are revealed; there is no limit to the mysteries of nature and to our desire to understand them. The study of complexity offers an opportunity to stand back and consider the global interactions of fundamental units – atoms, elementary particles, genes – to create a synthesis that crosses the borders of scientific disciples, to see a grand vision of nature.

References

Alexander, A.B., Chai, H., Creer, T.L., Miklich, D.R., Renne, C.M. & Cardoso, R. (1973). The elimination of chronic cough by response suppression shaping. *Journal of Behavior Therapy and Experimental Psychiatry*, 4, 75–80.

Ball, P. (1999). *The self-made tapestry. Pattern formation in nature.* Oxford: Oxford University Press.

Bandura, A. (1977). Self-efficacy: toward a unifying theory of behavioral change. *Psychological Review*, 84, 191–215.

Bandura, A. (1986). *Social foundations of thought and action. A social cognitive theory.* Englewood Cliffs, NJ: Prentice-Hall.

Bandura, A. (1997). *Self-efficacy. The exercise of control.* New York: W.H. Freeman and Company.

Blumberg, B. (1995). Forward. In: P. Coveny & R. Highfield, *Frontiers of complexity. The search for order in a chaotic world.* New York: Ballantine Books.

Carver, C.S. & Scheier, M.F. (1998). *On the self-regulation of behavior.* New York: Cambridge University Press.

Charles, C., Whelan, T. & Gafni, A. (1999). What do we mean by partnership in making decisions about treatment? *British Medical Journal*, 319, 780–782.

Christopher, K.L., Wood, R.P. II, Eckert, R.C., Blager, F.B., Raney, R.A. & Souhrada, J.F. (1983). Vocal-cord dysfunction presenting as asthma. *New England Journal of Medicine*, 308, 1566–1570.

Cilliers, P. (1998). *Complexity and postmodernism. Understanding complex systems.* New York: Routledge.

Collins, F.S. (1999). Microarrays and microconsequences. *Nature Genetics*, 21, 2.

Coveney, P. & Highfield, R. (1995). *Frontiers of complexity. The search for order in a chaotic world.* New York: Ballantine Books.

Creer, T.L. (1970). The use of a time-out from positive reinforcement procedure with asthmatic children. *Journal of Psychosomatic Research*, 14, 117–120.

Creer, T.L. (1978). Asthma: psychological aspects and management. In: E. Middleton, Jr., C.E. Reed & E.F. Ellis (Eds), *Allergy: principles and practice* (pp. 796–811). St. Louis: C.V. Mosby.

Creer, T.L. (1979). *Asthma therapy: a behavioral health-care system for respiratory disorders.* New York: Springer Publishing.

Creer, T.L. (1983). Response: self-management psychology and the treatment of childhood asthma. *Journal of Allergy and Clinical Immunology*, 72, 607–610.

Creer, T.L. (1993). Medication compliance and childhood asthma. In: N.A. Krasnegor, L.. Epstein, S.B. Johnson & S.J. Yaffe (Eds), *Developmental aspects of health compliance behavior* (pp. 303–333). Hillsdale, NJ: Lawrence Erlbaum Associates.

Creer, T.L. (2000). Self-management and the control of chronic pediatric illness. In: D. Drotar (Ed.), *Promoting Adherence to Medical Treatment in Chronic Childhood Disease* (pp. 95–129). Hillsdale, NJ: Lawrence Erlbaum Associates.

Creer, T.L. & Christian, W.P. (1976). *Chronically-ill and handicapped children: their management and rehabilitation*. Champaign, IL: Research Press.

Creer, T.L. & Levstek, D. (1996). Medication compliance and asthma: overlooking the trees because of the forest. *Journal of Asthma*, 33, 203–211.

Creer, T.L., Renne, C.M. & Christian, W.P. (1976). Behavioral contributions to rehabilitation and childhood asthma. *Rehabilitation Literature*, 37, 226–232; 247.

Creer, T.L., Chai, H. & Hoffman, A. (1977). A single application of an aversive stimulus to eliminate chronic cough. *Behavior Therapy and Experimental Psychiatry*, 8, 107–108.

Creer, T.L., Ipacs, J. & Creer, P.P. (1983). Changing behavioral and social variables at a residential treatment facility for childhood asthma. *Journal of Asthma*, 20, 11–15.

Creer, T.L., Levstek, D.A. & Winder, J.A. (1998). Home monitoring of lung function measures. In: H. Kotses & A. Harver (Eds), *Self-management of asthma* (pp. 117–145). New York: Marcel Dekker.

Creer, T.L., Winder, J.A. & Tinkelman, D. (1999). Guidelines for the diagnosis and management of asthma: accepting the challenge. *Journal of Asthma*, 36, 391–407.

Falliers, C.J. (1970). Treatment of asthma in a residential center: a fifteen year study. *Annals of Allergy*, 28, 513–521.

Ford, D.H. (1987). *Humans as self-constructing living systems: a developmental perspective on behavior and personality*. Hillsdale, NJ: Lawrence Erlbaum Associates.

Ford, M.E. & Ford, D.H. (1987). *Humans as self-constructing living systems: putting the framework to work*. Hillsdale, NJ: Lawrence Erlbaum Associates.

Ford, D.H. & Urban, H.B. (1998). *Contemporary models of psychotherapy. A comparative analysis*, 2nd edn. New York: John Wiley & Sons.

Goerner, S. (1995). Chaos, evolution, and deep ecology. In: R. Robertson & A. Combs (Eds), *Chaos theory in psychology and the life sciences* (pp. 17–38). Mahwah, NJ: Lawrence Erlbaum Associates.

Hochstadt, N., Shepard, J. & Lulla, S.H. (1980). Reducing hospitalizations of children with asthma. *Journal of Pediatrics*, 97, 1012–1015.

Hyland, M.E. (1999). A connectionist theory of asthma. *Clinical and Experimental Allergy*, 29, 1467–1473.

Kazdin, A.E. (1989). *Behavior modification in applied settings*, 4th edn. Pacific Groves, CA: Brooks/Cole Publishing Co.

Klahr, D. & Simon, H.A. (1999). Studies of scientific discovery: complementary approaches and convergent findings. *Psychological Bulletin*, 125, 524–543.

Kneller, G.F. (1978). *Science as human endeavor*. New York: Columbia University Press.

Kushner, M. (1968). The operant control of intractable sneezing. In: C.D. Spielberger, R. Fox, & B. Masterton (Eds), *Contributions to general psychology: selected readings for introductory psychology* (pp. 513–517). New York: Ronald Press.

Levenson, R.W. (1974). Effects of thematically relevant and general stressors on specificity of responding in asthmatic and nonasthmatic subjects. *Psychosomatic Medicine*, 41, 28–39.

McFadden, E.R., Jr. & Stevens, J.B. (1983). A history of asthma. In: E. Middleton, Jr., C.E. Reed & E.F. Ellis (Eds), *Allergy: principles and practice*, 2nd edn (pp. 805–809). St. Louis: C.V. Mosby.

National Institutes of Health (1991). *Executive summary: guidelines for the diagnosis and management of asthma* (NIH Publication No. 91–3042A). Washington, DC: US Department of Health and Human Services.

National Institutes of Health (1997). *Expert panel 2: guidelines for the diagnosis and management of asthma* (NIH Publication No. 97–4051). Washington, DC: US Department of Health and Human Services.

Osler, W. (1892). *The principles and practice of medicine*. New York: D. Appleton.

Peshkin, M.M. (1930). Asthma in children. IX. Role of environment in the treatment of a selected group of cases: A plea for a 'home' as a restorative measure. *American Journal of Diseases of Children*, 39, 774–781.

Peshkin, M.M. (1959). Intractable asthma in children: rehabilitation at the institutional level with a follow-up of 150 cases. *International Archives of Allergy and Applied Immunology*, 15, 91–112.

Pirsig, R. (1974). *Zen and the art of motorcycle maintenance: an inquiry into values.* New York: William Morrow and Co., Inc.

Purcell, K., Brady, K., Chai, H., *et al.* (1969). The effect of asthma in children of experimental separation from the family. *Psychosomatic Medicine*, 31, 144–164.

Renne, C.M. (1982). *Asthma in families: behavior analysis and treatment* (Final report). National Institute of Heart, Lung & Blood. (Grant RO1-HL-22021).

Renne, C.M. & Creer, T.L. (1985). Asthmatic children and their families. In: M.L. Walraich & D.K. Routh (Eds), *Advances in developmental and behavioral pediatrics* (pp. 41–81). Greenwich, CN: Jai Press, Inc.

Renne, C.M., Creer, T.L., Wasek, G. & Chai, H. (1985). The family assessment project: direct observation of social interactions and asthma variables in home and laboratory. *CARIH Research Bulletin, No. 10.*

Rodenstein, D.O., Francis, C. & Stanescu, D.C. (1983). Emotional laryngeal wheezing: a new syndrome. *American Review of Respiratory Disease*, 127, 354–356.

Russo, D.C. & Varni, J.W. (Eds) (1982). *Behavioral pediatrics: research and practice.* New York: Plenum Publishing.

Skinner, B.F. (1953). *Science and human behavior.* New York: The Macmillan Co.

Sublett, J.L., Pollard, S.J., Kadlec, G.J. & Karibo, J.M. (1979). Noncompliance in asthmatic children: a study of theophylline levels in pediatric emergency room population. *Annals of Allergy*, 43, 95–97.

Thoresen, C.E. & Kirmal-Gray, K. (1983). Self-management psychology and the treatment of childhood asthma. *Journal of Allergy and Clinical Immunology*, 72, 596–606.

Varni, J.W. (1983). *Clinical behavioral pediatrics: an interdisciplinary biobehavioral approach.* New York: Pergamon Press.

Verbrugge, L.M. & Patrick, D.L. (1995). Seven chronic conditions: their impact on US adults' activity levels and use of medical services. *American Journal of Public Health*, 85, 173–182.

Waldrup, M.M. (1992). *Complexity: the emerging science at the edge of order and chaos.* New York: Touchstone.

Weiss, J.H., Lyness, J., Molk, L. & Riley, J. (1976). Induced respiratory change in asthmatic children. *Journal of Psychosomatic Research*, 20, 115–123.

Wilson, E.O. (1998). *Consilience. The unity of knowledge.* New York: Alfred E. Knopf.

Wolpe, J. (1958). *Psychotherapy by reciprocal inhibition.* Stanford, CA: Stanford University Press.

Wynn, C.M. (1997). Does theory ever become fact? In: J. Hatton & P.B. Plouffe (Eds), *Science and its ways of knowing* (pp. 60–62). Saddle River, NJ: Prentice-Hall.

Index

ABC analysis and decision making 159
acrivastine, psychological side effects 186, 187
action (in Self-Management Model) 161
  selective 166
action plan 342
  asthma 345–6
    childhood 51, 64–5, 70–1, 73–4
  CF 348
  COPD 347
  smoking 353–4
  TB 351
activities, *see* Life Activities Questionnaire for Adult Asthma; lifestyle
adherence/compliance (and nonadherence) 141, 197–231, 251–2
  asthma, *see* asthma
  CF, *see* cystic fibrosis
  COPD, *see* chronic obstructive pulmonary disease
  definition (of concept) and description 198, 200
    problems with definition 200–2
  in Health Counselling Model 152–3
  improving 221–5
  intentional vs unintentional 251–2
  measurement 203–7
  medication, *see* drug therapy
  patient factors 206–17
    decision making 164, 215–17, 241
    factors influencing patient compliance 208–15
  physician/practitioner factors 217–22
  QOL and 252
  significance of problem 198–9
  tuberculosis treatment 313
  see also relapse
adolescents
  asthma deaths, psychological/behavioral factors 48
  CF, psychological adjustment 259–60, 263
  compliance 212–13
advice, *see* education; information
African-Americans, *see* blacks
age
  asthma distribution 23–4, 292
  compliance and 212–13
  COPD distribution 292
air pollution (outdoor)
  asthma and 31, 291
  COPD and 29
airway(s)
  hypersensitivity/hyperresponsiveness (in asthma) 287–8
    assessment 120
    see also bronchoreactivity
  inflammation
    asthma 20, 287
    CF 257
  obstruction in asthma 122, 286–7, 287–9
    assessment, problems 130
    aware of but not bothered by 126
    induced (in investigations) 120, 122, 122–3
    intermittency and variability 287–9
    reversibility 286–7
  obstruction in COPD 289
  obstructive disease, chronic (=COPD), *see* chronic obstructive pulmonary disease
Alaskan Natives, asthma hospitalizations 25
albuterol 305
albuterol sulfate 305
  prolonged-release tablets 308
allergens/allergic disease and asthma 30, 292

allergic rhinitis, neuropsychological side effects of drugs 175–6, 183–92
alpha-1-antitrypsin deficiency and emphysema 90, 292
American Indians, asthma hospitalizations 25
American Thoracic Society definitions, COPD 86, 289
  chronic bronchitis 290
  emphysema 290
aminophylline 308
animals, pet, and asthma 63
antibiotics
  CF 257
  COPD 312
  TB, *see* antituberculosis drugs
anticholinergic drugs 305, 306–7
  side effects 307
    psychological 190–1
antihistamines, psychological side effects 72, 184–8
α_1-antitrypsin deficiency and emphysema 90, 292
antituberculosis drugs 312–13
  resistance 313
    multidrug 294, 303, 349
anxiety, asthmatic child 53
  with breathlessness 72
appointments, medical, compliance 207–8
asthma 3–9, 19–83, 117–38, 286–9, 291–3, 295–9, 302–3, 304–12, 343–6, 359–61, 378–89
  adherence/compliance issues 46–53, 61–2, 70, 202, 382–4
    medication compliance 206
  children with, *see* children with asthma
  chronic 86, 86–7
  COPD and, distinction 285
  definitions 20–1, 285, 286–9
  diagnosis 295–9
    incorrect, possible in children 387–9
    symptoms in 21–2
  emotional reaction, *see* emotional response
  epidemiology 19–44
    burden 22
    mortality 25–7
    prevalence 22–5
  family in, *see* family; parents
  genetics 29–30, 292–3
  health care, *see* health care
  illness perceptions 8–9
  learning theory 6–7
  prevention (of attacks) 294–5
    drugs used 308–12
  psychoanalytic theories 3–5
  psychological functioning, *see* psychological functioning
  psychological side effects of medications, *see* neuropsychological side effects
  psychomaintenance 7–8
  publication numbers in *Health Psychology* (1990s) compared to cardiovascular disease and cancer 2
  QOL 234–6
    activity interference 235, 239, 241
    children 235–6
    interaction of morbidity and psychology in 238, 239–40
    meaning of/perspectives on 248–50
    questionnaires specific to 242, 244, 245, 246
  research (psychological and behavioral) 359–62, 363, 378–89
    connectionist theory 376
    framing discussion of 378–81
    historical aspects 3–9
    Hyland's theory 378
    nonlinear variables in 381–9
  risk factors 30–4, 291–3
  self-monitoring 158
  severity 27–8
    classification 298–9
    variability 288–9
    see also status asthmaticus
  suggestion in 381–2
  symptom(s)
    activities interfered with by 235
    in diagnosis of asthma 21–2
    questionnaires (history-taking) 297
  symptom perception 117–38, 289, 344
    definitions 119–21
    improving 117–18, 131–2
    mechanisms 121–2
    methodologies in investigation of (and criticisms of them) 119–21, 130–1
    physiological factors influencing 122–4
    psychological perspective 124–30
    see also Index of Perceived Symptoms in Asthmatic Children
  as syndrome vs disease 289
  therapeutic behavior analysis 343–6, 355
  therapy/management 284, 302–3, 304–12
    drugs, *see* drug therapy
    goals 302–3, 343–4
    health care models 363
    multidisciplinary vs interdisciplinary approaches 359–61
    new strategies, development and introduction 361–2
    self-management, *see* self-management
  triggers/precipitating factors 5
    choosing to avoid 235
    environmental, *see* environmental factors
    in history-taking 297

Asthma Bother Profile 242, 243, 244
Asthma QOL Questionnaire 242, 244
atopy and asthma 30
atropine and its quaternary salts, psychological side effects 190
attention, symptoms affected by 237
attention deficit hyperactivity disorder, child with asthma 67
attitudes (patient) influencing compliance 214

beclomethasone 308
behavioral compliance 207–8
behavioral interventions/techniques (incl. behavior therapy)
  asthma 6–7
  CF
    chest physical therapy 273
    nutrition 271
  compliance influenced by 222–3
  COPD 12–13, 326–9
    muticomponent program 326–9
    smoking cessation and 321
  see also cognitive–behavioral approaches
behavioral medicine336-7, 356
beliefs influencing compliance 214–15, 216–17
beta-agonists 305, 306, 308, 310
  long-term 308, 310, 384
  short-acting 305, 306
  side effects 306, 310
    psychological 180
  see also sympathomimetics
bipolar disorder, pseudoephedrine-precipitated 192
birth factors, asthma 33
bitolterol 305
blacks (incl. African-Americans)
  asthma
    hospitalizations 25
    prevalence 23–4, 292
  COPD prevalence 292
breathing maneuvers (in asthma) influencing breathlessness 122
breathing problems (in asthma)
  recognition by caretaker 64
  response of caretaker/child to 64–5
Breathing Problems Questionnaire 242, 244, 247
  shortened version 243, 247
breathlessness, *see* dyspnea
bronchitis, chronic 86, 285, 290
  definitions 290
bronchoreactivity measurement (bronchoprovocation challenge)
  in asthma 21–2
  in COPD 320
  see also airway, hypersensitivity

caloric requirements, CF 271
carbon monoxide levels and smoking cessation in COPD 319, 321
caregivers/careproviders (non-professional)
  in asthma in children 56
    alternative 50, 62, 70
    primary, child as 66
    primary, medication adherence and 61
    psychiatric morbidity 68
    response to symptoms 50, 64, 70
  in CF, age of patient and transfer of treatment responsibilities from 274–5
  see also family; parents; Pediatric Asthma Caregiver's QOL Questionnaire
caregivers/careproviders (professional incl. physicians/practitioners)
  childhood asthma
    case illustration 70
    relationship issues 50, 56, 58–9, 59–60
  compliance issues 217–22
  patient communication, *see* communication
carotid body resection 117–18
cats and asthma 63
centriacinar emphysema 291
change in behavior, anatomy 338–41
chest physical therapy (CPT), CF 256, 272–3
  adherence 272–3
chest radiograph, TB 301
Child Assessment Schedule (CAS), CF 261–2, 262, 263, 264
Child Behavior Checklist (CBCL)
  CF 259, 260
  feeding and 272
  self-management and 276
Childhood Asthma Questionnaires 245
children
  allergic rhinitis, psychological side effects of drugs 183–91
  CF, *see* cystic fibrosis
  psychological functioning influencing compliance in 213
  see also adolescents
children with asthma 45–83, 378–89
  action plan 51, 64–5, 70–1, 73–4
  adherence issues, *see* adherence
  adherence/compliance 46–53, 61–2, 382–4
    case illustration 70
    with environmental triggers 50, 56, 62–4
    with medication 46–53, 61–2, 70, 382–4
    parental opinions and decision making 216, 252
  direct observation 378–81
  environmental factors, *see* environmental factors
  family/parents, *see* family; parents

children with asthma *continued*
integration of asthma into family life 51, 68–9, 71
knowledge/education issues, *see* education
prevalence 23–4
psychological functioning, *see* psychological functioning
psychological side effects of drugs, *see* neuropsychological side effects
QOL deficit 235–6
questionnaires 243, 245, 246
residential treatment, *see* residential treatment
responsibility issues 51, 56, 65–6, 71, 75
severe and/or poorly controlled 76
medication assessment 61
symptoms 58, 65
caregivers awareness/recognition of 50, 64, 70
parents' influence 385–8
parents'/child's response to 56, 58, 64–5, 70–1
Children's Asthma Research Institute and Hospital (Denver) 359–60
China, smoking in
deaths related to 353
stopping, obstacles 353–4
chlorpheniramine, psychological side effects 186
choices, making, *see* decision making
chronic obstructive pulmonary disease (COPD) 9–13, 85–116, 289–90, 291–3, 295, 299, 303, 317–33, 346–7
adherence/compliance issues 202
decision making 215–16, 217
health outcome and 108
medication 206
published guidelines for treatment 220
asthma and, distinction 285
behavioral interventions 90–7
variable explaining relationship between outcome and 106–11
causes 87
definitions 86, 285, 289–90
diagnosis 299
spectrum of diseases contributing to 86
genetics 87, 90, 292
neuropsychological functioning 12
papers published in *Health Psychology* (1990s) compared to cardiovascular disease and cancer 2
prevention 295
progression (hypothetical/typical case) 323–5
psychosocial consequences 10
psychosocial mediators of outcome 97–106, 113
public health impact 87–9
QOL 10–12, 99–101
questionnaires specific to 242, 244, 245
San Diego Program 95
survival and 99–101
rehabilitation, *see* rehabilitation
smoking and, *see* smoking
therapeutic behavior analysis 346–7, 355
therapy 89–90, 284, 303
compliance, *see subheading above*
goals 303, 346
health care models 363
medical treatment 89–90, 308–12
psychotherapy 12–13
self-management 1, 12, 13
smoking cessation in, *see* smoking cessation
surgical 90
chronic respiratory disease (in general)
compliance issues 210, 211–12, 220
QOL, *see* quality of life
self-management, *see* self-management
see also illness
Chronic Respiratory Disease Questionnaire 242, 245
cigarette smoke/smoking, *see* smoking
cities, inner, asthma 27
cognitive factors influencing compliance 209, 214–15
see also social cognitive learning theory
cognitive–behavioral approaches 240
COPD 13, 14
San Diego Program 95–6
smoking cessation 322
communication, patient–doctor, adherence and 218–19, 221
asthma and 383
see also information
complexity (and complex systems) 367–71, 390–1
characteristics 368–70
indispensable 370
definition 367–8
integration with social cognitive learning theory 373–6
mechanisms for action 376–8
compliance issues, *see* adherence
conduct disorder, child with asthma 67
connectionism 376–8
conscious awareness of asthma symptoms/breathlessness 124–5
consciousness raising (Health Counseling Model) 144–5
consequences (in Health Counseling Model), weighing 145–6
consultation, psychological, childhood asthma, referral for 54
context of behavior 381
asthma (suspected) in children and 388, 389

coping
  difficulties
    CF child 265
    CF child's parents 268
  strategies/methods 238
    CF family 274
  see also transactional stress and coping model
corticosteroids 307
  asthma 72–3, 307, 359
    inhaled 308, 309, 384
    oral/systemic 72–3, 307
  COPD 308
    needless prescription 220
  side effects 307, 309
    psychological 72–3, 180–3
cost(s)
  CF care 349
  smoking cessation in COPD 329
cost-benefit analysis, smoking cessation in COPD 329
cost-effectiveness
  Self-Management Model 162
  smoking cessation in COPD 329
cough in asthma 21
counseling/counselors, *see* health counseling
cromolyn sodium 308, 309–10, 384
  psychological side effects 183
cues and symptom perception in asthma, internal vs external 125
cystic fibrosis (predominantly children) 255–82, 347–9
  adherence/compliance issues 202, 268–77, 277, 278
    decision making and health beliefs and 216–17, 217
    environmental and behavioral prescriptions 208
    exercise programs 226–7
    medication 206, 269–70
    psychological functioning and 213
  medical overview 256–8
  psychological adjustment 259–68, 277
    children 259–65
    children's parents 265–8, 272
  therapeutic behavior analysis 347–9, 355
  therapy/treatment
    adherence, *see subheading above*
    costs 349
Cystic Fibrosis Family Education Program 276

deaths
  asthma 25–7
    children, psychological/behavioral factors 47–8, 67
  smoking-related 353
    WHO data 351, 353
  see also survival
decision making/making 215–17
  compliance and 164, 215–17, 241
    and parents of asthmatic child 216, 252
  in Health Counseling Model 146–7
  in Self-Management Model 160–1
    ABC analysis 159
    to stop self-management skills 164
decongestants, psychological side effects 186
  see also sympathomimetics
demographic factors influencing compliance 209, 212–13
depression
  asthmatic child 52, 69–72
  asthmatic child's parents 68
  CF child's mother 266
  COPD 109–11
  see also bipolar disorder
desensitization, systematic, asthma 6, 7
developing countries, smoking 353, 353–4
diet/nutrition
  asthma and role of 33
  CF patient's 258
    adherence 270–2
diphenhydramine, psychological side effects 185–6, 186, 187
direct observation
  asthma, children and family 378–81
  TB treatment 284, 303, 304, 350, 351
disability, COPD and, relationship between 91, 92
disability-adjusted life years (DALYs), COPD 88, 89
disease, *see* illness
doctors, *see* caregivers (professional)
drug therapy (medication)
  adherence 197–207
    asthma, children 46–53, 61–2, 70, 382–4
    drug assays (body) in assessment of compliance 203–4
    medication amounts assessed 203, 205
    patient attitudes to medication 209, 211–12
    tuberculosis 313
  allergic rhinitis 175–6, 183–91
  asthma (generally) 28, 304–12
    activity interference and impact of 239
    controller/preventive drugs 308–12, 384
    QOL issues 243, 251
    quick-relief drugs 304–7, 304–8
  asthma, children 46–53, 57–8, 72–3
    adherence issues 46–53, 61–2, 70, 382–4
    family understanding 56, 57–8
  CF 206, 269–70
  COPD 89–90, 308–12, 325–6

drug therapy (medication) *continued*
  multidrug regimens 283–4
  side effects 306, 307
    compliance and 221–2
    psychological, *see* neuropsychological side effects
  see also specific (types of) drugs
dysphoria with activity avoidance/interruption in asthma 235
dyspnea (breathlessness; shortness of breath)
  in asthma 118–19
    anxiety in children with 72
    assessment, criticisms 130
    cause 121
    conscious awareness 124–5
    lung function and 120
    physiological factors influencing 122–4
    psychological perspectives 126, 129
  in COPD 107
    behavioral intervention and its impact 107
    rehabilitation studies 97

education (knowledge)
  asthma (in child) 50, 60–1, 73, 74, 75
    case illustration 70
    NIH and, *see* National Institutes of Health
    parents 50, 56, 60–1
  CF 276
  compliance and 223, 223–4
  COPD
    rehabilitation program vs 97, 98, 110, 111
    smoking cessation, *see* smoking cessation
  in Health Counselling Model 148–9
  see also information
effectiveness
  of drug, vs efficacy 251
  Self-Management Model 162
  see also cost-effectiveness
efficacy vs effectiveness of drug 251
  see also self-efficacy
electronic monitoring of compliance 203
emotion(s), negative, asthma symptom perception and influence of 128–9
emotional functioning, asthmatic child's family 48–9
emotional precipitants of asthma in children, parents and 387, 388
emotional response to asthma and its symptoms 238
  family 51, 65, 70–1
emphysema 86, 285, 289–90
  centriacinar 291
  definitions 289–90
  genetic factors 90, 292
environmental boundary conditions in self-management 165–6
environmental factors (as triggers/precipitating factors) in asthma 30–2, 33–4, 291
  children 291
    case illustration 70
    change in environment from home to residential treatment centre 385–7
    family adherence with recommendations 50, 56, 62–4
    tobacco smoke, *see* smoking
  preventive strategies aimed at 294–5, 385–7
environmental factors (as triggers/precipitating factors) in COPD 291
environmental prescription in CF, compliance 208
enzyme replacement, CF 258
ephedrine, psychological side effects 188, 188–9, 189
ethambutol 313
ethnicity (race) and COPD/asthma 292
exercise (and exercise training/programs) 226–7
  in CF 257
    compliance with 226–7
  in COPD 107, 108
    compliance with 108
    depression and 110, 111
    San Diego Program 93–5
Expert Panel Report 2 Guidelines (NOH) 20, 302–3, 383

familial factors in asthma development 33
family
  asthma (childhood) and 45–83, 385–8
    direct observation of family 378–81
    family management approach 45–83
    in history-taking 298
  CF psychosocial factors and adherence and 273–4
  compliance and the 209, 213–14
  COPD, perceptions of illness 300
  see also caregivers (non-professional); father; mother; parents
Family Adjustment and Adaptation Response (FAAR) Model and CF 273–4
Family Asthma Management System Scale (FAMSS) 49–52, 54–69
  behavioral domains assessed 50–1, 59–69
  case illustration 69, 70–1
  interview 54–9, 77
family history-taking, asthma 298
family therapy, asthma 75–6
fat intake, CF 271
father of CF child, psychological adjustment 266–7, 272

see also family; parents
feedback/feedforward (in complex systems) 369, 374–5
feeding interventions, CF child, adherence 270–2
females
compliance 213
with COPD, social support satisfaction related to survival 101–2, 103
see also gender
FEV_1, asthma diagnosis 296
flunisolide 308
fluticasone 308
follow-up
educational value of follow-up visits affecting compliance 223
in Health Counselling Model 150–1
forced expiratory volume in one second (FEV_1), asthma diagnosis 296

gender
asthma (children) and 292
compliance and 213
COPD and, social support satisfaction related to survival 101–2
genetics
asthma 29–30, 292–3
CF 258
COPD 87, 90, 292
global distribution of asthma 23
goal selection and setting
in Health Counseling Model 147–8
in Self-Management Model 157–8
in therapeutic behavior analysis 341
asthma 343–4
CF 348
COPD 346
smoking 352
TB 350

habituation to asthma symptoms 127
health, role of behavior 336–8
see also illness
Health Belief Model of Behavior 216–17
health care/medical care
asthma
caregivers in, see caregivers/ (professional)
role 28
utilization 25
models of 362–4
see also treatment
health counseling (and Health Counseling Model) 141, 142–54, 168–9
expectations of health counselors in self-management 167
limitations of model 153–4
processes 143, 144–55
strengths of model 152–3
health education, see education
health-promoting behaviors, improving 225–7
heredity, see genetics
heuristics in decision making 160
Hispanic Americans, asthma prevalence 23
histamine-induced airways obstruction 122–3
historical aspects
asthma, psychological research 3–9
COPD care 93
history-taking (incl. questionnaires)
asthma 296, 297–8
COPD 299, 300
hospital use
asthma 25
children, overuse 384–5
COPD, smoking cessation program during 320–1
hypersensitivity/hyperreponsiveness, airway, see airway

illness and disease
chronic, see chronic respiratory disease
patient compliance and characteristics of 208–10
perceptions of, see also perception
positive consequences reported 249
role of behavior 336–8
Index of Perceived Symptoms in Asthmatic Children 245
individual differences and self-management 166
infections (respiratory)
asthma development and role of 32
in CF 257
in COPD, treatment 312
inflammation, airway, see airway
information (incl. instruction and advice)
acting on
in Health Counselling Model 149–50
in Self-Management Model 143
collection, in Self-Management Model 158
in compliance, practitioner role in provision and communication of 218–19, 221
asthma and 383
preparing patient to accept and act on, in Health Counseling Model 143, 144–9
processing and evaluation, in Self-Management Model 158–60
see also communication
informed model of health care 362
inhalation devices 240
compliance with 251
electronic monitoring 206
poor technique/incompetence influencing 211, 218

inheritance, *see* genetics
inner cities, asthma 27
instruction, *see* education; information
interdisciplinary vs multidisciplinary management, asthma 359–61
ipratropium bromide 305
 in COPD, smoking cessation and 322
 psychological side effects 190
isoetharine 305
isoniazid 312
 resistance 313
isoproterenol/isoproterenol sulfate 305

Jewish National Home for Asthmatic Children 386

lapse in behavior, *see* adherence/compliance; relapse
learned respiratory response, children with suspected asthma and 388–9
learning theory
 asthma 6–7
 social cognitive, *see* social cognitive learning theory
leukotriene modifiers 183, 308, 311–12, 384
life
 quality of, *see* quality of life
 valuation 248
  asthma 249
Life Activities Questionnaire for Adult Asthma 245
lifestyle (incl. activity)
 compliance with restrictions 207
 symptoms interfering with 238
  asthma 235, 239, 241
living situation in asthma
 history-taking 297–8
 hospital use and 385
Living with Asthma Questionnaire 242, 246
loratadine, psychological side effects 185–6
lung
 chronic obstructive disease, *see* chronic obstructive pulmonary disease
 infections, *see* infections
 transplantation, *see* transplantation
 volume reduction surgery in COPD 90
 see also National Lung Health Education Program
lung function, asthma, breathlessness and its relationship to 120
lung function tests/estimation
 asthma 132, 296, 296–7
  estimated vs actually recorded, comparison 121
 COPD
  San Diego Program 95, 97
  smoking cessation and 319–20
Lung Health Study (smoking cessation program) 318, 322, 326, 326–7
 components 326–7

males
 compliance 213
 with COPD, social support satisfaction related to survival 101, 102
 see also gender
manic–depressive (bipolar) disorder, pseudoephedrine-precipitated 192
medical appointments, compliance 207–8
medical care, *see* health care
Medical Compliance Incomplete Stories Index Test, CF 269
medical history-taking
 asthma 298
 COPD 300
medical monitoring of smoking cessation in COPD 328–9
medical treatment/management, COPD 89–90, 308–12
 smoking cessation and 319–21
 see also specific methods e.g. drug therapy
medications, *see* drug therapy
memory and QOL questionnaires 247
men, *see* gender; males
metaproterenol sulfate 305
methacholine challenge, COPD 320
methylprednisolone 305
methylxanthine drugs 308, 310–11
Missouri Children's Behavior Checklist (MCBC), CF 262, 263, 264
modeling improving compliance 224
montelukast 308
mood
 emotional reaction to asthma influenced by 238
 symptom perception affected by 237–8
mortality, *see* death
mother of CF child
 psychological adjustment 261, 262, 266, 267, 267–8
  family dynamics and 274
  feeding and 272
 psychological adjustment of child reported by 264
 see also family; parents
motivation 238, 340
 in medical management of COPD 319–20
multidisciplinary vs interdisciplinary management, asthma 359–61
Mycobacterium spp.
 bovis 290
 culture 302
 direct identification 302
 tuberculosis 290, 302, 349–50
 see also tuberculosis

National Asthma Education/Education and Prevention Programs, *see* National Institutes of Health
National Cooperative Inner-City Asthma Study 23, 66
National Health and Nutrition Examination Survey (NHANES II), asthma 23
National Health Interview Study, asthma 23
National Institutes of Health 286
  National Asthma Education and Prevention Program's Expert Panel Report 2 Guidelines 20, 302–3, 383
  National Asthma Education Program (1991) 286
National Lung Health Education Program (NHELP) 225
NCICAS 23
nebulizers, instruction for use 218
nedocromil sodium 183, 308, 309–10
negotiation affecting compliance 222
neural networks (connectionism) 376–8
neural pathways/systems influencing breathlessness 121–2, 122–3
neuropsychological functioning, *see* psychological functioning
neuropsychological side effects of drugs 175–96
  allergic rhinitis 175–6, 183–92
  asthma 175–83, 191–2
    children 72–3, 176–9, 180, 181–2
NHANES II, asthma 23
NHIS, asthma 23
nicotine replacement therapy (NRT) in COPD 326, 327
NIH, *see* National Institutes of Health
nitrogen dioxide and asthma 31
nonadherence/noncompliance, *see* adherence
nonlinearity (with interactions between elements of complex systems) 369, 379
  asthma research and 381–9
  social cognitive learning theory and 374

obstructive lung disease, chronic, *see* chronic obstructive pulmonary disease
occupational factors, COPD 291
organismic boundary conditions in self-management 165
oxygen therapy, COPD 312
ozone and asthma 31

pancreatic enzyme replacement, CF 258
panic with asthma attacks 360–1
parallel distributed processing (connectionism) 376–8
parent(s)
  asthmatic child's 385–8
    decision making 216, 252
    education/knowledge 50, 56, 60–1
    interactions/relationships (incl. conflicts) with child 51, 66–7, 71, 75
    QOL issues 249–50
    resources 51, 67–8, 71
    responsibility issues 51, 56, 65–6, 71
    symptoms possibly influenced by 385–8
  CF child's 272
    chest physical therapy and 272–3
    feeding/nutrition and 271–2
    psychological adjustment 265–8, 272
  see also caregivers (non-professional); family; father; mother
Parenting Stress Index in CF 267
partners, QOL issues 249–50
paternalistic model of health care 362
peak expiratory flow (PEF) measurement 121, 132
  asthma diagnosis 296, 296–7
  Self-Management Model and 158, 159
Pediatric Asthma Caregiver's QOL Questionnaire 246, 250
Pediatric QOL Questionnaire 246
pediatric respiratory illness, *see* children
peer relationships, children with asthma 69
PEF, *see* peak expiratory flow
perception(s)
  of illness 8–9
    asthma, in history-taking 298
    COPD, in history-taking 300
  of symptoms
    in asthma, *see* asthma
    psychological factors affecting 237–8
perennial noncompliance 210
performance
  in compliance measurement, observation 203, 204
  in self-management, variability 166
personal (patient) factors
  compliance and 209, 212–15
  COPD and asthma occurrence and 292
personality and QOL questionnaires 248
pets and asthma 63
pharmacotherapy, *see* drug therapy
phenylpropanolamine, psychological side effects 188, 189
physical exercise, *see* exercise
physical therapy, chest, *see* chest physical therapy
physicians, *see* caregivers (professional)
pirbuterol sulfate 305
pollution, *see* air pollution
polymerase chain reaction, *M. tuberculosis* 302
post-traumatic stress disorder, asthmatic child 72
poverty and asthma 23, 25

practitioners, *see* caregivers (professional)
prednisolone 305
prednisone 305
  children 359
    psychological side effects 182
pseudoephedrine, psychological side effects 186, 187, 188, 188–9, 189, 192
psychiatric disorders
  asthmatic child's parents 68
  CF child 260
  drug-induced, *see* neuropsychological side effects
psychological adaptation/adjustment
  CF, *see* cystic fibrosis
  QOL questionnaires and 248
psychological factors in QOL deficits, interaction between morbidity and 236–42
psychological functioning (incl. neuropsychological functioning)
  asthmatic children 46–53
    secondary effects of asthma 69–73
  COPD 12
  drugs affecting, *see* neuropsychological side effects
  patient and family, compliance and 209, 213
psychological treatment/management
  asthma (child and family) 53–4
  COPD, San Diego Program 95–6
  QOL and 240
  see also specific methods
psychomaintenance, asthma 7–8
psychosocial dimensions
  CF child 259, 273–6
    diet/feeding and 271–2
  COPD, *see* chronic obstructive pulmonary disease
psychotherapy, COPD 12–13
public health impact/burden
  asthma burden 22
  COPD 87–9
pulmonary disorders/function/surgery/rehabilitation etc., *see* lung; rehabilitation
pyrazinamide 313

quality of life (chronic disease) 233–54
  asthma, *see* asthma
  compliance and 252
  COPD, *see* chronic obstructive pulmonary disease
  drug research and 243, 251
  interactions in deficits of
    between morbidity and psychology 236–42
    between QOL deficits 240–2
  meaning 233, 248–50
  number of articles on (=interest in topic) 233–4
  questionnaire assessment 242–50, 250
    problems with 247–50
quality of well-being scale (QWB) in COPD, survival and 99–100
questionnaires, *see* history-taking; quality of life

race and COPD/asthma 292
radiograph, chest, TB 301
receptor stimulation and symptom perception in asthma 122, 124
reciprocal determinism model 371–2
reductionism 366–7
referral in childhood asthma for psychological consultation 54
rehabilitation/pulmonary rehabilitation in COPD 13, 90–1, 112
  compliance 108
  depression and 110
  historical aspects 93
  San Diego Programs 93, 96–7
reinforcement
  for asthma-like symptoms exhibited by child 386–7
  compliance improved by 224
relapse/lapse in behavior
  in Health Counselling Model 150–1
  in Self-Management Model 164
    asthma 165
  see also adherence
relaxation training, asthma 6, 6–7
representation (in complex systems) 370
  social cognitive learning theory and 376
research, behavioral and psychological 359–93
  asthma, *see* asthma
residential treatment of childhood asthma 386
  Children's Asthma Research Institute and Hospital (Denver) 359–60
resources for persons (in therapeutic behavior analysis) 342
  asthma 345
  CF 348
  COPD 347
  smoking 352–3
  TB 350–1
Respiratory Illness QOL Questionnaire 242, 246
respiratory muscles causing breathlessness in asthma 121–2
responsibility issues
  CF 274–5
  COPD and asthma
    childhood asthma 51, 56, 65–6, 71, 75
    Self-Management Model and 162
rhinitis, allergic, neuropsychological side effects of drugs 175–6, 183–92
rifampin 312–13

St George's Respiratory Questionnaire 242, 246
salmeterol 308
San Diego Programs (COPD) 93–7
Satisfaction with Illness scale 250
seasonality, asthma 33–4
self-disclosure, asthma 8
self-efficacy (in COPD and asthma) 162, 164
  compliance and beliefs about 214–15
  COPD, related to survival 102–6
self-empowerment 240
self-instruction 161
self-management (self-care; self-control; self-directed behavior; self-help; self-regulation) in asthma and COPD 139–74, 224, 241
  asthma (specifically) 1, 7–9, 345–6
    children 59
    relapse 165
  CF 274, 276–7, 278, 348
  COPD (specifically) 1, 12, 13
  definitions 155, 156
  model 141, 154–8, 168–9
    limitations 165–8
    processes 143, 156–62
    strengths 102–5
  self-empowerment in 240
self-monitoring 224
  asthma 158
self-organization (in complex systems) 370–1
  social cognitive learning theory and 376
self-reaction 161–2
self-reported compliance 203, 204–5
sensory information associated with asthma symptoms, repression 126
sequences of events, behavioral patterns consisting of 380
sex, *see* gender
shaping (behavioral technique) 224
shared model of health care 363
signal detection methods, symptom perception investigation (in asthma) 120, 130
Silver Lining Questionnaire 250
skills required to achieve goals (in therapeutic behavior analysis) 342
  asthma 344–5, 345
  CF 348
  COPD 346–7, 347
  smoking 352, 353
  TB 350
skin testing
  allergen 30
  TB 301
smoking 225–6, 351–4
  causing COPD and associated diseases 87, 291
  cessation/control/reduction 352, 353
    in COPD, *see* smoking cessation in COPD
  environmental exposure triggering asthma 31, 291
    activity interference and 241
    children 63–4, 291
  therapeutic behavior analysis 351–4, 355
smoking cessation in COPD 225–6, 317–33, 346
  medical treatment and 319–21
    multiple risk factors impacting on 323–5
  programs 321–2, 325–9
    in hospitals 320–1
    ideal 325–9
    medical monitoring 328–9
social activities/relatinships (and their limitation), COPD 92, 101–2
social cognitive learning theory 371–6, 390
  connectionist systems and 378
  integration with complexity 373–6
  time and 380
social system, family (of child with asthma) as part of 49
sodium cromoglycate, *see* cromolyn sodium
spirometry in COPD 319–20
sputum testing, TB 301–2
status asthmaticus at Children's Asthma Research Institute and Hospital 359
steroids, *see* corticosteroids
Stop TB (WHO initiative) 350, 351
streptomycin 313
stress, parenting, in CF 267
  see also post-traumatic stress disorder; transactional stress and coping model
suggestion in asthma 381–2
sulfur dioxide and asthma 31
surgery, COPD 90
survival in COPD, psychosocial factors related to 99–106
  see also death
sympathomimetics, psychological side effects 72, 188–90
  see also beta-agonists; decongestants
symptoms
  asthma, *see* asthma; children with asthma
  COPD questionnaire 300
  psychological factors interacting with 237–8
  TB 300–1
systematic desensitization, asthma 6, 7

task demands in self-management 167–8
temporal factors, *see* time
terbutaline sulfate 305
theophylline 308, 361–2
  compliance, children 382–3
  psychological side effects 72, 176–80

therapeutic behavior analysis 341–54, 354–5
  of respiratory illnesses/conditions 353–4
therapy, *see* treatment
time
  complex systems and 379–80
  physician compliance and 220–1
tobacco industry, WHO information 352
  see also smoking
Tokelau/Tokelauans, asthma 29
transactional stress and coping model, CF 261
transplantation, lung and heart–lung
  CF 257–8
  COPD 90
treadmill endurance tests in COPD, San Diego Program 94–5
  outcomes 97, 98
treatment/therapy 283–316
  action plan, *see* action plan
  asthma, *see* asthma
  burden of
    in asthma 235
    tradeoff vs other forms QOL deficit 240–1
  CF, *see* cystic fibrosis
  complexity influencing compliance 209, 210–11
  COPD, *see* chronic obstructive pulmonary disease
  medical, *see* drug therapy; medical treatment
  psychological, *see* psychological treatment
  published guidelines for, compliance with 219–20
  responsibility issues, *see* responsibility issues
  surgical, *see* surgery; transplantation
  TB, *see* tuberculosis
  see also health care; self-management
triamcinolone 308
triprolidine, psychological side effects 186, 189
tuberculosis 290–1, 293–4, 295, 299–302, 303–4, 312–13, 349–51
  drug-resistant, *see* antituberculosis drugs
  prevention 295
  risk factors 293–4
  therapeutic behavior analysis 349–51, 355
  therapy 284, 303–4, 312–13, 350–1
    goals 303–4
twins studies in asthma
  genetics and 29–30
  suggestion and 381–2

vitamin supplements in CF 258
  adherence 270
vocal cord dysfunction vs asthma, children 389

weather and asthma 33
weight management with smoking cessation in COPD 328–9
western civilization, asthma as disease of 34
wheeze in asthma 21
WHO, *see* World Health Organization
women, *see* females; gender
World Health Organization (WHO)
  on smoking
    global market for tobacco 352
    initiatives 352
    morbidity/mortality data 351, 353
  on TB
    data 349
    Stop TB initiative 350, 351
  World Health Report 1999: Making a Difference 355–6
worldwide distribution of asthma 23

X-ray, chest, TB 301
xanthine drugs 308, 310–11

zafirlukast 183, 308
zileuton 183, 308